MEDICAL LABORATORY TECHNOLOGY

2nd Edition

A Procedure Manual for Routine Diagnostic Tests

Volume III

MEDICAL LABORATORY TECHNOLOGY

2nd Edition

A Procedure Manual for Routine Diagnostic Tests

Volume III

Chief Editor
Kanai L Mukherjee
Professor Emeritus
Fulbright Professor
Essex Community College, Baltimore, Maryland, USA

Co-editor
Swarajit Ghosh
University of Milwaukee, Wisconsin, USA

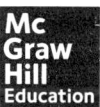

McGraw Hill Education (India) Private Limited
NEW DELHI

McGraw Hill Education Offices
New Delhi New York St Louis San Francisco Auckland Bogotá Caracas
Kuala Lumpur Lisbon London Madrid Mexico City Milan Montreal
San Juan Santiago Singapore Sydney Tokyo Toronto

McGraw Hill Education (India) Private Limited

Published by McGraw Hill Education (India) Private Limited
P-24, Green Park Extension, New Delhi 110 016

Third reprint 2014
RALACRDURCDAQ

No part of this publication may be reproduced or distributed in any form or by any means, electronic, mechanical, photocopying, recording, or otherwise or stored in a database or retrieval system without the prior written permission of the publishers. The program listings (if any) may be entered, stored and executed in a computer system, but they may not be reproduced for publication.

This edition can be exported from India only by the publishers,
McGraw Hill Education (India) Private Limited.

ISBN (13 digit): 978-0-07-007664-8
ISBN (10 digit): 0-07-007664-2

Vice President and Managing Director: *Ajay Shukla*
Executive Publisher: *R Chandra Sekhar*
Asst. Sponsoring Editor—S&T: *Simanta Borah*
Manager—Production: *Sohan Gaur*
Manager—Sales & Marketing: *S Girish*
Deputy Marketing Manger—Medical: *A. Rehman Khan*

General Manager—Production: *Rajender P Ghansela*

Information contained in this work has been obtained by McGraw Hill Education (India), from sources believed to be reliable. However, neither McGraw Hill Education (India) nor its authors guarantee the accuracy or completeness of any information published herein, and neither McGraw Hill Education (India) nor its authors shall be responsible for any errors, omissions, or damages arising out of use of this information. This work is published with the understanding that McGraw Hill Education (India) and its authors are supplying information but are not attempting to render engineering or other professional services. If such services are required, the assistance of an appropriate professional should be sought.

Typeset by Bukprint India, B-180A, Guru Nanak Pura, Laxmi Nagar, Delhi-110 092, and printed at Pashupati Printers Pvt. Ltd., 1/429/16, Gali No. 1, Friends Colony, Industrial Area, G.T. Road, Shahdara, Delhi 110 095

Cover Printer: SDR Printer

Cover Design: Kapil Gupta

Dedicated in memory of my wife

Bibha Mukherjee

*who inspired me to reach higher goals
and suffered most during the publishing of this book*

and

*to the **Medical Laboratory Technologists of India**
who motivated me to compile this book for them*

Foreword

I perused with interest the procedure manual compiled by Dr. Kanai L Mukherjee in collaboration with several Indian and American authors. Most of the sections are written jointly by a pathologist, a technologist and an instructor in medical technology. Thus, the content presents a blend of their rich and diverse practical experiences in clinical laboratory activities.

The manual, in three volumes, covers all the areas of medical laboratory technology with the minimum necessary theoretical foundation. The clinical significance of laboratory findings has also been discussed so that the technicians do not lose sight of the patient. Each chapter admirably deals with the care and use of laboratory equipment and the preparation of reagents. Haematology, blood banking, microbiology, serology, clinical pathology, clinical biochemistry, histopathology and cytology are well covered. All tests are described step by step with down-to-earth practical details to overcome errors. The narrative of the text reads as if the author is demonstrating the techniques to the reader; illustrations supplement the narration. A brief mention is also made of automation in haematology clinical biochemistry, and histology. The content can be easily understood by the technologists of developing countries.

Dr. Mukherjee has many years of experience in the supervision and training of medical laboratory technicians in the United States. Hence, he has a thorough understanding of the most suitable approach for training clinical laboratory personnel. Dr. Mukherjee has travelled widely in India as a Fulbright Visiting Professor in Medical Laboratory Technology (1983–1984) and has admirably tailored this manual to conditions in India and other developing countries by staying in close touch with the clinical laboratory technologists of India while writing this manual. This manual will serve not only as an indispensable work-bench reference book for the medical laboratory but will also be a valuable guide for the training of clinical laboratory personnel.

JAGANATHA REDDY, MD
Ex-President
Indian Association of
Pathologist and Microbiologists

Preface to the First Edition

This procedure manual has been designed to serve as a workbench reference book for the clinical laboratories of India and other developing countries. It can also be used as a textbook for competency-based education of students of medical laboratory technology and for in-service training of new employees in clinical laboratories. This publication caters to the long-felt need of documenting standard scientific procedures with the hope that it will facilitate quality control of laboratory findings.

The project of writing this procedure manual was undertaken when I visited India as a Fulbright Professor in Medical Laboratory Technology during 1983–1984. The basic material for this book was collected from 50 workshops conducted in different parts of India through the joint efforts of various educational institutions training medical technologists, All India Medical Laboratory Technologists' Association, Indian Association of Pathologists and Microbiologists, and the United States Educational Foundation in India. Looking to the special needs of clinical laboratory personnel, a number of contributors from India and the US joined this project with the goal of modernizing the clinical laboratories of developing countries and reducing the existing gap between medical practitioners, pathologists and technologists.

The present publication clearly differs from others existing in the market in its style of presentation. It is a job-oriented publication that emphasizes on the expected proficiency in performing routine diagnostic tests. It is written in a way that is understandable to the clinical laboratory personnel of developing countries. The ultimate goal of this book is to prepare the ground for the yield of reliable data for diagnosis of the patient's illness.

The book comprises 39 chapters, which are divided into nine sections: (I) Introduction, (II) Haematology, (III) Blood Banking, (IV) Microbiology, (V) Serology, (VI) Clinical Pathology, (VII) Clinical Biochemistry, (VIII) Histology and Cytology and (IX) Miscellaneous. Sections I–III are in Volume One, IV–VI in Volume Two and VII–IX in Volume Three. Except the first section, which prepares the groundwork for laboratory personnel, other sections deal with various diagnostic test procedures followed in different areas of the clinical laboratory. The last section of the book is a glossary of technical terms. Study questions are added at the end of each chapter, which will help the students review the materials presented. Two appendices are attached to Volume II and Volume III, respectively. Appendix to Volume II deals with the preparation of common culture media and Appendix to Volume III gives a bibliography along with a compendium of information useful for the laboratory workers.

This book does not claim to be an original contribution. It is a compilation of well-established procedures found satisfactory for the clinical laboratories of developing countries. Shortcomings are inevitable, and I welcome comments, which will improve the text in the future.

KANAI L MUKHERJEE

Preface to the Second Edition

The first edition of this book was an adventure. I travelled extensively in various parts of India, lecturing as a Fulbright Visiting Professor in the field of Medical Laboratory Technology (1983–1984). This gave me the opportunity to gather information about the operation of Medical Laboratories at various levels in a developing country like India. It also motivated me to write a textbook suitable for the needs of developing countries. I thank the publisher for accepting that script in its crude format and guiding me in every step of the process.

The result was unexpectedly positive. The book became popular in many developing countries (in spite of numerous typographical errors). The royalty from this book was distributed among many schools of medical technology and healthcare organisations.

The second edition is a consolidation of what we learnt from the first edition. Every chapter has been rewritten and reviewed by people who are experts in their field. Although India's progress over the past few decades has been phenomenal, the average man faces acute difficulty in understanding modern health science. Due to the high cost of modern medicine, it is only available to the affluent section of society, which can afford to pay for treatment. Medicine, both traditional and contemporary, looks for appropriate diagnosis before administering any course of treatment. Here the laboratory plays a vital role in guiding the physician toward appropriate therapeutic measures.

This is a practical book for quick reference and meant for laboratories with limited facilities. Our most important source of information is the publications from the World Health Organization (WHO). I am grateful to the Eskind Medical Library at Vanderbilt University at Nashville, Tennessee (USA) for providing support in my search for relevant literature for updating this book. I am also thankful to numerous educational institutions in India that critically evaluated this book before including it in their curriculum.

This book is the outcome of many hours of voluntary work involving those professionals and friends of mine, both Indian and American, who are genuinely interested in the progress of health care in developing countries. I am grateful to all of them.

The second edition of this book is dedicated to my deceased wife, Bibha Mukherjee, Ph.D., whose quiet contribution and support have all along been the main inspiration for me to do my best for the people of India. I am grateful to Dr. Swarajit N. Ghosh, MD, co-editor, for his assistance in preparing the material.

Proceeds of this book are humbly donated to the Kiran Centre, Varanasi (India), for their dedicated service to physically challenged children and youngsters, irrespective of their social, cultural and religious backgrounds.

Kanai L Mukherjee

Acknowledgements to the Second Edition

The first edition of the book, published in 1988, was received very well, beyond our expectations. The publisher was happy and so were the students.

After 22 years of its publication, the publisher requested me to work on a revision of the book, incorporating new information to keep up with the rapid advancement in medical technology. I suggested that they look for an editor in India so that the new content could focus on the special needs of developing countries. The publishers made an honest attempt to find an editor for more than a decade, but an editor with desktop publishing skills is hard to find. Such skills were necessary to keep the cost of production low.

Realising the need for an updated edition after the remarkable success of the first, Mr. R. Chandra Sekhar of Tata McGraw Hill Education Private Limited of India approached me and requested me to revise the book with the help of my friends and colleagues in the USA and India, who cherish a global spirit. I was hesitant in the beginning as it involved a considerable amount of work. Finally I agreed, with the assurance from my co-editor, Dr. S. Ghosh—a young physician with medical training in India, work experience in England, research experience in the USA and well-versed in modern publishing technology.

Once the decision was made that the revision will be done in the US with help of WHO, using modern facilities of communication, doors opened for many to contribute: Indian and American physicians from all spheres—professors of big universities to small-town practitioners, research workers, laboratory technicians and prospective Indian medical students or these aspiring to enter into the medical field. They all pitched in with great enthusiasm to update the information. They were all volunteers, genuinely interested in extending their help to the global underprivileged population, for the sake of humanity. I took up the job of organizing the new material, based on my years of clinical laboratory experience in India and the USA. Focussed on the needs of the developing countries, the authors rewrote each chapter, updating the material. The young budding physicians provided technical information, library search and, best of all, taught me the skill of desktop publishing. I am so very thankful to each one of them.

KANAI L MUKHERJEE

Acknowledgements to the First Edition

Compilation of such a comprehensive manual cannot be done single-handedly. My job was much simplified by my colleagues and friends in India and in the United States who contributed individual chapters. They all agreed to work on the raw material provided by the technologists of India and to accept changes recommended by the reviewers. Dr Sarah Israel helped me maintain uniformity and continuity in the text. Her experience in working with developing countries proved to be a valuable asset.

This project was initiated by Dr B. S. Narang, Professor of Pathology, All India Institute of Medical Sciences, New Delhi. His demise two years ago was a personal loss, but it reinforced my commitment to complete this manual. I received overwhelming support from the All India Medical Laboratory Technologists Association (AIMLTA) through Mr. Manindra Choudhuri. I am also thankful to Dr. N. C. Das, Director of the Adult Education Centre, Jadavpur University, Calcutta, for introducing a continuing education programme for the laboratory workers of India for whom this manual is written. The support for the continuing education project will come from the royalty earned from this publication.

I am indebted to the United States Educational Foundation in India (USEFI) for awarding me a Fulbright Visiting Professorship and for financial assistance (1983–1984). USEFI also organised workshops in different parts of India that formed the foundation of this book. I am thankful to my employer, the Essex Community College, Baltimore (USA), for granting me sabbatical leave and for allowing me to use their facilities. Clinical laboratories of the University of Maryland (USA) and the Johns Hopkins University (USA) provided moral and academic support.

I am indebted to the many manufacturers mentioned in Appendix III, and particularly to Dr P. K. Desai, Director of Span Diagnostics, for encouraging me at every step. Dr Jaganatha Reddy has obliged me by writing the Foreword; his comments are of great value to elevate the professional morale of laboratory workers.

It is difficult for me to express my gratitude towards my wife, Dr. Bibha Mukherjee, who endured five years of financial and emotional stress while I was deeply engrossed in preparing this book.

KANAI L MUKHERJEE

Contents

Foreword	*vii*
Preface to the Second Edition	*ix*
Preface to the First Edition	*xi*
Acknowledgement to the Second Edition	*xiii*
Acknowledgement to the First Edition	*xv*
Contributors and Reviewers (Second Edition)	*xxiii*
Contributors and Reviewers (First Edition)	*xxv*
Abbreviations Commonly Used in Medical Laboratories	*xxvii*

SECTION VII: CLINICAL BIOCHEMISTRY

29. Biochemical Processes of the Body Under Normal and Pathogenic Conditions — 821
Ashim K. Bhattacharya
Normal and Abnormal Biochemical Processes of the Body *821*
Basic Physiology and Biochemistry of the Body *822*
Interrelated Metabolic Processes of the Body *828*
Functions of Various Body Organs *829*
Biochemical Changes in the Body under Pathologic Conditions *832*
Basic Clinical Biochemistry *834*
Diagnostic Biochemical Profiles *834*
Review Questions 839

30. Specimen Collection and Processing for Biochemical Analyses — 840
Swarajit Ghosh
Blood *841*
Urine *847*
Cerebrospinal Fluid *848*
Review Questions 849

31. Application of Analytical Techniques in Clinical Biochemistry — 850
Salil Das
Basic Analytical Techniques in Clinical Biochemistry *851*
Basic Steps in Analytic Chemistry *851*
Application of Analytical Techniques in Clinical Biochemistry *852*
Review Questions 871

32. Automation in Clinical Biochemistry — 872
Kanai L Mukherjee, Dipto Chakravarty and Aurin Chakravarty
Classification of Automated Systems 873
Steps of Automation in Biochemical Analyses 874
Computers in the Clinical Laboratory 877
Automated Analysers in Developing Countries 885
Point-of-Care Testing: A New Approach 891
Time-Saving Devices and Kits 892
Automation in Developing Countries 892
Review Questions 893

33. Routine Biochemical Tests — 894
Shanker Mukherjee
Determination of Blood Glucose 896
Determination of Serum Protein 906
Determination of Blood Urea 911
Determination of Creatinine 914
Determination of Bilirubin 916
Diagnostic Enzymology 919
Lipid Profile 935
Electrolytes 939
Acid–Base Balance and Blood Gases 945
Review Questions 951

34. Biochemical Test Profiles — 952
Subir Paul
Analytes Commonly Tested in Chemistry Profiles 953
Protein (for General Checkup) 953
Electrolytes 955
Mineral Metabolism 955
Kidney (Renal) Function Tests 956
Liver Function Tests 957
Cardiac Function Tests 958
Lipid Metabolism 959
Carbohydrate Metabolism 960
Thyroid Function Tests 960
Other Tests of Organ Function 960
Gastric Function Tests 962
Pancreatic Function Tests 965
Test for Malabsorption 967
Review Questions 970

Contents xix

35. **Clinical Toxicology and Therapeutic Drug Monitoring** 971
    Kaushik Kundu and Sanket Nayyar
    Role of Toxicology Laboratory *972*
    Analytical Approach in Toxicology *973*
    Drug Screening *980*
    Heavy Metal Poisoning *985*
    Review Questions *987*

SECTION VIII: HISTOLOGY AND CYTOLOGY

36. **Introduction to Histotechnology and Cytotechnology** 991
    Papreddy V. Kashireddy and Rohini Chakravarthy
    Introduction to Histology and Cytology Laboratories *991*
    Basic Terminology *993*
    Laboratory Reagents and Equipment *994*
    Laboratory Supplies *1002*
    Preparation of Reagent Solutions *1004*
    Review Questions *1005*

37. **Laboratory Techniques in Histology** 1007
    Venk Mani
    Logging in of Specimens *1008*
    Preparation of Tissues *1009*
    Processing of Tissues *1015*
    Preparation of Sections *1021*
    Routine Staining Procedure in Histotechnology *1025*
    Special Stains and Staining Techniques *1030*
    Stains for Particular Substances *1037*
    Stains for Microorganisms *1043*
    Frozen Section Technique *1050*
    Handling and Embedding of Small Tissue Fragments *1053*
    Review Questions *1053*

38. **Laboratory Techniques in Diagnostic Exfoliative Cytology** 1054
    Krishna Mallik
    Collection of Specimens and its Clinical Significance *1055*
    Preparation of Specimens for Cytological Evaluation *1056*
    Identifying Characteristics of Benign and Malignant Cells *1062*
    Review Questions *1063*

SECTION IX: MISCELLANEOUS INFORMATION

Medical Terminology, Glossary of Technical Terms and Appendices   1067
Rohini Chakravarthy and Kanai L Mukherjee
   Prefixes Commonly Used in Medical Terminology   *1067*
   Suffixes Commonly Used in Medical Terminology   *1068*
   Glossary of Technical Terms   *1068*
   Appendix A: Sources of Information and Readings   *1096*
   Appendix B: Comments on Reporting of Test Results   *1100*
   Appendix C: Miscellaneous Information   *1103*
   Appendix D: Conversion of Conventional Units to International (SI) Units   *1104*
   Appendix E: Table of Panic Values   *1105*
   Appendix F: Diagnostic Test Panels   *1106*
   Appendix G: Professional Organizations Connected with Indian Clinical Laboratories   *1107*
   Appendix H: Suppliers of Clinical Laboratory Products   *1107*

Index   I.1–I.5

Contents of Volume I

SECTION I: INTRODUCTION

1. Human Health and Clinical Diagnosis in Developing Countries	1
2. Introduction to Clinical Laboratories	11
3. Laboratory Safety and First Aid	21
4. Introduction to Laboratory Equipment and Basic Laboratory Operation	44
5. Specimen Handling and Laboratory Records	130
6. Units of Measurement and Preparation of Reagent Solutions	181
7. Good Laboratory Practices and Statistical Quality Control	196

SECTION II: HAEMATOLOGY AND COAGULATION

8. Introduction to Haematology	213
9. Basic Laboratory Procedures in Haematology	220
10. Routine Haematological Tests	227
11. Special Haematological Tests	286
12. Interpretation of Laboratory Findings in Haematology	310
13. Introduction to Haemostasis and Haemostatic Disorders	315
14. Laboratory Investigation of Bleeding Disorders	325

SECTION III: IMMUNOHAEMATOLOGY OR BLOOD BANKING

15.	Introductin to Blood Transfusion Therapy	351
16.	Collection and Processing of Blood for Transfusion	371
17.	Routine Laboratory Procedures in Blood Bank	398
18.	Blood Transfusion Services and Clinical Approach to Haemolytic Disease of the Newborn	437
	Index	*I.1–I.17*

Contents of Volume II

SECTION IV: MICROBIOLOGY

19.	Introduction to Diagnostic Microbiology	449
20.	Identification of Pathogenic Bacteria	505
21.	Laboratory Diagnosis of Mycotic Infections	595
22.	Laboratory Diagnosis of Parasitic Infections	624

SECTION V: SEROLOGY

23.	Introduction to Immunology and Serodiagnostic Tests	669
24.	Laboratory Procedures in Serology	688

SECTION VI: CLINICAL PATHOLOGY

25.	Urine Analysis	731
26.	Laboratory Examination of Miscellaneous Body Fluids	771
27.	Semen Analysis	796
28.	Stool Examination	805
	Index	*I.1–I.14*

Contributors and Reviewers (Second Edition)

Alex Alexander, MD
Retired Medical Officer,
(Reviewed Ch. 1)
Veteran's Affairs, USA

Bibhas Bandy, MD
Surgeon,
Washington County Hospital,
Hagerstown, MD 21740, USA

Mukul Banerjee, PhD
Professor Emeritus (Physiology),
Mehery University Medical Centre,
Nashville, TN, USA

Bruce Basch, MD
Practicing Physician,
Allentown, PN, USA.

Tapendu Basu, MD, FRCP (C), FACP
Consultant and Nephrologist,
Carroll Hospital Center,
Westminster, MD, USA

Ashim Bhattachary, PhD, DSc
Professor (Health Sciences),
Louisiana State University,
New Orleans, LA, USA

Aloka Chakravarthy, PhD
Chief Statistician (in charge),
Central Drug Administration,
Washington, DC, USA

Ashish Chakravarthy, MD
Specialist (Emergency Medicine),
Nashville, TN, USA

Anuradha Chakravarthy, MD
Associate Professor (Radiation Oncology),
Vanderbilt University Medical Centre,
TN, USA

Aurin Chakravarty
Research Investigator (Medical Technology),
Washington, DC, USA

Dipto Chakravarty, MS
Specialist (Computer Technology),
Washington, DC, USA

Monisha Chakravarthy
Research Investigator (Medical Technology),
University of Pennsylvania, USA

Rohini Chakravarthy
Research Investigator (Medical Technology),
Nashville, TN, USA

Satyabrata Chatterjee, MD
Cardiologist, St. Joseph's Hospital,
London, KY, USA

Salil K. Das ScD, DSc
Professor of Cancer Biology, Meharry Medical
College, TN, USA

Satyajit Das, BS
Research Investigator (Medical Technology),
Nashville, TN, USA

Volkmar Dierolf, PhD
Professor (Physics)
Lehigh University,
Allentown, PA, USA

Abhijit Ghosh, PhD
Retired from Department of Agriculture,
Government of India
(Surveyor of Health Report from India)

Swarajit Ghosh, MD
Research Leader,
Medical Research Center,
University of Milwaukee, WI, USA

Alan Junkins, PhD
Microbiologist,
University of Iowa Medical Center,
Iowa City, IA, USA

Ashoke Khanwalkar, BS
Research Investigator (Medical Technology),
University of Harvard,
Boston, MA, USA

Vivek Khanwalkar, BS
Specialist (Information Management),
Philadelphia, PA, USA

Papreddy V. Kashireddy MD, PA (ASCP)
Northwestern Memorial Hospital,
Chicago, IL 60611, USA

Kaushik Kundu, MD
Physician (Internal Medicine),
Saint Luke's Hospital,
Allentown, PA, USA

Krishna Mallik, MD
Specialist (Orthopaedic Surgery and
Arthroscopy Reconstruction), Mountain Vista
Medical Center, Mesa, AZ, USA

Venk Mani, MD
Pathologist,
Dickson Medical Associates, TN, USA

Shanker Mukherjee, MD
Practising Physician (Nephrology),
Allentown, PA, USA

Kanai L Mukherjee, MT, PhD
Fulbright Professor,
Emeritus Director of MLT Program, ECC,
Baltimore, MD, USA

Sanket Nayyar, BS
Medical student,
Meharry University Medical Centre,
Nashville, TN, USA

Ian M. Smith, MD
Retired Professor (Internal Medicine),
University of Iowa, IA, USA

Ekarshi N. Ojha, MS
Research Assistant (Genetic Medicine),
Vanderbilt University, USA.

Indrani D. Ojha, PhD
Department of Education,
State of Tennessee, Nashville, TN, USA

Subir Paul, MD
Practising Physician (Nephrologist),
Alabama, GA, USA

Pampee Paul Young, MD, PhD
Blood Bank and Transfusion Services,
Vanderbilt University Medical Centre,
Nashville, TN, USA

Contributors and Reviewers (First Edition)

Richard L. Angerer, MS
Associate Professor (Chemistry), Essex Community College, Baltimore, MD, USA

Chayya S. Angadi, MSc
Lecturer (Microbiology), SNDT Women's University, Mumbai, India

Elizabeth Bastio, MS, C(ASCP)
Specialist (Clinical Chemistry), Instruction, Villa Julie College Baltimore, MD, USA

Belur Bhagwan, MD
Pathologist-in-chief, Sinai Hospital, Baltimore, MD, USA

H. M. Bhatia, PhD
Director, National Institute of Immunohaematology, KEM Hospital, Mumbai, India

Ashim K. Bhattacharya, PhD
School of Medicine, University of Louisiana, New Orleans, LA, USA

Barbara Carr, MT, MS
Associate Professor, Catonsville Community College Baltimore, MD, USA

Meeta Chattoraj, MS
School of Graduate Studies, Department of Chemistry, University of Chicago, USA

Willie Q. Cartwright, MT, MS
Assistant Professor, University of Maryland Baltimore, MD, USA

Anuradha Chakravarthy, MD
Mayo Clinic, Rochester, MM, USA

Ashish Chakravarthy, MD
Department of Pathology, University of Maryland, Baltimore, MD, USA

Neil T. Constantine, MT, PhD
Assistant Professor, University of Maryland, Baltimore, MD, USA

Pradip K. Desai, MD
Director, Span Diagnostics, Surat, India

Deepa Dutta, MD
Head, Microbiology Section, Sinai Hospital, Baltimore, MD, USA

Satish K. Ganju, PhD
Professor, Uday Pratap College, Gorakhpur University, Varanasi, India

Meera Ghosh, PhD
Research Officer (Environmental Sciences), Jawaharlal Nehru University, New Delhi, India

B. K. Goel, MSc
Supervisor, Clinical Biochemistry Lab., All India Institute of Medical Sciences, New Delhi, India

Shyamal Das Gupta, PhD
Head, Division of Pharmacology, Defence Research and Development, Gwalior, India

John Hangasky, PA
Assistant Professor, Physician,
Assistant Program, Essex,
Community College, Baltimore,
MD, USA

N. Kandasamy,
Technical Assistant,
Madras Medical College, Madras, India

Bibha Mukherjee, PhD
Professor, Morgan State University,
Baltimore, MD, USA

Kanai L Mukherjee, MT (ASCP), PhD
Fulbright Professor,
Director, MLT Program, Essex Community
College, Baltimore, MD, USA

B. S. Narang, MD
Associate Professor (Pathology),
All India Institute of Medical Sciences,
New Delhi, India

William H. Neal, Jr, BS
Assistant Professor, Emergency Medical
Technology Program, Essex Community
College, Baltimore, MD, USA

Vinayak B. Pawar, MT, PhD
Assistant Professor, University of
Maryland Baltimore, MD, USA

Diana Powlowski, AA
American Red Cross, MLT Instructor in
Blood Bank, Essex Community College,
Baltimore, MD, USA

S. Ramakrishnan, PhD
Professor of Biochemistry, Jawaharlal Institute
of Postgraduate Medical Education and
Research, Pondicherry, India

Terry R. Reynolds, MT
Instructor, University of Maryland,
Baltimore, MD, USA

Usha Rusia, MD
Lecturer, Department of Pathology,
University College of Medical Sciences,
New Delhi, India

Virginia Schurman, MS
Associate Professor (Microbiology),
Essex Community College, Baltimore,
MD, USA

Robert J. Solomon, PA, MS
Associate Professor, Physician Assistant
Program, Essex Community College,
Baltimore, MD, USA

S. K. Sood, MD
Professor of Pathology University,
College of Medical Sciences,
New Delhi, India

Joseph Testa, PhD
Professor (Chemistry),
Essex Community College, Baltimore,
MD, USA

Jagan N. Thupari, MD, DCP
Immunology Research Lab.
Francis Scott Key Medical Center,
Johns Hopkins University, Baltimore, MD, USA

Harold Woods, MT (ASCP)
Chief Technologist of Blood Bank,
Veterans Hospital, Baltimore, MD, USA

Abbreviations Commonly Used in Medical Laboratories

Abbreviation	Expanded version	Abbreviation	Expanded version
A	absorbance	CK	creatine kinase
Ab	antibody	CLL	chronic lymphocytic leukaemia
ACT	activated clotting time		
AFB	acid-fast bacillus	CLS	clinical laboratory scientist
Ag	antigen	CLT	clinical laboratory technician
AHG	antihuman globulin	cm	centimetre
AIDS	acquired immunodeficiency syndrome	CNS	central nervous system
		CO	carbon monoxide
ALL	acute lymphocytic leukaemia	CO_2	carbon dioxide
ALP, AP	alkaline phosphatase	CPD	citrate-phosphate-dextrose
ALT	alanine aminotransferase (formerly, SGPT)	CPK	creatinine phosphokinase
		crit	haematocrit
AML	acute myelogenous leukaemia	C & S	culture and sensitivity
ANA	anti-nuclear antibody	CSF	cerebrospinal fluid, colony stimulating factor
APTT	activated partial thromboplastin		
		cu mm	cubic millimetre/mm^3
AST	aspartate aminotransferase (formerly SGOT)	DAT	direct antiglobulin test
		DIC	disseminated intravascular coagulation
BA	blood agar		
BBP	blood borne pathogen	Diff	differential count of WBC
BP	blood pressure	EBV	epstein-Barr virus
BSI	body substance isolation	EDTA	ethylenediaminetetraacetic acid
BT	bleeding time		
BUN	blood urea nitrogen	EIA	cerebrospinal fluid
C	Celsius, centigrade	EMB	enzyme immunoassay
CBC	complete blood count	ESR	erythrocyte sedimentation rate
cc	cubic centimetre		
CGL	chronic granulocytic leukaemia	EU	Ehrlich units
		F	Farenheit
chol	cholesterol	FBS	fasting blood sugar

Abbreviation	Expanded version	Abbreviation	Expanded version
FDP	fibrinogen degradation products	LPF	low power field
		m	metre
FUO	fever of unknown origin	M	molar
G	gravitational force in dynes/cm	MCH	mean cell haemoglobin
g, gm	gram	MCHC	mean cell haemoglobin concentration
GGT	gamma glutamyl transferase		
GI	gastrointestinal	MCV	mean cell volume
GTT	glucose tolerance test	µg	microgram
GU	genitourinary	µL	microlitre
HAV	hepatitis A virus	µmol	micromole
Hb, Hgb	Haemoglobin	mEq	milliequivalent
HBV	hepatitis B virus	mg	milligram
hcg	human chorionic gonadotropin	MI	myocardial infarction
		mIU	milli International Unit
HCO_3^-	bicarbonate	mL	milliter
Hct	haematocrit	MLT	medical laboratory technology
HCV	hepatitis C virus		
HDL chol	high density lipoprotein cholesterol	mm	millimetre
		mmol	millimole
HDN	haemolytic disease of the newborn	mol	mole
		MT	medical technologist
H & H	haemoglobin and haematocrit	nm	nanometre
		OD	optical density
HIV	human immunodeficiency virus	OGTT	oral glucose tolerance test
		PCV	packed cell volume
HLA	human leukocyte antigen	pH	hydrogen ion concentration
ICU	intensive care unit	PMN	polymorpho-nuclearneutrophil
Ig	immunoglobulin		
IgG	immunoglobulin G	POCT	point-of-care testing
IgM	immunoglobulin M	ppm	parts per million
IM	infectious mononucleosis	PRC	packed red cells
ITP	idiopathic thrombocytopenic purpura	PT	prothrombin time
		QA	quality assessment
IU	international unit	QC	quality control
IV, i.v.	intravenous	qs	quantity sufficient
Kg or kg	kilogram	RA	rheumatoid arthritis
L	litre	RBC	red blood cells
LD, LDH	lactate dehydrogenase	RF	rheumatoid factors
LDL chol	low density lipoprotein cholesterol	RhIG	Rh immune globulin
		RIA	radioimmunoassay

Section VII
Clinical Biochemistry

Abbreviation	Expanded version	Abbreviation	Expanded version
RNA	ribonucleic acid	STS	serological test for syphilis
RPM	Revolution per minute	TIBC	total iron binding capacity
RPR	Rapid plasma reagin	TLC	total leukocyte count/thin layer chromatography
sed rate	Erythrocyte sedimentation rate	UA	urinalysis/uric acid
SGOT	serum glutamic oxaloacetic transaminase	UP	universal precaution
		UTI	urinary tract infection
SGPT	serum glutamic-pyruvic transaminase	UV	ultraviolet
		VD	venereal disease
SI	international unit	VDRL	Venereal Disease Research Laboratory
sp.gr.	specific gravity		
staph	*Staphylococcus*	VLDL	very low density lipoproteins
Stat	immediately	vWF	von Willebrand factor
STD	sexualiy transmitted disease	WBC	white blood cell
STI	Sexually transmitted infection	XDP	fibrin degradation product
		>	more than
strep	*Streptococcus*	<	less than

29

Biochemical Processes of the Body Under Normal and Pathogenic Conditions

♦

Ashim K. Bhattacharya

Chapter Outline

- ♦ *Normal and Abnormal Biochemical Processes of the Body*
- ♦ *Basic Physiology and Biochemistry of the Body*
- ♦ *Interrelated Metabolic Processes of the Body*
- ♦ *Functions of Various Organs*
  - *Liver, kidney, heart, pancreas, endocrine glands, lung, brain*
- ♦ *Biochemical Changes in the Body under Pathological Conditions*
- ♦ *Basic Clinical Biochemistry*
  - *Chemistry profiles*
  - *Types of specimens for chemical analyses*
  - *Units of measure in clinical chemistry*
  - *Reference (normal) ranges*
- ♦ *Diagnostic Biochemical Profiles*
  - *Protein, electrolytes, kidney function panel, liver function panel*
  - *Cardiac function panel, lipid profile, thyroid function profile*
  - *Mineral metabolism*
- ♦ *Review Questions*

NORMAL AND ABNORMAL BIOCHEMICAL PROCESSES OF THE BODY

The clinical biochemistry laboratory analyses the chemical constituents of various body fluids, notably serum (or plasma), urine and spinal fluid. Most of these analyses reflect the biochemical malfunction of various organs of the body such as the liver, heart, kidney, brain and pancreas and the endocrine system. Thus it becomes imperative for any beginner to understand the basic biochemical setup of the body and the role of various organs to maintain homeostasis (chemical balance) in the body. This understanding helps in the diagnosis of a diseased state on the basis of specific biochemical changes.

BASIC PHYSIOLOGY AND BIOCHEMISTRY OF THE BODY

The human body is an incredible machine that requires fuel to run, is capable of eliminating waste products, coordinates various biochemical processes occurring inside the body and has the unique capability of reproduction. The food that the body consumes (carbohydrates, fats and proteins) acts as the fuel that supplies energy and in addition, participates in building the structure of the body (protein).

The materials that the body consumes are classified in chemical terms as **organic** and **inorganic**. The inorganic compounds are salts, water, acids, bases and others. These inorganic compounds (e.g. sodium chloride, NaCl or common salt) do not have carbon atom and do not originate from living matter. The organic compounds, however, have carbon atoms as their essential constituent and are often related to living material. The intake of organic food, water, inorganic salts and vitamins leads to the synthesis of a variety of organic substances inside the body that play a vital role in its sustenance. A few of the important functions are building of body structure, supply and storage of energy (e.g. glycogen, fats, etc.), regulation of biochemical processes at the cellular level (e.g. enzymes) and regulation of interrelated activities of various organs (e.g. hormones). The **inorganic salts** control many physical processes of the body such as osmotic pressure, enter into the structures of various organic compounds and are closely related to different physiological functions of the body (Fig. 29.1). **Water** metabolism and **pH** (an expression of active acidity and alkalinity) play a significant role in numerous biochemical processes. These will be discussed in subsequent sections.

Ethane (increasing carbon chain)

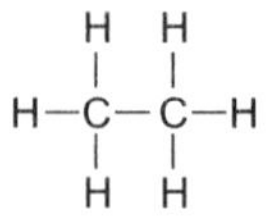

DERIVATIVES OF HYDROCARBON

Ethyl alcohol (with hydroxyl group attached)

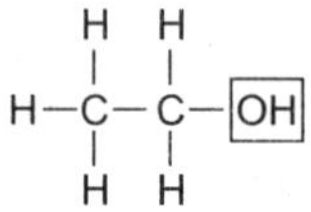

Acetaldehyde (with carbonyl group attached at end)

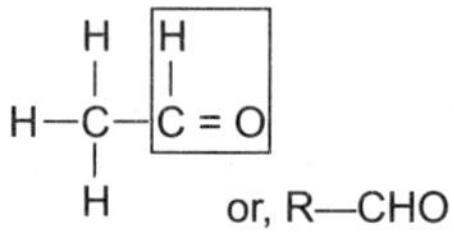

Acetone (a ketone, with carbonyl group attached at intermediate position)

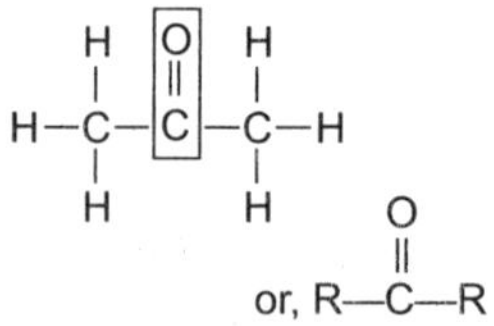

Acetic acid (vinegar, with carboxyl group attached at the end, which is carbonyl group + hydroxyl group)

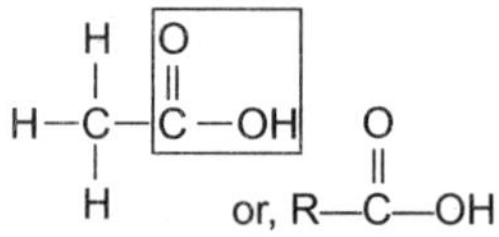

Amino acid (glycine, with carboxyl group and amino or NH_2 group attached to same carbon atom)

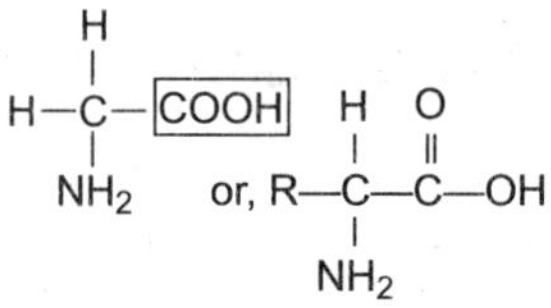

Fig. 29.1 *Some important chemical structures that form the basis of various organic compounds of the body (R, alkyl group with varying numbers of carbon atoms).*

The basic physiological functions of the body are carried out by a few organs (Fig. 29.2). These can be broadly divided as the digestive system, circulatory system, respiratory system, excretory system and reproductive system. The **digestive system** breaks down the complex organic molecules of food into simpler molecules, which are then absorbed in body circulation. The excretory system helps to eliminate the materials that the body cannot absorb. The heart functions in the transport of materials through the circulatory system by acting as a pump. The lungs help the body to pick up oxygen from the air and put it into the circulatory system so that it can be transported to various parts of the body. The lungs also help to eliminate the gaseous waste and carbon dioxide. The kidneys help in filtering the blood; thereby the unwanted metabolites are rejected and the essential ones are taken back into circulation. There are other vital organs in the body that participate in the synthesis and excretion (liver) and digestion (pancreas).

The endocrine glands regulate many physiological processes of the body by sending chemical messengers to the active sites; these are called **hormones**. The **enzymes**, on the other hand, regulate the intracellular biochemical activities of the body. The characteristic functions of various vital organs of the body (liver, heart, kidney, pancreas, etc.) are closely related to their enzymatic composition. When these organs are in distress, the intracellular enzymes are released into the blood stream. Hence, a search for the elevated level of specific enzymes in the serum forms the basis of **diagnostic enzymology** in identifying the malfunctioning organ. The brain is connected to the spinal cord. Activities of the brain and the reflex action of the spinal cord seem to work jointly in governing the physical activities of the body and allow the body to make judgements on the basis of its past experiences. This can be compared with the function of a central computer system of the body.

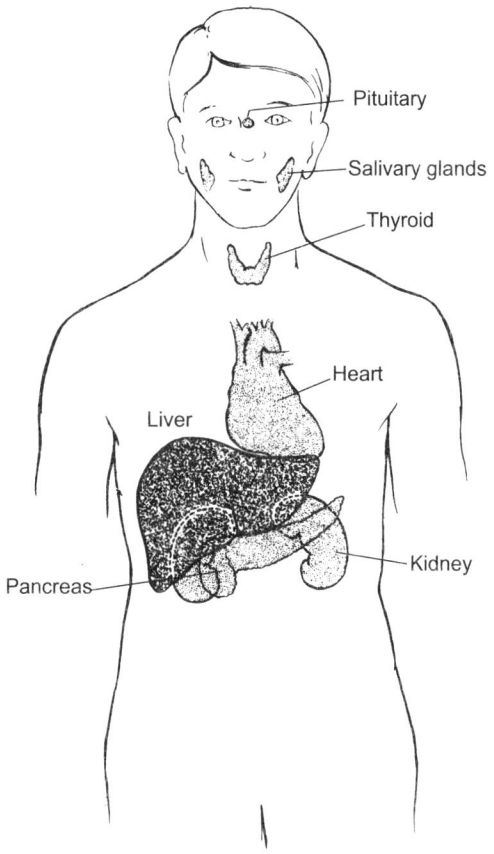

Fig. 29.2 *Location of some of the important organs of the body.*

The chemical structures of some of the basic organic compounds connected with the physiology of the body are shown in Fig. 29.3. These and many other organic compounds enter into the structure of the body and govern its complex physiological functions.

Carbohydrates are a class of organic compounds with the elements carbon (C), hydrogen (H) and oxygen (O) that form the principal source of energy for the body. Sugars are carbohydrates, which are classified as **monosaccharides** or simple sugars, such as glucose, fructose and galactose, **disaccharides**, such as maltose and sucrose, and **polysaccharides**, such as starch and glycogen, which are complex carbohydrates formed by the union of monosaccharides. Hydrolysis is a chemical reaction by which complex organic compounds such as starch are broken down to simpler components (Fig. 29.3). Water molecules enter into the process of cleavage. Polysaccharides are hydrolyzed to sugars, proteins to amino acids and fats to fatty acids and glycerol. Digestion of food in the digestive tract is largely a process of hydrolysis accomplished by various digestive enzymes that break down carbohydrates, fats and proteins.

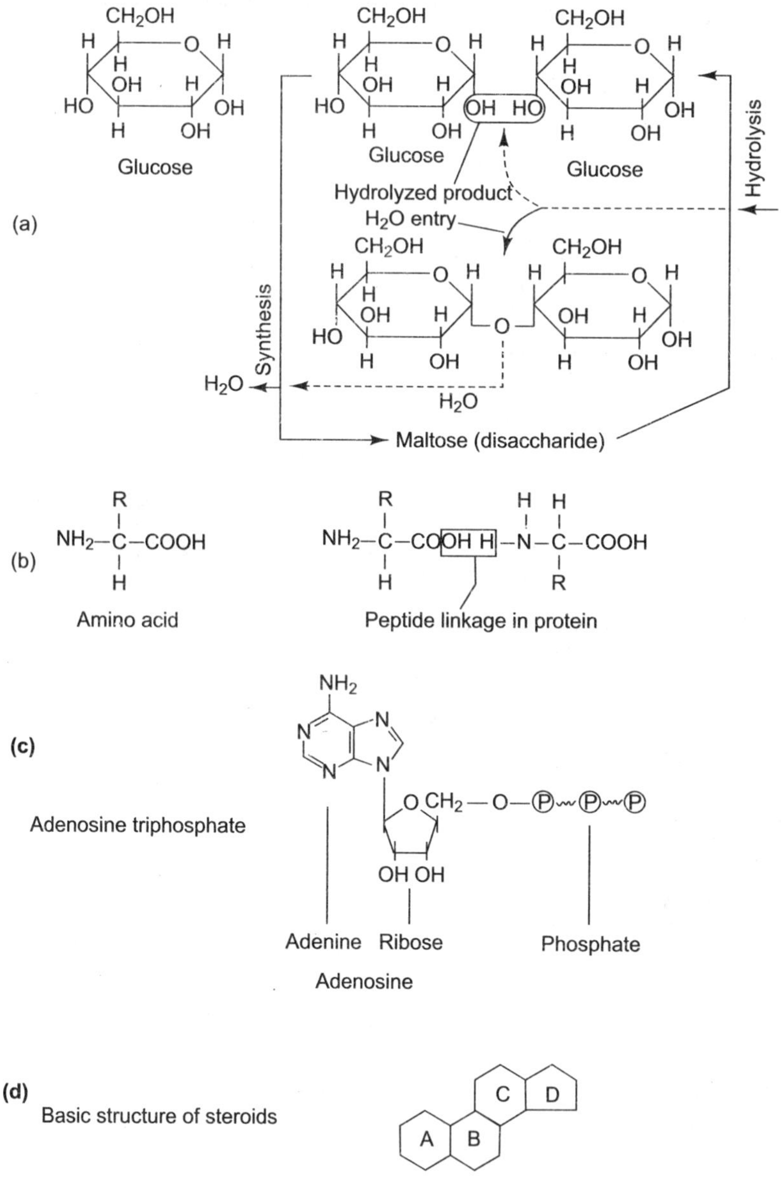

Fig. 29.3 *Chemical structures of some of the important biochemical constituents of the body: (a) carbohydrate, (b) protein, (c) nucleotide and (d) steroids.*

Proteins are organic nitrogenous compounds of the body made of amino acids (principally), which are linked by peptide bonds (Fig. 29.3). The elemental composition of proteins includes carbon, hydrogen, oxygen and nitrogen, and occasionally sulphur, phosphorous, iron and other metals. Proteins form the basic structural component of the body. They may act as a secondary source of energy from the oxidation of their hydrolysed product, the amino acids. Serum proteins include albumin and four components of globulin—alpha$_1$, alpha$_2$, beta and gamma. Proteins are classified as simple or conjugated. On hydrolysis, the simple proteins (albumin, globulin) reduce to only amino acids. Conjugated proteins, on the other hand, produce other organic compounds along with the amino acids. Some of the conjugated proteins are haemoglobin, nucleoprotein, phosphoprotein and lipoprotein.

Amino acids, the building blocks of protein, are formed by the amination of carboxylic acids. The basic formula for the amino acids is NH_2–CH(R)–COOH where R stands for various organic compounds, either **aliphatic** or **aromatic** (Fig. 29.3). When amino acids are used as a source of energy by the body, the amino group (NH_2) is first removed through the process of **deamination**. The ammonia generated by the deamination process is converted to urea ($CO[NH_2]_2$) in the **liver** through the ornithine cycle (Fig. 29.4). The remaining organic acid then enters into the Krebs cycle and is oxidized (Fig. 29.9). There are about 22 amino acids generally found in the living body, of which 10 are essential. Numerous combinations in the amino acid sequence lead to the existence of an unlimited number of plant and animal proteins. Amino acids can well be considered as the alphabets of the language of life.

Non-protein nitrogenous compounds are also important constituents of the body, as discussed further. These include urea, uric acid, creatinine, bilirubin, urobilinogen and nucleic acids.

Urea is synthesized in the liver from ammonia and carbon dioxide (Fig. 29.4). It is eliminated through the urine, which protects the body from ammonia toxicity. Uric acid is the product of purine metabolism and is a result of nucleoprotein breakdown. Uric acid cannot be metabolized by the body and is eliminated through the urine. Accumulation of uric acid in the blood results in renal failure.

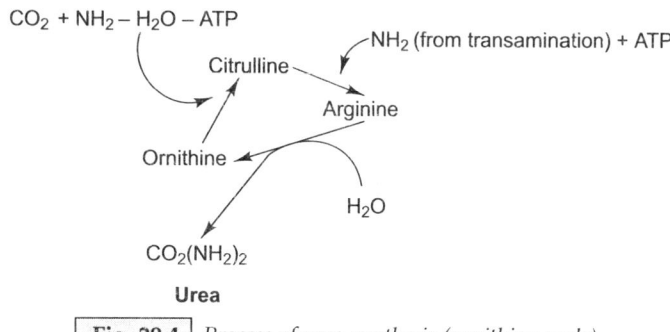

Fig. 29.4 | *Process of urea synthesis (ornithine cycle).*

After the elimination of water molecule from creatine, it generates **Creatinine**. Creatine is associated with the anaerobic phase of muscle contraction and energy transfer. Creatinine is maintained at a constant level in the body and eliminated through the urine.

Bilirubin is a pigmented non-protein nitrogenous compound of the body that originates from the breakdown of haemoglobin (Fig. 29.5). Haemoglobin consists of a complex organic compound haeme (iron + protoporphyrin, a non-iron pigment) and globin (a protein). During the degradation of haemoglobin in the reticuloendothelial cells (particularly in the spleen), the protoporphyrin forms free bilirubin (Fig. 29.5). Free bilirubin is insoluble in water and is transported to the liver as bilirubin–albumin complex. In the liver, free bilirubin is conjugated with glucoronic acid, forming conjugated bilirubin. The conjugated bilirubin is soluble in water and is excreted from the liver into the duodenum through bile. In the intestine, bilirubin is converted into urobilinogen by the action of bacterial enzymes. Most of the urobilinogen is eliminated through the faeces, and a part of it is reabsorbed from the intestine into the circulation and then excreted through the urine or re-excreted in the bile along with the conjugated bilirubin.

Nucleic acids are another group of complex organic nitrogenous compounds that are found in the cytoplasm and nucleus. The most important nucleic acids are **ribonucleic acid** (RNA) and **deoxyribonucleic acid** (DNA). In higher animals, DNA is the carrier of **genetic information** from the parent to the offspring through the mediation of chromosomes. **Purines** and **pyrimidines** are products of nucleoprotein and nucleic acid breakdown. Adenine and guanine are the purines, whereas uracil, cytosine and thymine are the pyrimidines.

Nucleotides are the structural units of nucleic acids, which are composed of phosphoric acid, a sugar and a nitrogenous base (purine or pyrimidine). Adenosine is the most important nucleotide and is formed of adenine and a ribose sugar molecule—a pentose with five carbons. Adenosine diphosphate (ADP) and adenosine triphosphate (ATP) are examples of nucleotides that participate in the energy transfer process of the body (Fig. 29.6). Energy is trapped in the chemical bond of various organic compounds and when the latter break down through oxidation or other processes, energy is released. The released energy is picked up by the phosphate bond and added to ADP. The energy is stored like a battery in ATP. The ATP can transport energy to different parts of the body as an organic molecule; when the body needs energy, the ATP is tapped and energy is released from the high-energy phosphate compound. The latter is converted to the low-energy phosphate compound, ADP, which is ready to pick up a new energy package again.

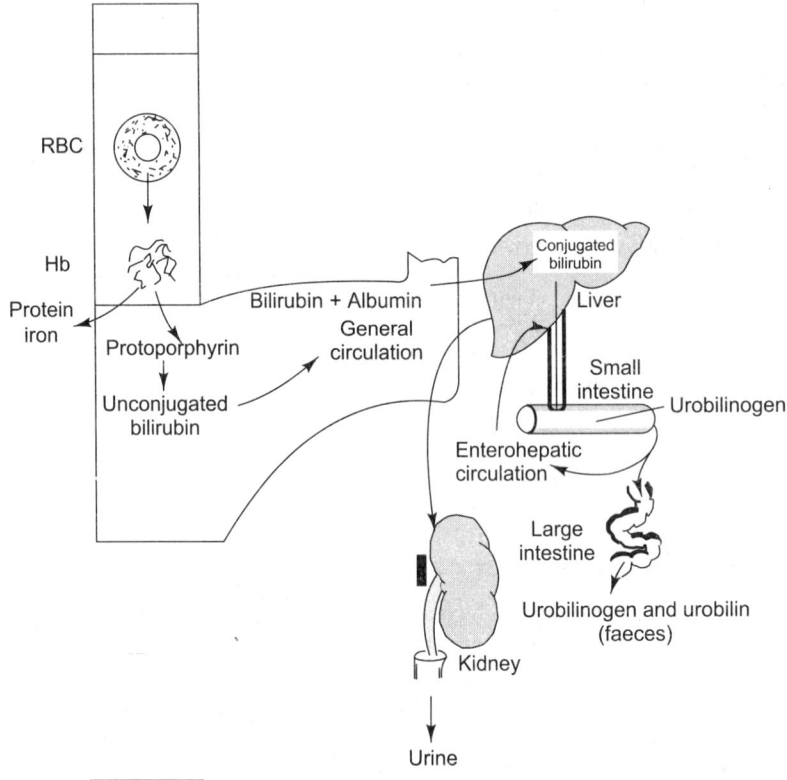

Fig. 29.5 *Haemoglobin degradation and bilirubin metabolism.*

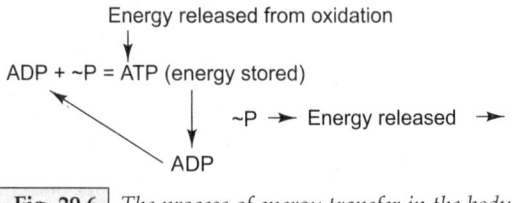

Fig. 29.6 *The process of energy transfer in the body.*

Lipids make up the fourth most important group of organic compounds after carbohydrates, proteins and non-protein nitrogenous compounds. They are insoluble in water but soluble in organic solvents such as chloroform, ether and alcohol. In chemical terms, lipids are esters of fatty acids with the basic elemental composition of C, H and O. Although the same elements form the basic structure of carbohydrates as well, the lipids are in a more reduced state; in other words, they have more hydrogen and thus can store more energy (calories). Complex lipids may include phosphorus and nitrogen to form phospholipids and lipoproteins. Esters are formed by the chemical reaction of fatty acids with an alcohol (contains OH group). This is similar to the formation of salt by the reaction of an acid with a base or alkali (this also contains an OH group).

$$HCl + NaOH = NaCl + H_2O$$
$$Fatty\ acid + Glycerol = Ester + H_2O$$

Triglyceride is a simple lipid that is formed by the union of glycerol and three fatty acids—stearic, oleic and palmitic (Fig 29.7). Complex lipids are also esters but they include other chemical groups (phosphate to form phospholipids, protein to form lipoproteins and glucose to form glycolipids). In sphingolipids, the glycerol is replaced by an amino alcohol called **sphingosine**. Vitamins A, D, E and K are fat soluble, and bile pigments (bilirubin), waxes, carotene and fatty acids are soluble in organic solvents; hence, they are also classified as lipids. Most dietary **fats** are first digested by the fat-digestive enzyme lipase, which hydrolyses the fat into fatty acids and glycerol. The latter is soluble in water and absorbed directly into the body from the digestive tract, whereas fatty acids, which are not soluble in water, are absorbed by the body from micelles (colloidal suspension) produced in the digestive tract with the help of bile salts (sodium glycocholate and sodium taurocholate). **Glycerol**, other than from the dietary origin, is also a metabolic product of glucose breakdown. Thus the body can re-synthesize its own fat from the basic ingredients—fatty acids and glycerol. The liver plays an important role in the synthesis of body fats. Fat is transported in the body by the lipoproteins, which are synthesized in the liver and small intestine. In the body, the lipids can serve as structural and functional elements (e.g. plasma membrane), as precursors of many essential substances as a secondary energy source and as an insulator.

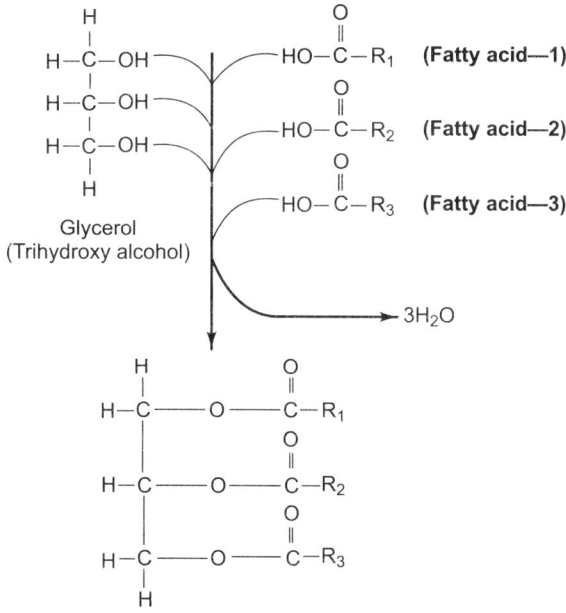

Fig. 29.7 *Formation of triglyceride from glycerol and fatty acids through dehydration synthesis (opposite of hydrolysis).*

Sterols have fatlike properties (insoluble in water but soluble in organic solvents). Steroids are chemically related to sterols (e.g. steroid hormones, vitamin D and bile acids). Steroids have a characteristic chemical structure (Fig. 29.8). Cholesterol is one of the important sterols of the body and is the precursor of a number of steroid hormones. Body cholesterol can be in the form of free cholesterol or esterified cholesterol. Esterification of cholesterol occurs in plasma with the aid of an enzyme, lecithin-cholesterol acyltransferase (LCAT), produced in the liver. Cholesterol is present in all lipoproteins and two-thirds of the plasma total cholesterol is esterified with long-chain fatty acids, with linoleic acid being the predominant fatty acid in man. The cholesterol esters in the plasma are in a state of constant turnover because of their continual hydrolysis and re-synthesis. It is suggested that esterified cholesterol is easy to transport through the plasma, from the tissues to the liver—the seat of body-cholesterol synthesis.

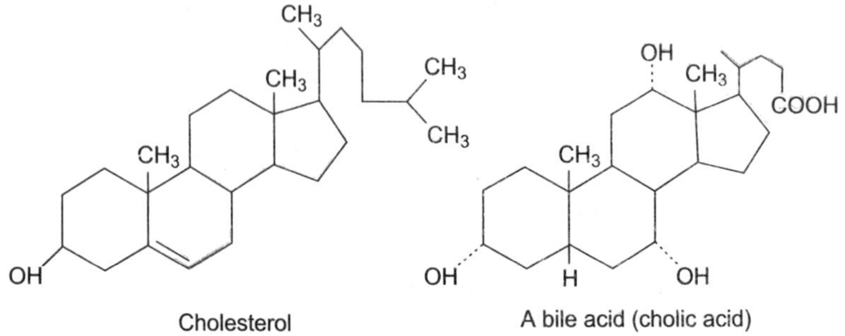

Fig. 29.8 Chemical structures (steroids) of cholesterol and bile acid.

Ketone bodies include three organic compounds—acetone, acetoacetic acid and beta-hydroxybutyric acid. These are the products of fat degradation through incomplete oxidation.

INTERRELATED METABOLIC PROCESSES OF THE BODY

The body performs a number of synthetic (anabolic) and degradative (catabolic) metabolic processes that are closely interconnected. For the synthesis of complex organic compounds from simpler compounds, energy is required. Some of the important synthetic reactions of the body are formation of glycogen from glucose, proteins from amino acids, fats from fatty acids and glycerol and urea from ammonia and carbon dioxide. Conversely, the degradation processes yield simpler products from complex organic compounds. Digestion and oxidation are the two most common degradation processes. Simpler products of digestion are oxidized aerobically (oxygen consumed) to the ultimate molecules of water and carbon dioxide. Energy released by the breakdown of chemical bonds is available for the growth and development of the body. Mitochondria, present in cells, are the seat of the Krebs cycle.

The interrelated metabolic processes, involving carbohydrates, fats and proteins, are shown in Fig. 29.9. Dietary glucose is stored by the liver as glycogen (animal starch) which is a polysaccharide. When the body needs energy, glycogen is first converted into glucose. In the following biochemical steps glucose is anaerobically degraded (the process is called glycolysis and does not require oxygen) to pyruvic acid (3-C compound). Glucose-6-phosphate is one of the intermediate products of glycolysis which is capable of supplying energy to red cells without the aid of oxygen; the metabolic pathway belongs to the hexose monophosphate shunt. Pyruvic acid is the end product of glycolysis that may either lead to the formation of lactic acid under anaerobic conditions, or may lose one carbon (C), forming acetate (2-C compound, acetylcoenzyme A, acetyl-coA) prior to its entry into the Krebs cycle. The acetate thus acts as the junction box for the metabolic products of carbohydrates, fats and proteins in order to supply energy for the growth and development of the body. At the final stage of oxidation, the acetate enters the Krebs cycle and oxidatively 'burns out' with the intake of oxygen and releasing carbon dioxide, water molecules and energy as the end products.

FUNCTIONS OF VARIOUS BODY ORGANS

The function of the human body is regulated by its various organs. These organs do not function independently but coordinated by a network of chemical communication. In the following sections we will elaborate some of the most important organs of the body, their normal functions and signs of abnormalities.

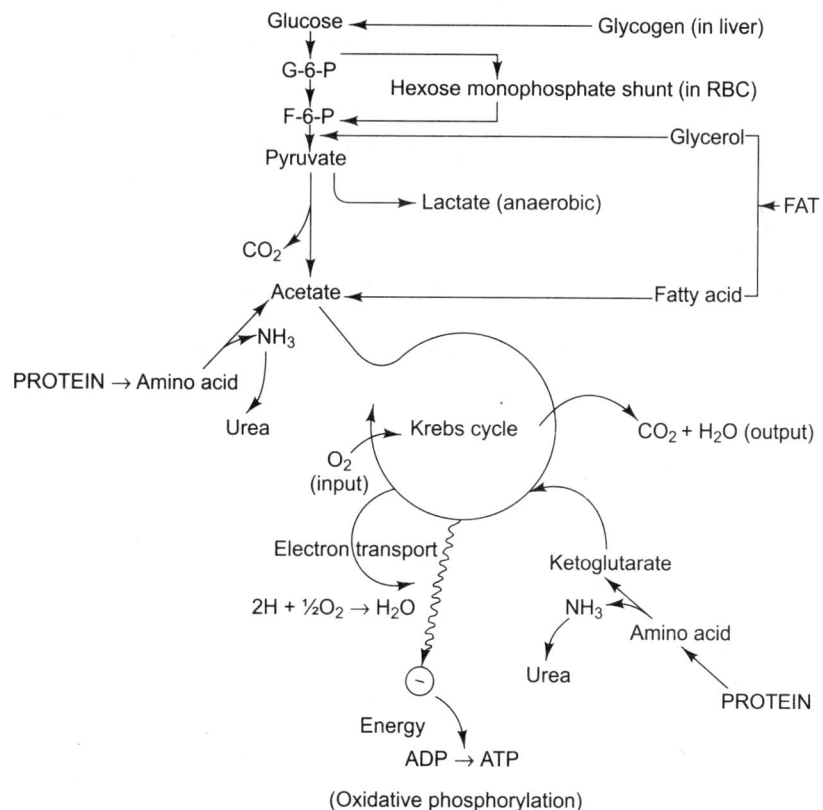

Fig. 29.9 *Interconnected biochemical processes of the body leading to aerobic respiration.*

Liver

The liver plays a vital role in the metabolic processes of the body. These processes can be broadly classified as synthesis, storage and excretion. The liver **synthesizes** a variety of organic compounds—albumin, fibrinogen, urea, uric acid, prothrombin, lipoprotein, transferrin, glycoprotein, hippuric acid, cholesterol and other lipids. Glucose is **stored** in the liver as glycogen and is returned to the blood circulation when the glucose level decreases. Other than glycogen, the liver stores fat-soluble vitamins (A, D, E and K) and vitamin B. The **excretory** and detoxifying functions of the liver are evident from the process of removal of free bilirubin, the product of haemoglobin breakdown. Free bilirubin is conjugated in the liver and excreted as bile pigment into the intestine. Many other toxic substances are similarly removed from blood circulation through the bile duct; many of these substances are insoluble in water and hence cannot follow the kidney route.

Jaundice, hepatitis, cirrhosis (degeneration), fatty liver, infection (abscess) and amyloidal condition are some of the pathologic conditions of the liver. Diagnostic test results for the assessment of liver function include increased serum transaminase activity, fall of blood urea nitrogen (BUN), fall of serum albumin, increased prothrombin time (PT) in coagulation, increased ammonia concentration in blood, decreased levels of conjugated bilirubin and esterified cholesterol in serum (Table 29.1). Fructose and galactose are converted to glucose by the liver when they are present in serum. Thus when these sugars are injected into the body, during the tolerance tests, they are not readily removed from the blood in case of liver disorders. The detoxification action of the liver is assessed by administering bromosulphophthalein (BSP), 95% of which is removed from blood within 15 min when the liver is normal.

Table 29.1 Routine clinical chemistry profiles

Ordering physician:	Name of patient:			
Date:	Date of birth:			
	Outpatient		Ward (Location)	
			Nurse	
General Profile	Glucose Protein Phosphorus AST A/G ratio	BUN Albumin Uric acid LDH Globulin	Bilirubin Calcium Alkaline Phos. Cholesterol T4	Date of specimen collection: Time of specimen collection: Technician collecting specimen:
Kidney (renal) Profile	Sodium Chloride Creatinine	Potassium Glucose	CO_2 BUN	Date of reporting result: Time of reporting result: Technician reporting: Other comments:
Liver (hepatic) Profile	Bilirubin total Albumin Serum LDH ALT	Bilirubin direct Alk. Phos. A/G ratio Gamma GT	Protein AST Globulin Liver LDH	
Cardiac Profile	AST	LDH	CK (CPK)	
	CK isoenzymes: Only done if CK is elevated			Laboratory supervisor:
Lipid Profile	Cholesterol	Triglyceride	HDL	
Thyroid Profile	T3	T4	TSH	
Iron Profile	Total iron Total iron binding capacity Unsaturated iron binding capacity			

Kidney

The primary function of the **kidney** is to filter blood but it also reabsorbs the essential ingredients from the filtrate, which results in urine formation. Thus the kidney is closely related to the maintenance or homeostasis of the body which reflects on the water and electrolyte balance, and production of certain hormones. The chemistry panel for kidney function test is given in Table 29.1. This includes glucose, BUN, creatinine, uric acid and electrolytes. Renal failure is diagnosed by the increased level of serum creatinine, and urea. The glomerular filtration rate (GMR) for creatinine clearance is a reliable index to assess kidney diseases.

Heart

The heart is another important organ of the body and is the centre of the circulatory system. Heart diseases are caused by a number of agents. The clinical chemistry laboratory assesses the condition of the heart through enzyme assays of creatine kinase (CK), AST and lactic dehydrogenase isoenzymes (Table 29.1).

Pancreas

The pancreas releases digestive enzymes (e.g. amylase, lipase) into the digestive system. This is referred to as external secretion. The pancreas also secretes insulin, an endocrine hormone, from the islets of Langerhans which are tiny isolated masses of ductless glands located in the pancreas. This secretion is referred to as an **internal secretion**. Thus, the pancreas has both an external and an internal secretion. A pathologic state of the pancreas is diagnosed in the laboratory by the assay of digestive enzymes in serum and in urine.

Endocrine Glands

Endocrine glands are ductless glands that produce internal secretion or hormones which act as chemical messengers. The brain, hypothalamus and pituitary act in concert to control the body functions through the mediation of several target organs. The target organs are triggered by the hormones released by the conductors of the orchestra—the brain, hypothalamus and pituitary.

Hormones are mostly steroids, proteins and amines. They regulate the interdependent metabolic processes of the body and its overall development. The latter includes the reproductive system, personality, ability to meet conditions of stress and resistance to disease. Insulin plays an important role in the carbohydrate metabolism and its deficiency leads to hyperglycaemia (increased glucose concentration of blood) and glucosuria (glucose excretion in urine). Thyroid hormones—triiodothyronine or T_3 and thyroxine or T_4—are intimately connected with the carbohydrate metabolism of the body and regulate several other metabolic processes.

There are two components of the **pituitary**—anterior and posterior. The **posterior** pituitary is connected with only one hormone vasopressin or anti-diuretic hormone (ADH). ADH controls water absorption from the intestine and the kidney. The anterior pituitary, on the other hand, releases a number of hormones that trigger several target organs. The target organs respond by releasing appropriate hormones to meet the physiological needs of the body. Abnormal levels of these hormones, high or low, may cause a number of pathophysiological problems which will be discussed in detail in the subsequent pages.

The following are some of the examples of anterior pituitary-controlled hormones which are of clinical significance.
1. **Thyroid-stimulating hormone** (TSH): controls the release of thyroid hormones T_3 and T_4.
2. **Adrenocorticotropic hormone** (ACTH): stimulates the adrenal gland cortex, which secretes corticosteroids (e.g. aldosterone, 17-hydroxy corticosteroids and 17-ketosteroids) and androgens.

3. **Gonadotropins**: They stimulate the testes to release testosterone and 17-ketosteroids, and the ovary to release oestrogen and progesterone.

The following are the examples of those hormones which are **pituitary-independent**:
- **Adrenal medullary hormones**: epinephrine and norepinephrine (catecholamines). Hypersecretion of catecholamines is seen in pheochromocytoma, a vascular tumour of chromaffin tissue of the adrenal medulla.
- **Insulin** from the pancreas.
- **Parathormone** from the parathyroid gland.
- **Serotonin** (5-hydroxytryptamine): 5-hydroxyindoleacetic acid (5-HIAA) is produced during serotonin metabolism. Increased discharge of 5-HIAA in urine is diagnostic of certain intestinal tumours.
- **Human chorionic gonadotrophin** or HCG: This is released from the placenta in pregnant women.

The chemistry panel for the thyroid function includes T_3, T_4 and TSH (Table 29.1).

Lung

The lung governs the gaseous exchange in the body. It supplies oxygen to remote cells of the body and removes carbon dioxide produced in the cells during the metabolic processes. Haemoglobin acts as a carrier of these gases (CO_2 and O_2) between the lungs and the cells. The pathologic states of respiratory acidosis and alkalosis originate from the fluctuation of the partial pressure of carbon dioxide in blood. Metabolic acidosis and alkalosis, on the other hand, are governed by the serum bicarbonate level, which is regulated by the kidney. Metabolic disorders like **ketosis** may also lead to metabolic acidosis.

Brain

The brain is the primary centre for regulating and coordinating various activities of the body. Pathologic states of the brain (infection, tumour, haemorrhage) can be assessed from the laboratory study of cerebral spinal fluid (CSF) and by other methods. CSF connects the brain with the spinal cord and physical and chemical changes of the spinal fluid signal meningeal problems.

BIOCHEMICAL CHANGES IN THE BODY UNDER PATHOLOGIC CONDITIONS

A delicate biochemical balance (homeostasis) is maintained by the body under normal conditions. When this is disturbed, a pathologic state is suspected. As the chemical composition of the body is greatly dependent on the functions of various organs and endocrine glands, a study of the chemical changes can be helpful in speculating on the source of trouble.

We will consider here the abnormal carbohydrate metabolism of a patient with diabetes mellitus, caused by insulin deficiency, in order to illustrate the interrelated biochemical processes of the body (Fig. 29.10). *Note:* Diabetes insipidus is caused by ADH deficiency. The commonly referred diabetes is diabetes mellitus.

The four main abnormalities in diabetic patients are listed as follows:
1. Glucose is not readily removed from the circulation for storage in the liver as glycogen.
2. The Krebs cycle does not function efficiently and thus glucose is not burnt out.
3. Non-availability of glucose to meet the body's need for energy, results in the degradation of fats. The degradation, however, cannot go all the way to their oxidation in the Krebs cycle because the latter is inhibited by the lack of insulin.
4. As a result, formation of ketone bodies (ketosis), metabolic acidosis and increased anion gap accompany untreated diabetes.

Abnormal chemical composition of serum reflects the dysfunction of some of the vital organs of the body. Biochemical test profiles for various disorders of organs are presented in Chapter 34 in this Volume. Thus, decreased protein concentration (particularly albumin), decreased PT, increased bilirubin concentration and increased transaminase activity are some of the indications of liver disorder. On the other hand, increased protein level will guide the physician towards the possible diagnosis of infection and lymphoproliferative disorders. This is because lymphocytes and plasma cells are responsible for the synthesis of antibodies (globulin) which is raised under the aforesaid pathologic conditions. Similarly, abnormality of the kidney will result in the building up of waste materials in the body and is recognized by the elevated urea level in serum and a corresponding increase in serum creatinine and levels of inorganic ions. Other laboratory information such as the presence of casts in urine (urine analysis) and decreased GFR will support the initial diagnosis of renal failure.

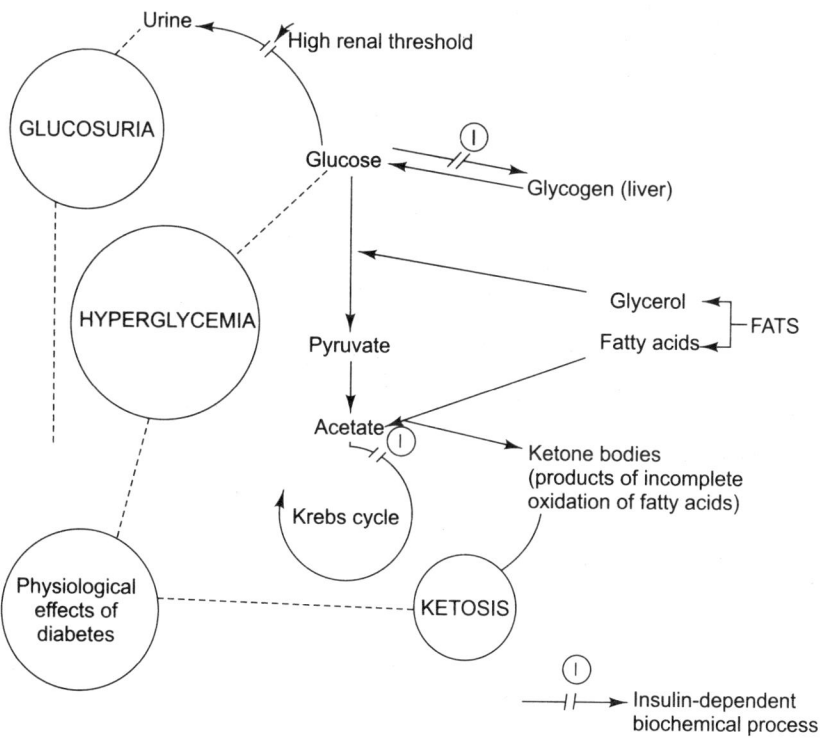

Fig. 29.10 *Metabolic disorder in diabetes mellitus.*

In recent years, accurate analysis of **serum enzymes** has greatly assisted in locating the organ with abnormal function. Most organs of the body have the predominance of some specific enzymes in their cells in order to carry out their biochemical functions. For example, the liver contains a high concentration of transaminases for carrying out transamination activities. If the organ is in distress, its cellular enzymes are released into the blood stream. Thus the elevation of specific enzyme levels in blood may indicate the organ of their origin to be in a pathologic state. To cite an example, increased amylase and lipase activities in serum indicate pancreatic disorder, and increased transaminase activity suggests liver disorder. These will be further discussed in the following sections.

BASIC CLINICAL BIOCHEMISTRY

Chemistry Profiles

Blood chemistry tests are classified as 'routine' or 'special'. The **routine tests** are those which are frequently ordered. Chemistry profile, or metabolic profile, is a group of tests performed simultaneously on a patient specimen to provide an assessment of the patient's general condition. This has been discussed earlier with the functions of organs. The physician can use the results of the chemistry profile, in conjunction with the physical examination and history, to assess the overall health of the patient (Table 29.1). Many automated chemistry analyzers are capable of performing various chemistry profiles in a group.

Tests that are ordered less frequently, such as hormone or certain drug levels, may be performed occasionally and are sometimes referred to as special tests. They are carried out in special laboratories.

Types of Specimens for Chemical Analyses

Specimens arriving at the desk of the chemistry laboratory include blood, urine and less commonly CSF and synovial, pleural or pericardial fluid. Specimens, other than blood and urine, are collected by the physician. Some specimens require patient preparation such as fasting glucose or after-meal (postprandial) and the patient must be instructed accordingly in order to obtain reliable result while others require routine handling. The technician collecting the specimen, however, must be aware of the tests to be performed so that the specimens are collected and processed appropriately. Many of the specimens (e.g. urine) changes its chemical composition upon standing and a fast handling of these specimens is recommended.

Units of Measure in Clinical Chemistry

Clinical chemistry test results are usually reported in metric units or SI units (Table 29.2). Commonly used units are milligrams (mg) or micrograms (μg) per decilitre (dL), millimoles per litre (mmol/L) or in the case of enzymes, enzyme activity units per litre (U/L). In developing countries, however, the older units may still be in use and, hence, a conversion factor has been provided in Table 29.2 for reporting these results in modern units (SI).

Reference (Normal) Ranges

The reference (or normal) range of a substance is determined by measuring the level of the substance in a portion of the general population and applying statistical methods to the data. The reference range is not universal. Hence each hospital should maintain its own reference range. The process of establishing the reference range has been discussed in Chapter 7 of Vol. I. Table 29.2 gives the reference range of commonly tested analytes in a chemistry laboratory. If the result of the patient is beyond the normal range, it must be highlighted (or flagged) in order to draw the attention of the physician. If the results have reached the panic value, the physician or the ward nurse should be informed immediately.

DIAGNOSTIC BIOCHEMICAL PROFILES

Biochemical profiles are group of tests performed in the biochemistry laboratories which are used to assess the general function of the body or for the diagnosis of specific organ disorders (Table 29.2). Measurement of the protein level of serum and electrolyte concentration is included in most routine chemistry profiles and hence they are discussed separately.

Table 29.2 Clinical chemistry reference values in conventional and SI units

Test (Substance measured)	Conventional Unit	Conversion Factor	SI Unit
Alanine aminotransferase (ALT)	3–30 U/L	1	3–30 U/L
Albumin	3.8–5.0 g/dL	10	38–50 g/L
Alkaline phosphatase (AP)	20–130 U/L	1	20–130 U/L
Aspartate aminotransferase (AST)	10–37 U/L	1	10–37 U/L
Bicarbonate (HCO_3^-)	22–28 mEq/L	1	22–28 mmol/L
Bilirubin (Total)	0.1–1.2 mg/dL	17.1	2–21 µmol/L
Bilirunin (Direct)	0–0.3 mg/dL	17.1	0–6 µmol/L
BUN	8–18 mg/dL	0.357	2.9–6.4 mmol/L
Calcium	8.7–10.5 mg/dL	0.25	2.18–2.63 mmol/L
Chloride	98–108 mEq/L	1	98–108 mmol/L
Cholesterol (Total)	140–200 mg/dL	0.026	3.6–6.5 mmol/L
Creatinine	0.7–1.4 U/L	88.5	62–125 umol/L
Creatinine kinase	30–170 U/L	1	30–170 U/L
Gamma glutamyltransferase (GGT)	3–40 U/L	1	3–40 U/L
Glucose	70–110	0.05	3.9–6.2 mmol/L
Iron	65–165	0.18	11.6–29.5 µmol/L
Lactic Dehydrogenase (LD)	110–230 U/L	1	110–230 U/L
Phosphorus	3.0–4.5 mg/dL	0.32	0.96–1.44 mmol/L
Potassium	3.5–5.4 mEq/L	1	3.5–5.4 mmol/L
Sodium	135–148 mEq/L	1	135–148 mmol/L
Thyroid stimulating hormone (TSH)	0.35–5.0 µIU/mL	1	0.35–5.0 mIU/L
Total protein	6.0–8.0 g/dL	10	60–80 g/L
Triglycerides	10–190 mg/dL	0.011	0.11–2.15 mmol/L
Uric acid	3.5–7.5 mg/dL	0.06	0.21–0.44 mmol/L

Protein

Two major groups of serum proteins are **albumins** (60%) and **globulins** (40%). Albumin is made in the liver while globulins, particularly immunoglobulin, are made by lymphocytes and plasma cells.

Total protein is commonly measured in serum, but it can also be measured in urine and CSF, where the concentration is normally low. In the laboratory serum total protein and albumin are directly measured by the colorimetric procedures while the concentration of globulin is computed (total protein − albumin = globulin). The reference value of serum protein is 6.0–8.0 g/dL (60–80 g/L) and represents the sum of many different proteins. Decreased levels of **albumin** can occur in liver disease, starvation, impaired amino acid absorption, increased protein catabolism, or protein loss through the kidney or gastrointestinal tract. The ratio of albumin and globulin (A/G) has diagnostic significance and can be computed and reported.

Electrolytes

In clinical chemistry, the term electrolytes refer to the major **cations**—sodium (Na^+), potassium (K^+) and the major **anions**, chloride (Cl^-) and bicarbonate (HCO_3^-). These four ions have a great effect on hydration and acid–base balance (pH), as well as heart and muscle function. Electrolyte measurement is included in most routine chemistry profiles and renal profiles.

Of the two cations present in serum, sodium is of higher concentration 135–148 mmol/L (mEq/L) than potassium 3.5–5.4 mmol/L (mEq/L). In case of the balancing anions, chloride is of higher concentration—98–108 mmol/L (mEq/L) and bicarbonate is at a lower range, 22–28 mmol/L (mEq/L).

Kidney Function Panel

Proper kidney function is necessary in order to maintain water and electrolyte balance of the body (homeostasis, Table 29.1). Creatinine is excreted by the kidney. It is the waste product of creatine phosphate, a substance stored in muscle and used for energy. The reference range for serum **creatinine** is 0.7–1.4 mg/dL (62–125 μmol/L). When renal function is impaired, blood creatinine level rises, but more than 50% of kidney function must be lost before this happens. Creatinine level is not affected by diet or hormone levels. Thus kidney panel tests include serum concentrations of creatinine, BUN and uric acid (Table 29.2). They all increase when there is an impairment of urine formation or excretion, which occurs in renal disease, shock and water imbalance or ureter blockage.

In mammals, surplus amino acids are converted to **urea** and excreted by the kidneys. This surplus is measured as blood urea nitrogen, or **BUN**. The reference range of **BUN** is 8–18 mg/dL (2.9–6.4 mmol/L). BUN concentrations, unlike creatinine, are influenced by diet, hormones and kidney function. Therefore, BUN level is not as good an indicator of kidney disease as is the creatinine level. BUN levels can be low during starvation, pregnancy and a low-protein diet. Increased BUN concentration can occur during a high-protein diet, after administration of steroids and in kidney disease.

Uric acid is formed from the breakdown of nucleic acids and is excreted by the kidneys. It has low solubility and tends to precipitate as uric acid crystals or urates. Uric acid measurement is principally used to diagnose and treat gout, a disease in which uric acid precipitates in tissues and joints, causing pain. Uric acid levels can also increase after massive radiation or chemotherapy because of increased cell destruction. Many laboratories do not include uric acid as a part of kidney function test. The reference range of serum uric acid is 3.5–7.5 mg/dL (0.21–0.44 mmol/L).

Liver Function Panel

The liver is both a secretory and excretory organ and has numerous metabolic functions (Table 29.1). The liver functions in carbohydrate metabolism, synthesizing glycogen from glucose. Most plasma proteins are made in the liver, including albumins, lipoproteins and transport proteins, and blood coagulation proteins such as fibrinogen. The liver is also important in lipid metabolism and is one source of cholesterol. It is also a storage site for glycogen, vitamins and many other substances. Numerous tests are used to estimate liver function. Most clinical laboratories include bilirubin and a number of liver enzymes, in their liver function panel. But these tests are not considered as specific for a particular disease. They only reflect liver tissue damage or liver dysfunction. In addition, significant liver function must be lost or impaired before some laboratory tests show abnormality.

Most laboratories include total protein, albumin, globulin, A/G ratio, bilirubin (total and direct) and a number of liver enzymes in their **liver function test panel** (Table 29.1). Clinical significance of the levels of total **protein**, albumin levels in serum has been discussed earlier.

Bilirubin is a waste product from the breakdown of haemoglobin, formed in the liver and excreted in the bile. In the liver, most bilirubin becomes bound to glucuronide and is then excreted into the bile—this is called conjugated or **direct bilirubin**. Bilirubin that is not conjugated is called indirect bilirubin. The terms direct and indirect come from the way the bilirubin is determined in the laboratory. Bilirubin assay usually measures both **total bilirubin** and direct bilirubin while **indirect bilirubin** is calculated from those two numbers. The reference range of total serum bilirubin (Table 29.2), or bilirubin in short, is 0.1–1.2 mg/dL (2.0–21.0 µmol/L) and that of direct bilirubin is 0–0.3 (0–6 µmol/L). Serum bilirubin is measured to assess liver function and gall bladder dysfunction. An increase in the bilirubin level may indicate excessive destruction of haemoglobin such as in the haemolytic anaemias, impaired excretion by the liver such as in biliary obstruction (more increase in direct bilirubin) or gall bladder disease, or impaired bilirubin processing as in hepatitis.

Various metabolic activities of liver are accomplished by its intracellular **enzymes**. When the liver cells are damaged, these enzymes are released in circulation and can be recognized by its serum assay. Some enzymes, however, are widely distributed in many body tissues, whereas others are found in only a few tissues. Hence, the measurement of enzyme levels is not always specific for damage to a particular organ but is most helpful when used with other tests, clinical symptoms and patient history. The **diagnostic enzyme assays** for monitoring liver function include alkaline phosphatase (ALP), lactate dehydrogenase (LDH), gammaglutamyl transferase (GGT) and alanine aminotransferase (ALT) and aspartate aminotransferase (AST). Generally, only one enzyme need be measured, as levels tend to mirror each other.

The reference range of **ALP**, also called AP, is 20–130 U/L (Table 29.2). Its sharp rise in the serum level may be related to liver tumours and lesions and a moderate increase is often associated with hepatitis. Serum levels of aminotransferases (ALT and AST) increase with the damage of liver cells and come down as recovery occurs. ALT was formerly called serum glutamic-pyruvic transaminase (SGPT) or GPT, in short. ALT level is low in cardiac tissue and high in liver tissue. This enzyme usually rises higher than AST in liver disease, with moderate increases (up to 10 times normal) in cirrhosis, infections, or tumours, and increases up to 100 times normal in viral or toxic hepatitis. The reference range of serum ALT is 3–30 U/L.

AST was formerly known as serum glutamic oxaloacetic transaminase (SGOT) or GOT. This enzyme is also present in many other tissues, particularly cardiac, muscle and not confined to liver. Hence it can be elevated after myocardial infarction, as well as in liver disease. The reference ranges of these enzymes are given in Table 29.2.

GGT is found in kidney, pancreas, liver and prostate tissue. GGT can be more helpful than AP in determining liver damage because GGT remain normal in bone diseases while AP may rise with bone disease as well. It is also more helpful than AST because it remains normal in muscle disorders. GGT measurement is a standard practice to monitor the recovery from hepatitis. The reference range for serum GGT is 3–40 U/L.

LDH is widely distributed in tissues. Serum LDH increases with liver disease as well as in case of myocardial infarction (heart attack). Haemolysis also causes a rise in the serum LDH level as this enzyme is also present in the red cells. The reference range for the serum LDH is 110–239 U/L.

Cardiac Function Panel

Although cardiac function test panel include AST (formerly called SGOT) and LDH but CK, also called creatine phosphokinase (CPK), is more helpful in the diagnosis of myocardial infarction (Table 29.1). Although CK is present in large amounts in muscle and the brain, and in small amounts in organs such as liver and kidneys, but its pattern of rise and fall in case of heart attack is very typical. An increase in the serum CK level (normal range, 30–170 U/L) may be related to skeletal muscle damage and brain injury. In case of heart attack, CK is released from the damaged heart muscle and rises five to eight times the upper limit of normal. It, however, falls rapidly back to normal levels within 3–4 days. When the CK is high, its isoenzymes assay should be called for in order to confirm myocardial infarction.

Lipid Profile

Lipids are closely associated with cardiovascular diseases (CVD) which includes blood pressure and cardiac problems. Lipids are synthesized in the body from dietary fats. The most commonly measured lipids are cholesterol, triglycerides and high-density lipoprotein (HDL).

Cholesterol is present in all body tissues, and serum concentrations tend to increase with age. Elevated cholesterol levels can increase the risk of coronary artery disease. It is recommended that total serum cholesterol levels be maintained below 200 mg/dL (normal range, 140–250 mg/dL). Cholesterol fractions such as low-density lipoprotein (LDL), HDL and very low density lipoprotein (VLDL) are also measured for various diagnostic reasons. Triglycerides are the main form of neutral lipid.

Thyroid Function Profile

The thyroid gland synthesizes a number of hormones that stimulates metabolism. Tyrosine, an amino acid and iodine are necessary ingredients for the synthesis of these hormones. Excessive secretion of thyroid hormone (hyperthyroidism), as it happens in Grave's disease, or insufficient secretion of thyroid hormone (hypothyroidism), as it happens in myxedema, are both pathological states that disturbs the normal function of the body. Two major thyroid hormones are thyroxine, also known as T_4, and triiodothyronine, or T_3. Thyroid profiles or endocrine panels will include measurement of free or total T_4, free or total T_3 along with TSH, thyroid stimulating hormone. TSH is an anterior pituitary hormone that regulates thyroid gland activity. The reference value of TSH is 0.35–5.0 µIU/mL (Table 29.2). Measurement of thyroid hormones is usually not included as part of a routine chemistry profile.

Mineral Metabolism

Minerals are necessary for good health. The more important ones are sodium, potassium, calcium, phosphorus (phosphate) and iron, whose concentrations are frequently measured as part of the chemistry profile. **Sodium** is the chief cation (positively charged ion) of extracellular body fluids that stays outside the cell. **Potassium**, on the other hand, is the chief cation of intracellular fluid (within cell). **Calcium** and **phosphorus** are necessary for proper bone and tooth development. Calcium is also needed for coagulation. Most phosphorus in the body is in the form of inorganic phosphate and hence the terms, phosphorus and phosphate are used interchangeably in this text. Pure phosphorus per se is highly unstable.

The reference value of serum **calcium** is 8.7–10.5 mg/dL (2.18–2.63 mmol/L). Of all the minerals in the body, calcium is present in the highest concentrations. Approximately 99% of this, however, is bound in calcium complexes in the skeleton and is not metabolically active. The calcium assay measures only the unbound metabolically active ions of calcium. Calcium is required for blood coagulation and for normal neuromuscular excitability. The calcium balance is influenced by vitamin D, and several hormones. These hormones control dietary absorption of calcium, calcium excretion by the kidneys, and calcium movements in and out of bone. Increased blood calcium concentration (hypercalcaemia) may be related to hormone disorders, bone malignancies, excessive vitamin D and acidosis. This may lead to kidney stone formation. Decreased level of calcium (hypocalcaemia) can be life-threatening and should be reported to the physician immediately

Reference range for the serum **phosphorus** is 3.0–4.5 mg/dL (0.96–1.44 mmol/L). Approximately 80% of the phosphorus is in the bone and the rest is mostly in high-energy compounds such as ATP. Phosphorus levels are influenced by calcium and certain hormones.

Iron is needed for haemoglobin synthesis and is an integral component of some enzymes. Normally the serum iron is in the range of 65–165 µg/dL (11.6–29.5 µmol/L). Iron is absorbed from dietary sources and is highly conserved by the body. In blood iron is transported by a serum protein, called **transferrin**. Iron deficiency leads to anaemia which indicates poor haemoglobin concentration. The deficiency can be due to insufficient iron in the diet, poor iron absorption, impaired release of stored iron, or increased iron loss due to bleeding. Serum iron levels can be elevated with haemolytic anaemia, increased iron intake, or blocked synthesis of iron-containing compounds, such as occurs in lead poisoning.

Review Questions

1. Give the characteristic features of the following organic compounds found in the body and how they originate: carbohydrate, protein, lipids (fats), urea, bilirubin and creatinine.
2. Discuss the following metabolic cycles: Krebs cycle and ornithine cycle.
3. What are purines and pyrimidines? How do they form in the body?
4. What are the various breakdown products of haemoglobin? How are they discarded by the body?
5. With the help of a diagram show the metabolic processes involved in the formation and elimination of bilirubin by the body.
6. What is a simple lipid? How is this different from compound lipid?
7. What are the functions of liver, brain, kidney, pancreas and heart?
8. Which are the two major types of serum proteins and what are their major functions?
9. What three enzymes are useful in diagnosing liver disease?
10. What is the significance of bilirubin assay? What is the difference between direct and indirect bilirubin? What is conjugated bilirubin?
11. What are endocrine glands? How do they control and coordinate the functions of the body?
12. What is insulin? What is its clinical significance?
13. Discuss the abnormal carbohydrate metabolism of diabetic patients.
14. What patient preparation is needed before drawing blood for lipid profile?
15. A doctor ordered the following chemistry tests for a patient: Creatine kinase (CK), AST and cholesterol fractions. Which of the following the doctor is trying to diagnose:
    (a) Heart disease   (b) Renal disease   (c) Liver disease   (d) Thyroid disease?

30

Specimen Collection and Processing for Biochemical Analyses

◆

Swarajit Ghosh

Chapter Outline

- ◆ Blood
  - Patient preparation and timing of specimen collection
  - Collection of blood specimen
  - Specimen transport, storage and preservation
  - Problems associated with specimen collection and processing
  - Unacceptable specimen for testing
  - Preparation of serum specimen for biochemical analyses
  - Preparation of protein free filtrates
  - Safety precautions
- ◆ Urine
  - Types of urine specimens
  - Procedure of specimen collection
- ◆ Cerebrospinal Fluid
- ◆ Review Questions

Biochemical data are as good as the specimen which is analysed. Collection, preservation, handling, storage, identification, recording and other steps are accessory to the accuracy of test procedure. In this chapter, our primary focus is on the handling of specimens submitted for biochemical analysis in order to provide reliable and meaningful information to the physician. The technician should also be aware of the conditions that make the specimens unsuitable for the analysis. We will concentrate on three types of specimens—blood, urine and cerebrospinal fluid (CSF), which are submitted for routine biochemical analysis. Occasionally, however, other body fluids such as pleural, synovial and pericardial fluids are also submitted to the biochemistry laboratory for their biochemical assays. Blood and urine are collected by the technician or phlebotomist but other body fluids are collected by the physician. They are highly precious and hence marked as 'STAT' for immediate attention.

Special attention must be paid to the type of specimen required for each test and to the handling and processing of the specimen. Laboratory analyses can only produce useful results if they are performed on a specimen that has been properly collected and maintained in an appropriate environment until the test is performed. General comments about the collection, care and disposal of specimens after analysis, have been discussed earlier (Chapter 5 in Vol. I). In this chapter, we will concentrate on the specific requirements of the biochemistry laboratory.

BLOOD

Blood for chemical analysis can be capillary, venous or sometimes arterial (for blood gas measurement). Some modern methods can use whole blood, serum or plasma for testing while others may require one particular type of specimen, such as heparinized plasma.

Serum is the specimen used for most clinical biochemistry analyses. Serum is the fluid portion that remains after blood has been allowed to clot. Hence, blood is collected in a tube without any anticoagulant, allowing the blood to clot, centrifuging the clotted specimen, and removing the liquid (serum). Many modern laboratories are now using serum separator tubes that contain a substance that forms a barrier between the serum and cells during centrifugation. **Plasma**, on the other hand, is obtained by removing the liquid portion of anticoagulated blood following centrifugation. The serum or the plasma to be used for testing must be separated as soon as possible from the blood's cellular portion. This prevents the exchange of substances between the cellular and liquid portions, which could alter test results.

Whole blood is sometimes the specimen of choice for certain analyses. In many modern methodologies whole blood is acceptable, which makes it easier and faster. Such specimens are ideal for point-of-care testing on the bedside. Blood specimens from infants are drawn by capillary puncture. Heparinized capillary tubes are used to prevent clotting. If the blood is drawn by venipuncture, it must be collected in an anticoagulant tube, such as heparin or EDTA, to prevent clotting. The tube of whole blood must be mixed well immediately before testing.

Patient Preparation and Timing of Specimen Collection

In certain tests **patient preparation** is as important as the specimen in order to get reliable and meaningful results. Some body fluid constituents are affected by meals, medications or the time of the day. Each test procedure contains specimen collection and handling instruction that must be strictly followed. Most blood constituents, however, do not change significantly after eating, so blood used for these can be collected at any time. However, concentrations of constituents such as glucose, inorganic phosphate, triglycerides and cholesterol will change after eating, and specimens for these tests are usually collected when the patient is fasting, generally in the morning before breakfast. Water intake may not be restricted during this period.

Specimens collected from patients with lipid metabolism disorder (lipaemia) or shortly after a patient has eaten may appear **lipaemic**. Since lipaemic serum or plasma is milky or cloudy, it can interfere with certain tests, particularly those that use photometry. Hence, a fasting specimen is recommended. If the laboratory receives a lipaemic specimen, the lipid can be removed from the top, after centrifugation, with the help of a Pasteur pipette. Sometimes, placing the specimen in the refrigerator (at 4°C) overnight also helps.

In some diseases, certain blood constituents follow patterns of increase or decrease that make the collection time very important. For example, **creatine kinase**, an enzyme measured to detect heart attacks (myocardial infarctions), rises rapidly after a **heart attack** and falls back to normal levels in the 3–4 days following the attack. If this enzyme is not measured during this critical period, a heart attack can go undiagnosed. Similarly, iron and corticosteroids show a tendency to change with the time of day (diurnal variation). Hence, it is important, therefore, to note the collection time of specimens for these tests and to consider this when interpreting test results.

During therapy the drug level increases after the administration of the medicine. Hence for therapeutic drug monitoring, specimens must be drawn at set time intervals before or after administering medications.

Collection of Blood Specimen

Blood is collected by **venipuncture** (Fig. 30.1). Arterial blood is recommended for the analysis of blood gases and the specimen is collected by the physician. The blood specimen submitted for blood gases must be heparinized and sealed in order to avoid gaseous exchange between the specimen and its environment, and also it should be kept in ice. A serum specimen is mostly required for the biochemical analysis of blood; hence, anticoagulant is not added to the specimen container during blood collection. If plasma is required for the analysis (e.g. in case of blood gases), **heparin** is recommended (20 U/mL). Heparin is least interfering in biochemical analyses, but is expensive. Hence, heparin should be used only when an alternative anticoagulant is not available, e.g. in the analysis of blood gases and pH. Heparin is the only anticoagulant which is neutral and does not affect the pH. EDTA-anticoagulated whole blood is used for the determination of glucose-6-phosphate dehydrogenase of red blood cells. Plasma anticoagulated with fluoride-citrate can be used, instead of serum (recommended), for reporting blood glucose level as '**reducing substance**'. This is done when a delay is expected in glucose analysis. Fluoride inhibits glycolysis and thus prevents the loss of glucose during the lag period between specimen collection and glucose analysis. Fluoride is a weak anticoagulant and hence, it is combined with citrate (Chapter 5 in Vol. I). Addition of fluoride, however, prevents the use of the enzymatic method for the glucose assay (e.g. glucose oxidase method), which is required for the reporting of '**true glucose**' value. Table 30.1 gives the list of additive or anticoagulant used for various chemistry tests and those sent to other laboratories.

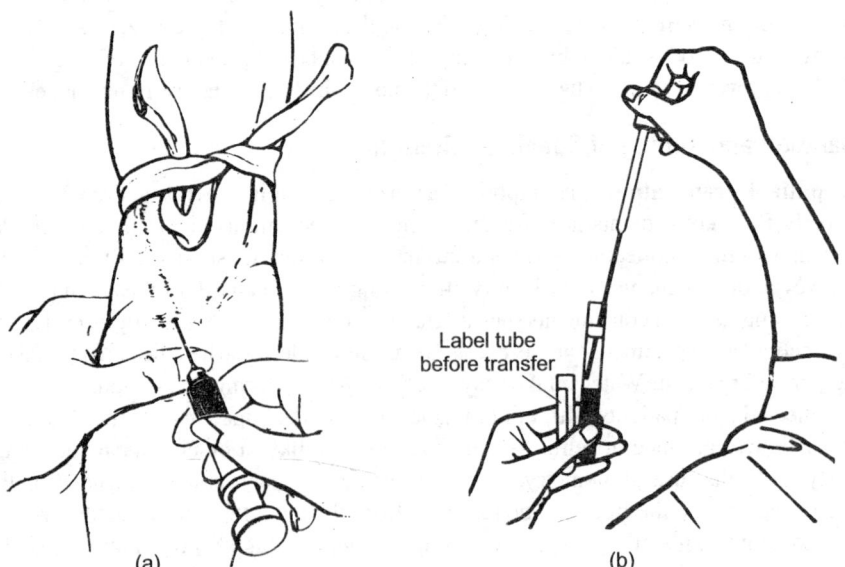

Fig. 30.1 *Preparation of serum for biochemical analysts: (a) collect blood by venipuncture (b) in a container without anticoagulant. Allow the blood to clot at room temperature for 1 h and then separate the serum for biochemical tests.*

The specimen container used for blood collection in the biochemistry laboratory must be clean, free from detergent and bleach. After washing thoroughly with tap water, the containers should be finally washed with deionized water, and must be dried (preferably in an oven). The syringe used for blood collection should also be dry and the needle should be removed before transferring the blood held in the syringe. This prevents haemolysis. Haemolysed blood is unsuitable for most chemical analyses and physical damage of red cells or presence of water may lead to their lysis. Many of these problems are now eliminated by the use of vacuum tubes.

Table 30.1 Use of additive or anticoagulant for various tests of chemistry and for other laboratories

Additive or anticoagulant	Usage
None	Serum, blood chemistries and blood banking
Polymer gel/silica activator	Serum separation, blood chemistries
Lithium heparin	Whole blood, plasma, blood chemistries
Glycolytic inhibitor + anticoagulant	Glucose determination
None or sodium heparin	Trace metals
EDTA	Whole blood, haematology and blood banking
3.2% or 3.8% sodium citrate	Coagulation tests
ACD solution	Blood banking studies
Buffered sodium citrate	Westergren ESR

Specimen Transport, Storage and Preservation

Specimen transport is one of the greatest challenges in developing countries. They not only have limited means of transportation but the weather can be hostile and the infrastructure of business may be far from satisfactory. The method of transportation is determined by the distance. Specimens for point-of-care testing (in physician's office or on the bedside of the hospital) require no transport. This technology is fast developing.

Within hospital premises, usually a distribution team transports the specimen to appropriate laboratories with minimum delay. Holding the specimen in leak-proof, impact-resistant containers is recommended in order to avoid biohazards. Occasionally, courier services are available to transport specimens to another laboratory, perhaps located in different city. Air transport is always desirable for prompt analysis. Regardless of the transport methods used, specimens must be packaged in secure containers to avoid contamination (use strong zippered plastic bags with biohazard signs printed outside). These must also be transported in an environment that meets biosafety regulations and protects the quality of the specimens.

For most routine tests to be performed **within an hour**, the specimen can remain at room temperature until testing. However, if the testing is to be delayed for a few hours, keep the specimens in the refrigerator at 4°C temperature. Do not freeze them unless instructed. Some specimens, however, should be immediately frozen after collection to prevent the loss of enzyme activity. Specimen for bilirubin determination should be stored in the dark as it degrades with exposure to light.

Problems Associated with Specimen Collection and Processing

It is repeatedly emphasized that reliable test results can only be obtained if the technologist has a proper specimen to work with. Improperly collected or handled specimen can cause misguiding erroneous test results. It is estimated that nearly 50% of the laboratory time is spent on specimen preparation and hence, it becomes extremely important that it is done correctly the first time. Some of the most important problems and the ways to avoid them are listed below:

Haemoconcentration

Defective technique of blood collection may affect the result by concentrating certain blood constituents. If the tourniquet is left on too long (more than 1–2 min) during venipuncture, this may likely to occur.

Haemolysis

Haemolysed blood cannot be used for most biochemical analyses. Intracellular enzymes and minerals are released (K^+, LD, AST) which contaminates the serum sample. The result does not represent the true picture of patient's circulatory status. Haemolysis can be caused by over centrifugation, excessive shaking of the sample, freezing of red cells, poor venipuncture technique or contact with water.

Over centrifugation

During serum separation, blood specimen without anticoagulant should remain undisturbed for 20–30 min at room temperature for the formation of clot. It should then be centrifuged to separate the serum from blood cells. Serum should be removed from the clotted blood as soon as possible after centrifugation. This is now been done conveniently with the use of special gel (serum separator vacuum tube), but that may not be available in developing countries (Fig. 30.2). To obtain plasma, the anticoagulated specimen can be centrifuged immediately after collection.

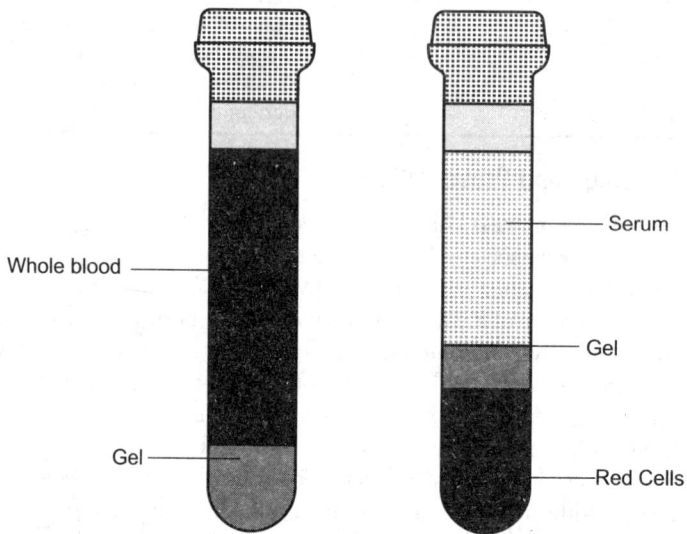

Fig. 30.2 *Serum separator tube: (a) before centrifugation, following collection of blood and (b) after centrifugation of the collected blood. Serum is at the top, ready to be taken out for testing. The gel separates red cells from serum.*

Remember:
- Never freeze serum or plasma with the red cells. Freezing will cause cell lysis.
- Keep the cap on the blood collection container until the test is done. Evaporation may give false results. Gas exchange can also occur which will alter the pH and bicarbonate concentrations.
- Use clean glassware and pipettes for transferring specimens. The containers should be dry and clean in order to avoid contamination.
- Collect blood in the sequence of 'without anticoagulant' followed by 'with anticoagulant'. Accidental contamination of the needle with anticoagulant, during blood transfer, may affect the results.

Unacceptable Specimen for Testing

Following are some of the examples of criteria that must be met for a specimen to be acceptable for laboratory testing:
- Label must be complete (name, date, time of collection and name of person collecting the specimen) and attached in the proper place.

- Blood specimen must be free of haemolysis.
- Anticoagulated blood specimens must be free of clot. (Lack of mixing, immediately after collection, may cause this problem.)
- Specimen must be delivered to the laboratory within the specified time after collection.
- Outer surface of specimen container must have no visible contamination.
- Specimen must be stored properly until the time of testing.
- Blood specimens cannot be drawn from a site above an intravenous line.
- Specimens collected in anticoagulant must have the proper blood anticoagulant ratio.

Preparation of Serum Specimen for Biochemical Analyses

Serum must be separated promptly from the clotted blood. This is easy when the blood is collected in a centrifuge tube.

1. Allow the blood to clot for 15 min at room temperature (do not refrigerate). If the clotting period is prolonged (1 h) it produces a greater quantity of serum and minimizes haemolysis.
2. Remove the clot that is adhering to the wall of the centrifuge tube by '**ringing**'. Ringing is a common laboratory term that means a gentle sweep around the inside walls of the tube with an applicator stick or glass rod in order to dislodge the clot from the wall. Excessive ringing is not necessary.
3. Centrifuge at 2500 rpm for 5 min.
4. Separate the supernatant (serum) within 2 h from the time of specimen collection. If the serum is not separated promptly, intracellular fluid is excreted, which produces erroneous findings for such analyses as potassium. Serum glucose level is also found to fall more rapidly due to glycolysis, if the cells are in contact with the serum. While separating the serum avoid contamination with red cells.
5. Keep the serum in labelled tubes at room temperature. If delay is anticipated, refrigerate the serum specimen. Protect the specimen from strong light (Sun) and heat which will lead to faster deterioration of the serum constituents sought in the analysis. Refrigerated specimens can be analysed within 24 h.

Precautions:
- Before taking the aliquot for analysis, the serum specimen must be brought to room temperature; otherwise the volume of the aliquot will be inaccurate.
- Specimens for bilirubin analysis must be promptly processed and protected from direct light. Conjugated bilirubin is very sensitive towards light and leads to false low values if the specimens are not kept in the dark.
- Haemolysed serum is unsuitable for many biochemical analyses. As a result of haemolysis, constituents of red cells are released into the serum which leads to false elevated values of serum for those constituents which are found in higher concentration inside the red cells, e.g. potassium, protein and cellular enzymes of red cells—acid phosphatases, lactic dehydrogenase and transaminases. False low values may also result due to dilution of the serum and the cellular contents of red cells—cholesterol, sodium, chloride and others. Haemoglobin may directly interfere in some of the analyses such as lipase, bilirubin and enzymatic, glucose determination.
- Before the results of the biochemical analysis are finally accepted by the physician, possible interference in the biochemical analyses by the drugs that the patient is taking, must be considered.

Preparation of Protein-Free Filtrates

Albumin and globulin are the primary proteins present in serum. These **proteins precipitate** when the serum specimen is treated with various reagents during analysis and thus interfere in photometric measurements. Manual methods of analysis often require 'protein-free filtrate' (Fig. 30.3). Details of the procedure, however, will be discussed further with the individual analysis.

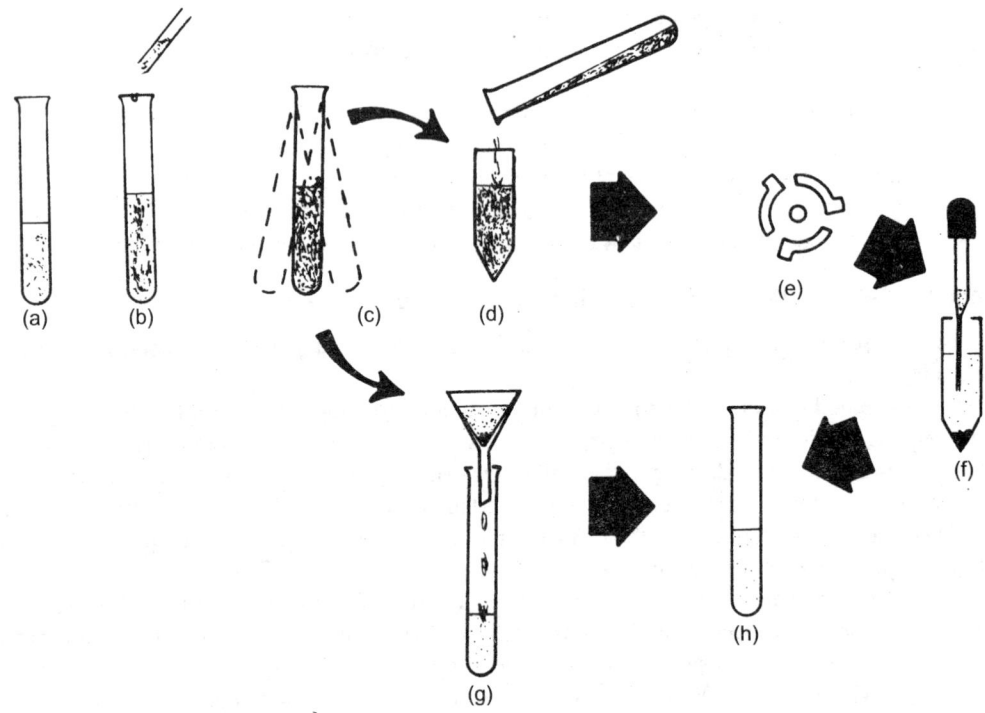

Fig. 30.3 *Preparation of protein-free filtrate.*
Take an aliquot of serum specimen in a test tube and mix it with a known quantity of protein precipitating reagent (a–c). The precipitated protein is then removed either by centrifugation (d–f) or by filtration (g, h). The protein-free filtrate (h) is needed for certain analyses.

For preparing protein-free filtrate, add appropriate **precipitating reagent** to a known quantity of serum and note the dilution (multiply the final result with the dilution factor). The precipitated protein is removed either by centrifugation or by filtration. The supernatant or filtrate is then taken for biochemical analysis. The three commonly used methods are as follows:

Folin–Wu method

This method uses sodium tungstate and sulphuric acid. The filtrate is acidic and is used in the analysis of creatinine, urea and uric acid.

Somogyi method

This method uses zinc sulphate and barium hydroxide. The alkaline filtrate is specially used for glucose determination as 'reducing substance'. Glucose reported by the Somogyi method is close to 'true glucose' value determined by the enzymatic method.

Trichloroacetic acid (TCA) method

This method uses 3–5% TCA and the filtrate, after removing the protein precipitate, is used for the determination of glucose, urea and other blood constituents.

Caution: Trichloroacetic acid is **corrosive**. Use it with care.

Most new methods, however, are more sensitive and require small quantities of specimens. Thus the interference due to precipitation is minimal and the serum protein need not be removed. In the automated systems, the use of certain chemicals and dialysis has eliminated the protein removal step. In case of protein and enzyme determinations, or when the proteins do not interfere in the analysis, preparation of a protein filtrate is not necessary.

Safety Precautions

Technician should always be cautious in handling blood specimen. All specimens must be considered as infectious. Accidental exposure to blood and body fluids is more likely to occur during collection and processing of specimens than during specimen analysis. Standard precautions must be observed at all times. Some of the important precautions are as follows:

- Use appropriate protective equipment such as gloves, face protection (when needed), fluid resistant laboratory coat, frequent hand washing and changing of gloves.
- Use safety devices to avoid mouth pipetting, disposal needles, etc.
- Stay updated on specific procedures to handle patient with contagious disease.
- The technician should be aware of uncapping vacuum tubes containing specimens. This presents the potential hazards of aerosol creation, splatters and tube breakage.
- Modern laboratories use plastic tubes in order to prevent breakage and cleaning. The laboratory must have arrangement for their safe disposal.

URINE

Urine specimens are routinely analysed for the diagnosis of renal and metabolic disorders. They can also be used in toxicology investigation. Qualitative screening of a single discharge can provide an overall picture of renal disorder and diabetic condition (glucosuria), but quantitative biochemical analysis of a urine specimen is done for hormonal assays and diagnosis of endocrine-related problems.

A urine specimen is relatively easy to collect, but for quantitative analysis of a 24-h specimen, the patient's cooperation in collecting 24-h urine is very important along with the necessary attention of the nursing staff to refrigerate the specimen during collection. A composite sample of the urine discharged through the 24-h period is necessary because many of the constituents exhibit diurnal variation (e.g. most of the hormones). The 24-h urine gives a total picture which is fairly reproducible.

Types of Urine Specimens

A **morning specimen** of urine, collected before breakfast, is considered to be ideal for the chemical screening of a '**single-specimen**'. A random urine specimen can also be used for screening. For urobilinogen analysis with a single-specimen, an afternoon specimen is preferred. The specimen should be collected between 2 p.m. and 4 p.m. The laboratory should provide labelled clean containers for the collection of urine (Chapter 5 in Vol. I). For collecting a **24-h specimen**, the container should be of about 4-L capacity with appropriate preservative (Table 30.2). The bottle must have a proper label with the name of the patient, hospital, date of collection, starting time and finishing time. Write in bold letters; **DO NOT DISCARD** (24-h urine collection, refrigerate promptly). Refrigeration is needed during 24-h urine collection. Inadequate amount of preservative, loss of voided specimens or inclusion of two morning specimens in a 24-h period are common sources of error in specimen collection. The 24-h creatinine excretion stays constant for an individual and can be used as a guide to the adequacy of the 24-h collection. This is particularly useful if several 24-h urine specimens are collected from the same person.

Table 30.2 Collection of 24-hour urine for routine biochemical analyses

Test requested	Preservation procedure
Amylase, creatinine, uric acid, urea nitrogen, pregnanediol	Refrigerate during urine collection
Aldosterone, calcium, catecholamines	Add one of the acids to make pH 4.5 (acetic, boric, HCl) Refrigerate during urine collection
Corticosteroids, estrogens	Use boric acid (1 g/L of urine); refrigerate during urine collection
VMA	Acidify with HCl (5–10 mL); refrigerate during urine collection
Porphobilinogen	Collect in a dark bottle, with 5 g sodium carbonate to maintain alkaline pH; refrigerate during urine collection

Procedure of Specimen Collection

1. Ask the patient to empty the bladder and discard the first morning specimen.
2. Take a clean urine collection bottle with preservative and label. Fill in the information regarding the patient on the label. Note the time when the patient emptied the bladder. From this point urine will be collected for a 24-h period. Record the starting time on the label.
3. Collect all the urine discharged from the recorded time until the following 24-h period. At the end of the 24-h collection period the bladder is emptied and this urine specimen is added to those already collected. Refrigerate the specimen.
4. Measure the total volume and take a portion of well-mixed urine for biochemical analysis. Volume can be measured either from the markings on the bottle (if provided) or by pouring into a graduated cylinder. An easy way is by the weight method.
   (a) Weigh the container (W_c). Write the weight on the label.
   (b) Weigh the container with the 24-h urine specimen (W_{uc}).
   (c) Volume of the urine is $W_{uc} - W_c$. This method considers the specific gravity of urine to be 1, instead of greater than 1 (1.010 or higher), but the error is not very significant.

CEREBROSPINAL FLUID

Chemical analysis of CSF is needed to diagnose **meningeal problems** such as infection or development of a tumour. Routine chemical analysis of CSF is usually restricted to **protein** (globulin and total) and **glucose**. Details of specimen collection are discussed in Chapter 26 in Vol. II. Of the three tubes used in CSF collection, the third tube is taken for chemical analysis. This is least contaminated with blood cells. Presence of blood cells, especially haemoglobin, will lead to false high values of protein. One way to avoid contamination of red cells is to centrifuge the CSF (third tube) before taking the aliquot for protein assay.

Glucose analysis must be done promptly in order to avoid loss of glucose due to glycolysis. You can add sodium fluoride (0.5 mg/mL) to a portion of the CSF fluid, and then refrigerate.

Toluidine or glucose oxidase method, as described under serum glucose analysis (Chapter 33 in this Volume), can be used where protein-free filtrate is not necessary. Use 1 mL of diluted specimen (dilute 1 : 10, with distilled water) for the glucose assay.

The process of handling other body fluids such as pleural, synovial and pericardial fluids is also submitted to the biochemistry laboratory for their biochemical assays.

Review Questions

1. How do you prepare the serum specimen for biochemical analyses? Why are the haemolysed and lipaemic sera unsuitable for biochemical analyses?
2. What are the precautions taken for the specimens requested for bilirubin assay?
3. Which are the normal proteins present in the serum specimen? Why is it necessary to remove them prior to the biochemical analyses? How can this be avoided? Would you remove these proteins for the determination of total protein in serum?
4. When is the best time for collecting blood and urine specimens for routine biochemical analyses?
5. Why is it necessary to acidify the 24-h urine specimen collected for VMA analysis?
6. What is the recommended procedure for collecting 24-h urine specimen?
7. What is the clinical significance of collecting 24-h urine specimen?
8. What are the common biochemical analyses done with CSF specimen? If three tubes are used in CSF collection, which one should be used for biochemical analysis? Give reasons.

31

Application of Analytical Techniques in Clinical Biochemistry

Salil Das

Chapter Outline

- ◆ *Basic Steps in Analytical Chemistry*
- ◆ *Basic Principles of Analytical Techniques*
  - *Titrimetry*
  - *Photometry*
    - ❑ *Physical properties of light*
      - ○ *Light source*
      - ○ *Quality of light*
    - ❑ *Principles of absorption photometry (colorimetry)*
    - ❑ *Colorimeters and spectrophotometers*
      - ○ *Components of photometers*
    - ❑ *Basic technique of colorimetry*
      - ○ *Some commonly used terms*
      - ○ *Preparation of calibration curve*
      - ○ *Procedure of taking colorimeter readings*
    - ❑ *Reflectance photometry*
    - ❑ *Turbidometry and nephelometry*
  - *Electrochemistry*
  - *Immunochemistry*
    - ❑ *Radial immunodiffusion (RID)*
    - ❑ *Nephelometry*
    - ❑ *Labelled antibody techniques*
    - ❑ *Enzyme immunoassay (EIA)*
    - ❑ *Radioimmunoassay RIA)*
    - ❑ *Fluorescent antibody (FA) technique*
  - *Electrochemical technology*

- Electrophoresis
- Review Questions

BASIC ANALYTICAL TECHNIQUES IN CLINICAL BIOCHEMISTRY

Quantitative analysis of chemical constituents comes under the domain of analytical chemistry. Basic techniques such as centrifugation, filtration, heating, mixing, quantitative transfers and gravimetric procedures are described in Chapter 4 in Vol. I. In this chapter, we will concentrate on specific analytical procedures and instrumentation as applied to clinical biochemistry.

Nearly 30 tests are routinely done in clinical biochemistry and majority of these analyses are based on the principles of **photometry**, or the measurement of light. This includes colorimetry or absorption photometry, spectrophotometry, flame emission photometry and fluorometry. The technique of **electrochemistry** is used for the analysis of inorganic ions, pH and blood gases. The field of **immunochemistry** has expanded widely in recent years and has become an essential tool for the analysis of microquantities of drugs (drug monitoring), toxic compounds and the assay of hormones. We also have included **electrophoresis**, a technique used in separating closely related organic compounds such as haemoglobins and lipids. The technique of titrimetry has a limited application and does not fall within the aforesaid category of analytical chemistry. Its application in the preparation of a reagent has been discussed in Chapter 4 in Vol. I. Here, we mention its application in the analysis of a few analytes of clinical significance.

Our discussions in this chapter will focus on the specific technology and instrumentation that is best suited for non-urban laboratories in developing countries.

BASIC STEPS IN ANALYTIC CHEMISTRY

The basic steps in analytic chemistry consist of:

1. **Specimen processing**: Examples include separating serum from a whole blood specimen or the removal of a specific serum protein before running the test by a technique such as affinity chromatography.
2. **Chemical reaction**: A chemical reaction may be undertaken in order to measure the amount of the analytes present in the specimen. In the case of colorimetry, a chemical reaction with the substance sought generates a colour, the intensity of which is proportional to the quantity of the substance.
3. **A standard to compare**: A standard solution is an artificially made reagent solution of the substance to be assayed, which includes a known concentration of that substance. It is a reference solution to compare with the unknown, or the specimen. A control, however, is different from the standard solution. It is a specimen with a known value of the substance to be analysed. This is required for an internal quality **control**. Based on the derived standard curve for the assay, your internal control sample should have a reading equivalent to its known content of the substance.
4. **Calculation**: Calculate the concentration of the unknown in the specimen against the concentration of the standard (known). Usually an instrument is involved, which provides a numerical figure as a measure of the amount of the analyte under the given conditions, such as a specific wavelength. This value is used in the following formula for determining the concentration of the unknown

$C_u = \dfrac{IR_u}{IR_s} \times C_s$, where C_u is concentration of unknown, C_s is concentration of standard, IR_u is instrument response of unknown and IR_s is instrument response of standard.

APPLICATION OF ANALYTICAL TECHNIQUES IN CLINICAL BIOCHEMISTRY

Automation in biochemical analyses has proved to be of mixed blessing in developing countries. In the urban setting its use is widespread, and more and more laboratories are leaning towards automation. Using automation, the **turn-around-time** (TAT, the time taken between ordering the test and getting the results back to the physician) is greatly reduced. In addition, the results are more reliable than with manual methods, and a shortened TAT allows early diagnosis and treatment of patients. But automation requires that you have a large number of specimens to assay in order to make the process cost-effective. This is usually only possible in an urban setting. In villages spread out over the countryside with limited options for communication, automation seems to be beyond reach. The greatest hurdle is when the automation fails to function. The number of technicians, with the required hardware knowledge to get the machine back to normal, is limited.

Rather, the current trend of bringing handy instruments and analytical technology to the physician's office or the bedside is a relief for the more isolated facility. This point-of-care-testing (POCT) enables the physician to get the diagnostic information instantly. Thus blood glucose, blood urea nitrogen, blood gases, electrolytes and coagulation tests can now be done instantly at the bedside and trained laboratory personnel or nursing staff can perform these tests even though they may have limited knowledge of chemistry. Of course, controls must be run for all comparisons and data must be kept carefully for all analyses.

What instrument should a laboratory purchase in order to suit the needs of a developing country? Consider the following before making the decision:
- How many tests will be performed per day?
- Which tests are most helpful for the physician?
- Are trained personnel available to perform the test?
- What is the cost per test?
  Remember: Even an inexpensive instrument may need costly reagents and supplies.
- Should the instrument be purchased or leased? (If leased, the responsibility of maintenance and repair lies with the supplying company. In addition, the laboratory may be allowed to exchange an older model for a newer model when it arrives on the market.)
- What is the accuracy of the instrument?
  Note: An instrument that yields unreliable results is detrimental to patient care.

Most clinical laboratory instruments used in small laboratories in developing countries are discrete analysers. In other words, the tests are performed by applying each patient's sample to its own test cartridge, cassette, or reagent strip. After the patient's sample is applied to the test unit, the instrument must detect and quantitate the endpoint of the reaction. This is accomplished in different ways, depending on the design of the instrument. Four principles of instrumentation used in bench top or portable analysers are as follows:
- Titrimetry
- Photometry
- Reflectance photometry
- Ion-selective electrodes
- Electrochemical technology

We will also briefly mention other analytical techniques used in advanced laboratories in order to aware the students about some of the achievements made in this field.

Titrimetry

Titrimetric procedures are widely applied in the preparation of acid–base reagents and in determining the titrable acidity of gastric juice. Titrimetric analysis of calcium, chloride and bicarbonate also uses the same principle but the titration does not involve any acid or base. Instead, an appropriate reagent is used that will recognize the changes occurring in the titrating fluid as the titrant is mixed with the specimen. For calcium determinations, the titrant is ethylenediamine tetra-acetate (EDTA), which is a calcium binder. A fluorescent dye (Calcein) is used as an indicator and is added to the titrating fluid containing the specimen. The dye changes colour when calcium is removed from the system, and these changes are visible only under ultraviolet (UV) light. Titrimetric determination of chloride (Schales and Schales method) uses mercuric nitrate as the titrant and diphenylcarbazone as the indicator. Here the colour changes as soon as all of the chloride is removed.

Titrimetric determination of bicarbonate is now rarely done in clinical laboratories since the introduction of blood gas analysers. The mathematical relationship between total CO_2 and PCO_2 gives the value of bicarbonate (HCO_3^-). Titrimetric determination of acidity of gastric juice is based on the same principles but the procedure uses a special indicator (Topfer's reagent), and 0.1 N sodium hydroxide solution is used as the titrant.

Photometry

Photometry (photo = light; metry = measurement) is the most common analytic technique used in clinical biochemistry. The principle of photometry is based on the physical laws of radiant energy or light. In this method, the intensity of absorbed, transmitted, reflected or emitted light is measured and related to the concentration of the test substance. As colorimeters and spectrophotometers are widely used in clinical biochemistry laboratories, they are discussed separately.

Physical Properties of Light The visible range of the spectrum covers from 700 to 400 nm (Fig. 31.1). The wavelengths beyond the red end of 700 nm are the infrared and heat waves. The wavelengths below 400 nm are in the UV region and carry high energy and also deep penetrating actions. Hence, these are harmful for biological objects.

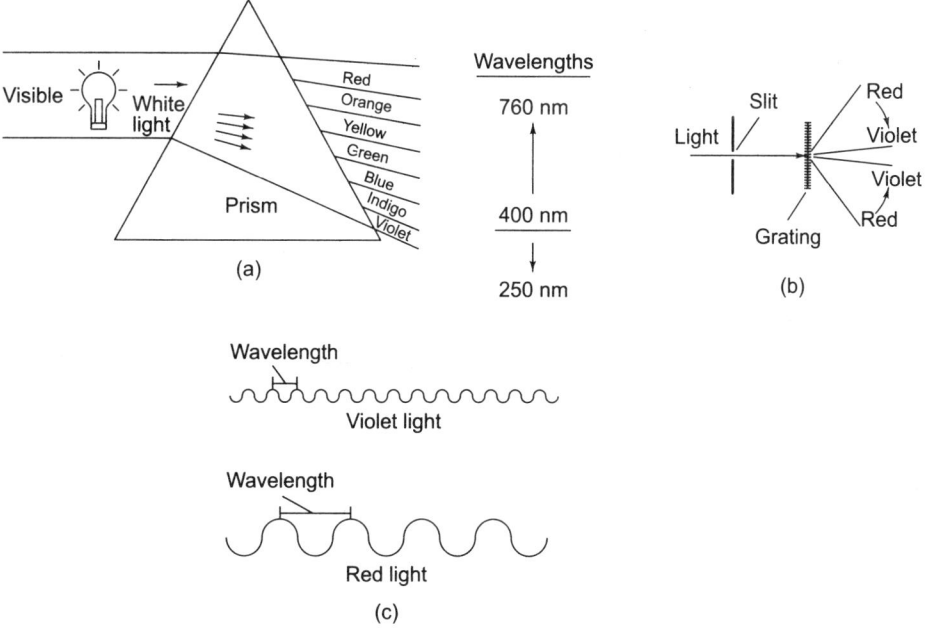

Fig. 31.1 *Components of white light. White light can be split by prism or diffraction grating (a and b). Violet light has shorter wavelength than the red light (c).*

Light source The light source provides the radiant energy for photometric determinations. In the case of the colorimeter, where a visible range of light is required, a tungsten lamp is the best choice. It emits a continuous spectrum of light in the visible range (420–760 nm). If the desired wavelength is in the UV region, a hydrogen lamp is used, which also gives a continuous spectrum in a range that extends from the lower visible to the lower UV range (600–250 nm), going down in the 'beyond-visible range'. The continuous spectrum gives the advantage of choosing any specific wavelength for the entire region—visible or UV. The xenon lamp emits high-energy UV rays and the mercury lamp gives discrete bands in the lower visible and UV range. These are mostly used in fluorometry where high energy is needed to excite an organic compound subjected to analysis. The hollow cathode lamp is another kind of lamp used in atomic absorption photometry, which emits only a single wavelength of light from a glowing metal. The wavelength emitted is specific for the metal (copper, selenium, zinc, lead and others) to be analysed.

Quality of light In order to increase the specificity and sensitivity of an optical measurement, a specific quality of light is allowed to enter the coloured solution. The quality of light is regulated by a monochromator in the case of spectrophotometers, which allows one to select a specific wavelength of light to pass through the test solution. The monochromator may be a prism or a diffraction grating (Fig. 31.2). Special coloured filters are used in a colorimeter, each of which has the limitation of providing a range of wavelengths near the desired wavelength (Table 31.1). The filter chosen for the colorimeter is usually complementary to the colour of the solution to be measured. The chosen wavelength should give the highest absorbance reading for the analysis. The height of the peak is proportional to the concentration of the substance in solution. The required wavelength is provided within the assay instructions.

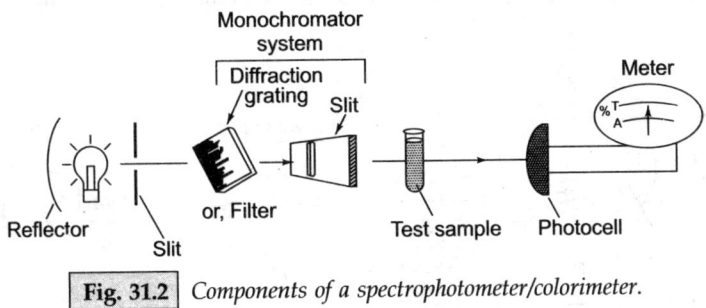

Fig. 31.2 *Components of a spectrophotometer/colorimeter.*

Table 31.1 Use of complementary filter

Colour of solution	Filter used	Peak transmission (nm)
Bluish-green	Red	680
Blue	Yellow	580
Purple	Green	520
Red	Blue-green	490
Yellow	Blue	470
Yellowish-green	Violet	430

Recently, in some automated systems, a dual wavelength measurement is introduced in order to eliminate the error due to the presence of protein, turbidity (e.g. lipaemic) or colour of the serum specimen (e.g. jaundiced).

Principles of absorption photometry

If a pencil of light is allowed to pass through a coloured solution, some amount of light will be absorbed while the rest of the light will be transmitted through the solution (Fig. 31.3a). The amount of light absorbed is proportional to the nature of the solution (expressed as extinction coefficient or 'a', a constant), the concentration of the solute or colour and the distance of the path of light. This is known as **Beer's Law** and can be expressed as follows:

$$A = a\,b\,c,$$

where A is absorbance, a is extinction coefficient (this is constant for the same analyte), b is distance of the path of light (constant, 1 cm) and c is concentration.

As 'a' and 'b' (1 cm) is constant, the new relationship can be expressed as

$$A \propto c.$$

This means that absorbance is a direct measure of concentration.

Since absorbance (A) is inversely related to transmittance (T)—more absorbed means less transmitted—the relationship of A and T (Fig. 31.3) is expressed as in the following equation

$$A = 2 - \log \%T.$$

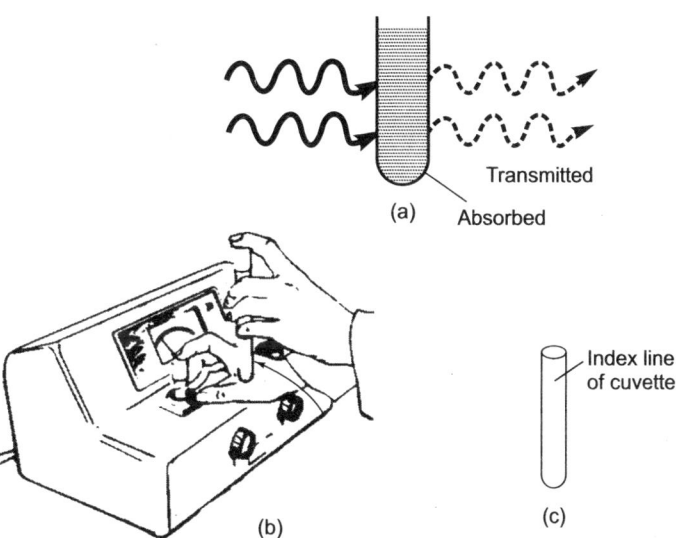

Fig. 31.3 *Principle of absorption photometry. (a) When light passes through a coloured solution part of it is absorbed and part of it is transmitted. (b) A modern spectrophotometer. (c) The index line on the cuvette which should be aligned with the marking given on the photometer so that the configuration of the cuvette does not change.*

The photo detector system, however, can only measure the transmitted light (Fig. 31.4a). If the scale of the photoelectric colorimeter is in %T, it should first be converted to absorbance (A), before using the values for the calculation of the concentration of the unknown (Figs 31.4b, c and 31.5).

$$\text{Concentration of unknown } (C_u) = \frac{A_u}{A_s} \times C_s,$$

where C_u is concentration of the unknown, A_u is absorbance of unknown (test solution), A_s is absorbance of the standard (known), C_s is concentration of the standard.

Note: The unit of the concentration (g/dL or mmol/L or mg/dL) will be the same as given for the standard.

Modern photoelectric colorimeters and spectrophotometers, however, provide the logarithmic scale of absorbance (*A*) along with the % transmittance, which is linear (Fig. 31.5). Thus, in setting the blank (e.g. water), the instrument must read 100% transmittance and have a '0' (zero) reading for absorbance.

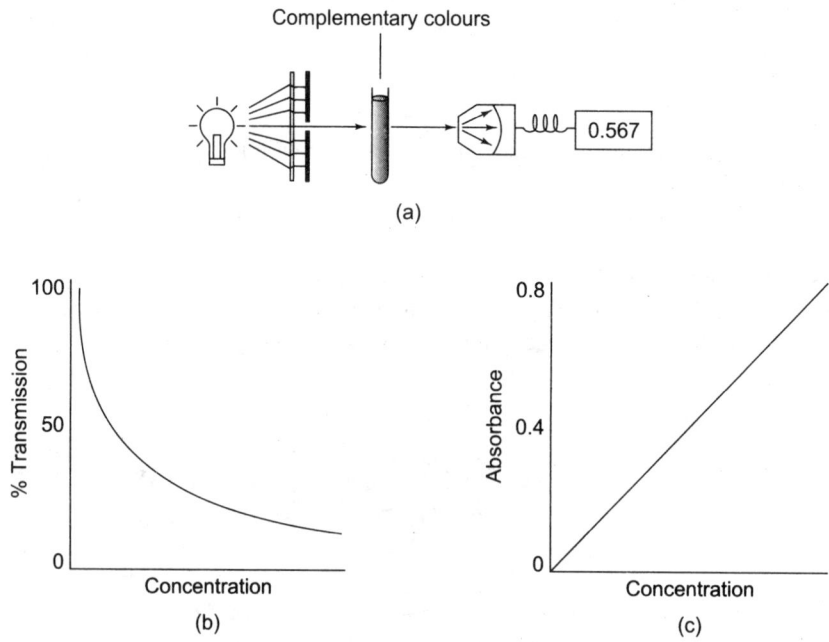

Fig. 31.4 *Application of Beer's law in absorption photometry. Use of complementary filter or wavelength of light to pass through the solution (red filter for blue solution) gives the best response. Concentration of the coloured solution is inversely proportional to percent transmittance (b) but directly proportional to absorbance (c). Hence standard curve on the linear graph should be made with the values of absorbance (c).*

Colorimeters and Spectrophotometers Colorimeters and spectrophotometers are closely comparable except that colorimeters use filters while spectrophotometers use prisms or a diffraction grating that yields a single selected wavelength of light. So we can say that spectrophotometers are only sophisticated colorimeters. These instruments can be stand-alone or part of an analyser that does multiple tests. As spectrophotometers are the single most important equipment in a clinical biochemistry laboratory, we will concentrate on the use and care of these instruments in the following pages.

Components of photometers The components of a modern spectrophotometer are shown in Fig. 31.2. A technician should understand the functions of each component in order to maintain them properly.

Light source: This provides the radiant energy. A tungsten lamp is used for the visible range and a hydrogen lamp for the UV and lower visible ranges.

Monochromator: These systems provide the desired quality of light by using **filters** (colorimeters) or a **diffraction grating** system (spectrophotometers). Spectrophotometers provide a narrower spectrum of light, thus making the test results more accurate. The diffraction grating has practically replaced the prism because they are inexpensive. Most of the analyses, however, are done by only a few preset wavelengths. For getting the best response for an absorbance reading, only complimentary colours are chosen to pass through the coloured solution (Fig 31.4a) in the cuvette—such as a red filter that is complimentary to a blue solution. Table 31.1 gives some of the most commonly chosen wavelengths of light.

Slit: The light emerging from the monochromator is then passed through a narrow slit that improves the quality of light by choosing a single wavelength. This is found in all spectrophotometers.

Cuvette: The cuvette holds the solution whose absorbance is to be measured. The cuvette is a part of the optical system; hence, extreme care must be taken in handling the cuvettes. The cuvette must be optically transparent, scrupulously clean, devoid of any scratch and free from contamination. The latter is of special significance when one is working in the UV range. Cleaning of the cuvette must be done with lens paper or soft tissue paper or toilet paper. Store the cuvette in a dry covered place; dust will scratch the cuvette. Never clean the cuvette in chromic acid; use only a mild good quality detergent.

Cuvettes are either round like a test tube or rectangular (often-called cells). The optical path within the cuvette is always 1 cm. Glass cuvettes are used for visible range spectrophotometry (or colorimetry) while quartz or silica cells are used for UV radiation. This is because glass absorbs UV light (does not pass through glass). Special plastic cuvettes (disposable) are now available, which are specially used for UV spectrophotometry. Cuvettes should not normally be replaced with a test tube. There will be a wide variation of the absorbance reading between the test tubes (use the blank for testing this). There are, however, exceptions to this general rule. Some simpler instruments make test tubes interchangeable with cuvettes, which makes the work easy. If this is done, try to choose one kind of test tube so that the reading of the blank remains constant.

Configuration (position in the holder) of the cuvette can affect the reading. In the case of cells, the side that allows the optical path to pass is clear while the other side is frosted. Specially made cuvettes are uniform and thus changing their configuration will not affect the absorbance reading. Some manufacturers provide a mark on the cuvette, which should be in line with the mark given on the colorimeter. For matching the cuvettes, number the cuvettes on a non-reading surface and fill them with water. Set the desired wavelength and take the absorbance for each cuvette. Never perform this match using empty cuvettes. Minor variations can be ignored but if the reading is more than 0.1, take a note of the error (+ or –) and make the adjustment in the final reading for samples. If several matched cuvettes are not available for keeping individual specimens, use two matched cuvettes, one for the blank and the other for the specimen. In this case, always rinse and drain the cuvette before pouring in new test solution or the standard.

Photodetector and galvanometer: The photodetector generates an electric current when light falls on it and then transmits it to the galvanometer. The needle of the galvanometer deflects as a consequence of the electric impulse and the deflection is proportional to the light intensity. The detector measures the transmitted light, which is reciprocally related to the absorbance. As Beer's Law shows the direct relationship between absorbance and concentration, the transmittance reading is first converted to the absorbance scale (Fig. 31.4) for preparing the standard curve. Modern colorimeters, however, provide the absorbance reading along with the transmittance reading on the scale provided. Note that the absorbance is read on a logarithmic scale, which is wider at low values and narrower at higher values. The highest reading of the absorbance is 2 (or infinity) while that of transmittance is 100. The '0' reading of the absorbance coincides with the 100% transmittance reading. An absorbance reading beyond '1' is used with caution as the error of the reading increases due to the compressed gradation of the scale in this region (Fig. 31.5).

Basic technique of colorimetry

The three basic steps of colorimetry or visual spectrophotometry are as follows:

1. **Chemical reaction:** This leads to the development of colour through a chemical reaction. If the test compound is a chromogenic substance, a chemical reaction may not be necessary.
2. **Physical measurement:** The detector measures the transmitted light (Fig. 31.2). The intensity of the colour is measured (A or $\%T$), both for the test solution as well as for the standard. The latter, with known concentration of the test compound, is treated identically as the specimen or test solution.
   Note: Use an appropriate filter to yield the desired quality of light.

3. **Calculation:** Results are either calculated by the mathematical formula or read from a calibration curve prepared from varying concentrations of the standard and the corresponding absorbance readings. If the readings are taken in %T, first convert the values to absorbance (A) before calculating the results (Fig. 31.5).

Some Commonly Used Terms

Blank solution: This is used to set the photometer to '0' absorbance (A) or '100%' transmittance (%T). This can be water or the reagent solution (if coloured), also referred to as a reagent blank.

Standard solutions: These are solutions of known concentrations, which range within the limits found in the specimen (normal and abnormal).

Test solution: This is the solution into which the specimen was added in order to develop a colour.

Control: This is identical to the specimen but, unlike the (unknown) specimen, the concentration of the analyte is known. A control is used to determine the accuracy and dependability of the test.

Preparation of Calibration Curve As with any other analytical technique, colorimetry requires the preparation of a calibration curve. The calibration curve shows the relationship between varying concentrations of the analytical compound sought and the instrument reading. In the case of photometry, the curve confirms that Beer's Law is obeyed. A slope of 45° is ideal for the calibration curve. It shows the balanced relationship between absorbance and concentration (Figs. 31.6a and b). In other words, for each increase in concentration, a satisfactory proportional increase in the absorbance reading is found. The same cannot be said for the other two curves shown (Figs 31.6c and d) against the ideal standard curve (Fig. 31.6a). If the curve is at an angle less than 45°, the sensitivity of the method is poor. In other words, a large change in concentration brings about only a small change in absorbance. On the contrary, if the calibration curve is at an angle greater than 45°, it indicates that the method cannot work on a wide range of concentrations of the substance to be analysed as the readings will vary too widely with a slight change in concentration. If the linear relationship is not observed (Fig. 31.5d) in the calibration curve, the technician must establish the limit of the linear relationship. It is a good policy to check the linear relationship and redraw the calibration curve whenever there is any change in the procedure or equipment performance, such as the changing of a bulb, a new standard, a new reagent, etc.

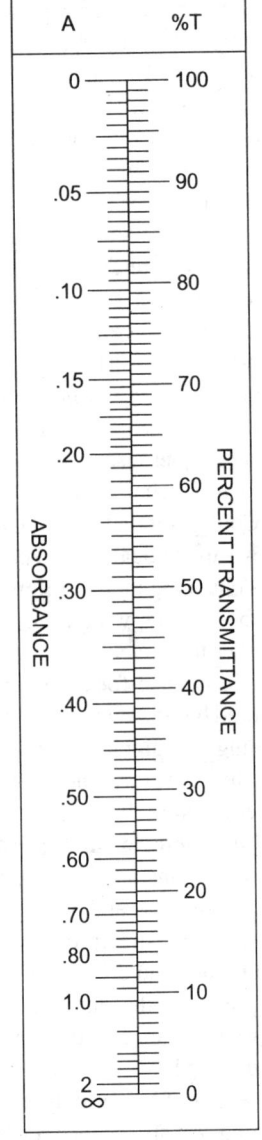

Fig. 31.5 *Conversion scales of transmittance (%) and absorbance.*

Procedure of Taking Colorimeter Readings The following procedure is taken from one of the manufacturer's instructions (Beckman Instrument Company, USA; Fig. 31.3b). Such instructions from similar photometers are available from other manufacturers as well (see Appendix at the end of this Volume).

Note: Read the manufacturer's instructions carefully before handling the instrument.

1. Set the instrument to 0%T setting (or μ setting of absorbance) with the help of the 'zero setting knob'. During the zero setting, light is not allowed to pass through the cuvette. In some instruments this is called 'dark current setting'.

2. Match two cuvettes after filling them with water and taking their absorbance readings. Record the error, if there is any. If the manufacturer supplies matched cuvettes, this will not be necessary.
   Note: The marking on the cuvette must be in line with the marking on the instrument so that the configuration of the cuvette remains identical while taking each reading (Fig. 31.3c).

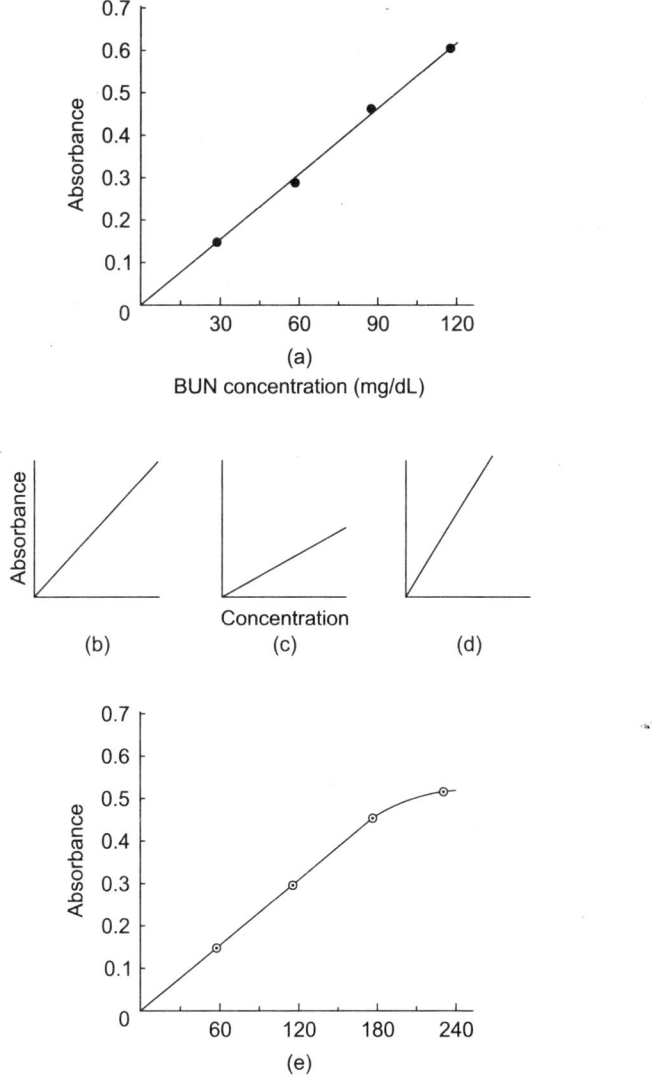

Fig. 31.6 *Significance of calibration curve. Typical calibration curve of BUN (a). Ideal calibration curve should have a slope of 45° between the absorbance and transmittance. Any deviation from the 45° slope (b) will result in an increased error (c and d). The calibration curve is good only up to the point where it shows linearity (e).*

3. Pour the blank into one of the cuvettes after taking out the water.
4. Set the instrument to $100\%T$ (or 0 absorbance) for the blank. Use the blank setting knob to set the other extreme of the galvanometer while light is passing through the blank.

5. Perform the required analytical procedures using various concentrations of the standard solutions.
6. Take the absorbance reading of each solution (variable concentrations). If a matched cuvette is used, rinse the cuvette each time and always start from the lowest concentration.
7. Record the readings in a tabular form—absorbance readings against the sequential concentrations of standards used.
8. Plot the calibration curve on linear graph paper for the absorbance readings (shown on the Y-axis) against the various concentrations of the standard (shown on the X-axis). See Chapter 4 in Vol. I for details.
9. The calibration curve should be at an angle of 45° and must be well labelled. Record the instrument and exact wavelength used. This is because the calibration curve varies between instruments and at different wavelengths.

Additional information

- If the calibration curve is not linear beyond a certain concentration (Fig. 31.6), the absorbance reading of the non-linear region should not be considered. The specimen should be diluted and rerun until the absorbance is in the linear region.
- In preparing serial dilutions of the standard, try to use larger quantities of a more dilute standard than very small quantities of a concentrated standard in the assay. The latter tends to increase the sample delivery error.
- Linear relationship of the calibration curve establishes the following mathematical formula

$$C_u = \frac{A_u}{A_s} \times C_s,$$

where C_u is concentrations of unknown, C_s is concentration of standard, A_u is absorbance of unknown and A_s is Absorbance of the standard.

The formula for calculating the concentration of the unknown (specimen) is applicable only when the relationship between absorbance and concentration is linear. Hence, the calibration curve should first be drawn before using the formula. If the curve is not linear and does not have a 45° slope, the results will not be reliable.

Note: The unit of concentration for the specimen will be the same as the standard.

Reflectance photometry

With the popularization of POCT, reflectance photometry is becoming handy as a part of solid-phase technology. The instrument does not need any liquid reagent and there are fewer breakdowns. The reagents are, however, more expensive but the results are reliable.

Reflectance photometers measure light intensity of a specific wavelength that is reflected by a coloured product (Fig. 31.7b). This reflected light is detected by a photocell, and the information is converted into the appropriate units. Instruments using solid-phase technology install reflectance photometry in their system, which is ideal for small laboratories. Technicians with limited training can handle most of these.

In solid-phase chemistry analysers (Fig. 31.7a), the reagents are in a dried form embedded in the test spot. One can use whole blood as the specimen. The blood sample is applied directly to the reagent strip, slide or cartridge that contains all the reagents needed for the analysis in the test area or reagent pad. The reagents are in multiple layers in a cartridge, with each layer having a specific function. The layers are capable of filtering the red blood cells, leaving only plasma to mix with the test reagents. The resulting colour of the final product is detected by reflectance photometry. The colour intensity is measured and converted to appropriate units for the test being performed. Different slides (or cartridges) are used for different tests. Nearly 30 different tests can be performed on a small desktop analyser.

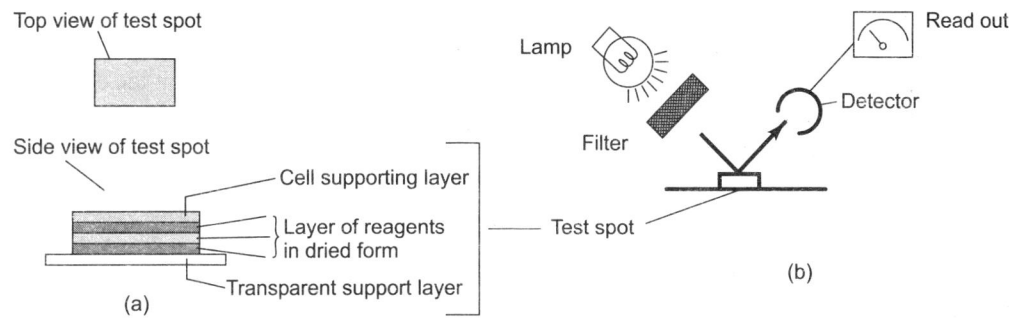

Fig. 31.7 *(a) Solid phase technology. Manufacturer provides reagents stacked on a spot, (b) specimen soaked in and the colour intensity measured by reflectance photometry.*

Urine strip analysers also operate by reflectance photometry. The reagent strip pads change colours depending on the composition of the urine. These colour changes are detected by the instrument and the results are displayed or printed.

Turbidometry and nephelometry

Turbidometry (Fig 31.8a) is classified under absorption photometry, but the radiant energy of light is intercepted by the solid particles, which are in a state of suspension in the liquid medium, rather than absorbed by the system. The machine measures the transmitted light. The method is difficult to standardize because the particle size is critical. This method is in use for several semi-quantitative assays, such as protein determination by a precipitation method and estimating the bacterial population before running an antibiotic sensitivity test (see Chapter 20 in Vol. II).

On the other hand, the method of nephelometry (Fig. 31.8b) measures the intensity of radiation scattered by a suspension. The procedure can be highly sensitive and has found its application in immunochemistry. If the antigen–antibody complex forms a fine suspension, this method of photometric assay can be applied in quantifying the immunochemical reaction.

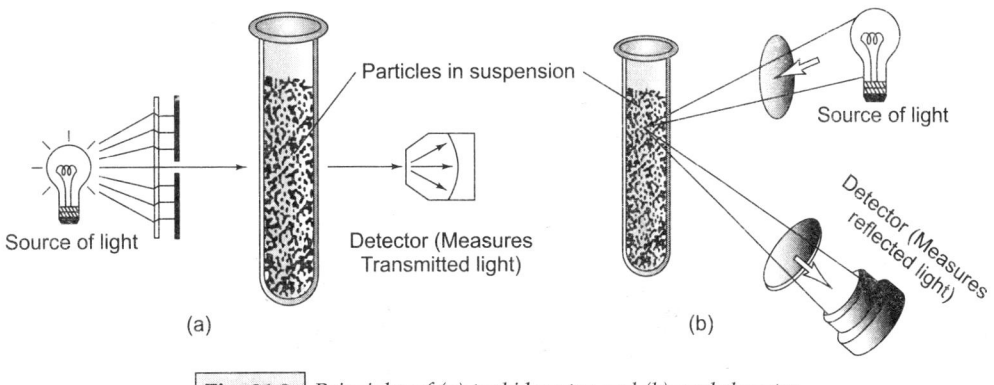

Fig. 31.8 *Principles of (a) turbidometry and (b) nephelometry.*

Electrochemistry

Electrochemical technology has suddenly become popular with the advent of hand-held glucose meters, which make it easy to monitor the serum glucose level of diabetic patients. Based on the same principle of measuring electrical energy—flow of current (**amperometry**), potential difference between electrodes (**potentiometry**) and others—various tests are now performed at ease. In some of the glucose meters, special electrodes measure the electrons generated when the sample and reagents react. Instruments based on the principle of amperometry measure glucose with the help of a disposable biosensor strip containing the electrode. When the sample interacts with the reagents in the biosensor strip, the current (electrons) generated is detected by the meter and converted into glucose units. It takes only a few seconds to complete the entire test.

Measurement of pH and various electrolytes are based on the principle of **potentiometry** (Fig 31.9). In simple words, it measures the potential difference between two electrodes that act as probes that are connected by the flow of ions in solution. A common use of electrodes in clinical chemistry is to measure the hydrogen ion concentration using a pH meter. **Ion-selective electrodes** selectively measure a particular ion in the presence of other ions. So a pH electrode is an ion-selective electrode for hydrogen (H^+). The pH meters are extensively used in clinical biochemistry laboratories for preparing various reagents and buffer solutions (Fig. 31.10).

Two electrodes are required for potentiometric analyses. One electrode contains a known concentration of the ion to be measured and is called the **reference electrode**. The other electrode, which is responsive only to

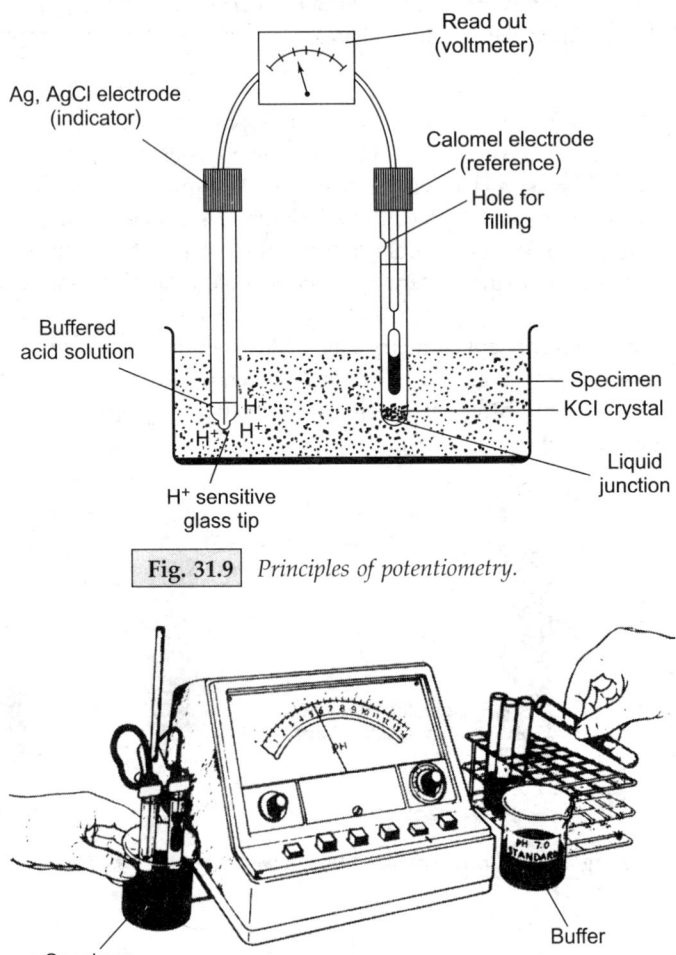

Fig. 31.9 *Principles of potentiometry.*

Fig. 31.10 *The pH meter is widely used in clinical biochemistry laboratories for preparing reagent solutions and buffers.*

the flow of current (amperometry) through the ion being measured, is exposed to the unknown solution. The difference between the concentration of ions in the reference electrode and the ions in the unknown solution causes an electrical potential to develop. This potential across a membrane in the electrode is proportional to the difference between the two concentrations. The potential, measured in voltage, is converted by the microprocessor into a number representing the concentrations of the ion in the unknown solution. Because each ion-selective electrode is responsive to a specific ion, the sodium (Na^+) electrode, for example, will measure only Na^+ ions in a sample. The technology of ion-selective electrodes is used in many clinical instruments and is particularly useful for measuring electrolytes.

Immunochemistry

Assay methods based on immunological principles are used in essentially all departments. In simple words, antibodies develop within our body through our defensive immune system as a result of invading foreign antigens (pathogens). The antibodies generated react with the antigens and make them inactive. This can be demonstrated in the laboratory through the agglutination of red blood cells, which carry the antigens on their surface. This has been discussed in Chapter 15 of Vol. I. The same principles are applied in the identification of various infectious agents, as will be presented in the chapter on immunology. Numerous other applications of immunology in the clinical laboratory include: tissue compatibility testing for grafting, identification of cells markers and evaluation of patients' immune function in the cases such as recurring infections, poor wound healing or other symptoms that indicate a possible problem with the immune response. We will confine ourselves here to the application of the same principles used in a chemical assay. Here the immunochemical methodology detects substances unrelated to the immune system, such as drugs or hormones, using antigen–antibody reactions.

While trying to focus on the application of immunochemical analytical procedures we will postpone our detailed discussion on the nature and types of antibodies, which are immunoglobulins, their structures and functions. This has been discussed in Chapter 23 of Vol. II and will be further elaborated in immunochemistry in the following sections.. Whether the laboratory is looking for the antibody in the patient's serum or circulating antigen (drug or hormone), the laboratory must be able to detect and quantitate the immunologic reaction. Commercially available latex particles carry the antigen or the antibody and the resulting immunologic reaction between the two can be visible (Fig. 31.11a). The lattice formation allows the precipitate to be visible to the naked eye (Fig. 31.11b). This process of agglutination leads to visible clumping or aggregation of cells or particles due to reaction with a specific antibody. Similar reactions are seen in blood typing. The test for rheumatoid arthritis is also based on this principle. Slide agglutination tests can give a qualitative or semi-quantitative result.

Radial immunodiffusion

The precipitation reaction of antigen and antibody is applied in a radial immunodiffusion (RID) test (Fig. 31.12) that measures the concentrations of various types of immunoglobulins (IgG, IgM or IgA) in patient's serum. Agar plates, about the size of a microscope slide, are commercially available and contain antihuman globulin or IgG (or antihuman IgA or IgM) diffused throughout the agar. The agar also contains small wells. Each well is filled with a patient's serum, a serum dilution, or a standard of a known amount of IgG. After setting up the plate, it is incubated for several hours. As the IgG in the serum or standard (kept in the well) diffuses out of the well and into the agar, it reacts with the anti-IgG in the agar and forms a white ring of precipitation around the well (Fig. 31.12). The diameter of the ring is proportional in the concentration of IgG in the sample. A standard curve is constructed using the diameters of the rings produced by the IgG standards. The concentration of the unknown is determined by comparing its precipitation diameter with the standard curve.

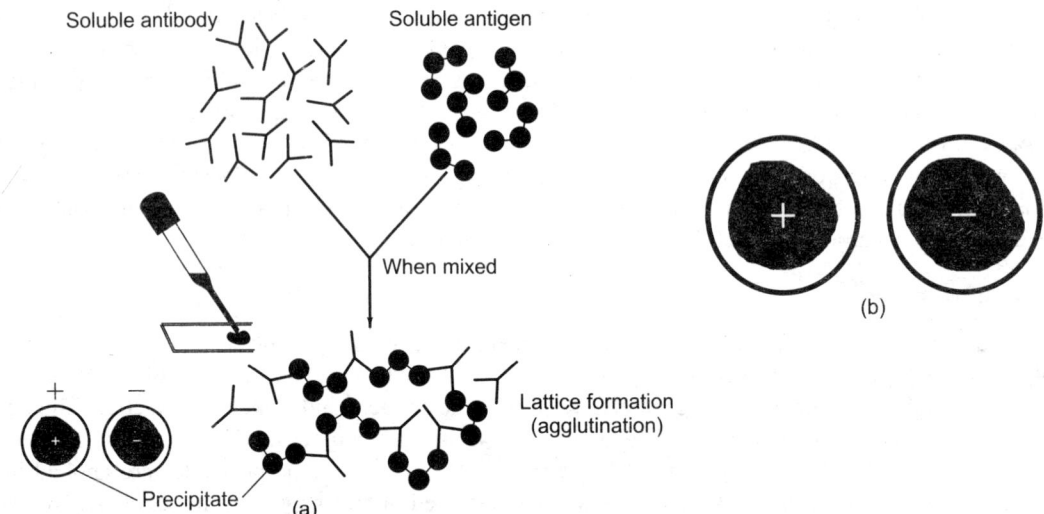

Fig. 31.11 *Immunological reaction of soluble antigen and soluble antibody may be visible by the clumping effect (agglutination) as a result of lattice formation of the antigen and antibody. The results could be used as a semi-quantitative assay.*

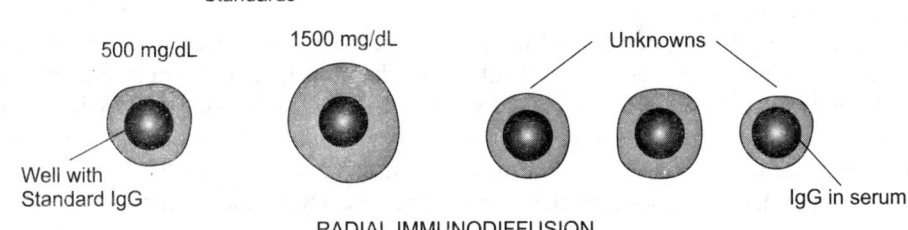

Fig. 31.12 *Illustration of agar precipitation technique (radial immunodiffusion) where rings of precipitation form when serum diffuses out of wells and reacts with specific antibody in agar. The size of the ring could give provide quantitative data for diagnosis.*

Nephelometry

When a specific antibody reacts with a soluble antigen, a suspension of very small particles forms, the concentration of which can be measured by a nephelometer. The use of nephelometry principles allows immunological tests to be automated. This is done by passing a beam of light through the suspension (Fig. 31.8) resulting from both the antigen–antibody reaction and the resultant precipitate formation. The light gets scattered. The scattered light is then collected electronically and measured for a quantitative report. The greater the amount of light scattered, the more concentrated is the suspension of the particles. This method has largely replaced the RID technique.

Labelled antibody techniques

Several types of immunological tests use labelled (or 'tagged') antibodies. These labelled antibodies are mostly antihuman globulins, which will recognize any antibody in the serum reacted with its corresponding antigen. Hence they are also referred to as anti-antibodies. The labelling can be done by the use of fluorescent dyes, enzymes or radioisotopes (Figs 31.13–31.15). The elements of an enzyme immunoassay (EIA) are depicted in Fig. 31.13. This figure shows the principles behind the application of both EIA and radioimmunoassay (RIA) in the determination of the concentration of various analytes. The fluorescent antibody (FA) technique, Western blotting, and flow cytometry are sophisticated versions of the labelled antibody technique. These methods are used in hormone assays, drug monitoring and to detect the presence of viral antigen (e.g. HAA) in serum.

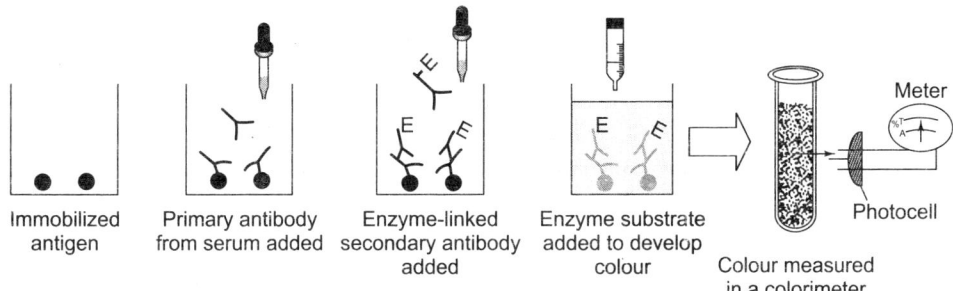

ENZYME IMMUNOASSAY

Fig. 31.13 *The technique of antibody labelling technique, using tagged-enzyme, in the quantitative assay of the amount of antibody present in the serum. The amount of antibody is detected by colorimetric method using substrate that yield colour. The non-labile antigen adhered to the wall of the container is available commercially.*

Enzyme immunoassay

EIAs use enzyme-labelled antibodies that result in a visible reaction (Fig. 31.13). This method utilizes less expensive equipment and therefore is becoming popular in developing countries. The test can be designed to detect either an antibody in a patient's serum, or a antigen (e.g. viral antigen) in circulation in a patient's body.

The process goes through four major steps. In the first step commercially available antigen-coated beads are taken in a container and incubated with the serum specimen of the patient. The antigen on the bead is the one, which is sought as the infectious agent. A patient's serum may have a primary antibody against the antigen sought. If the patient has the antibody against the antigen coated on the bead, it will become attached to the antigen. Subsequent washings in the following step do not take away the attached antibody on the bead. In the second step a secondary antibody, linked with an appropriate enzyme, is laid on the bead holding the primary antibody. The secondary antibody is an antihuman globulin, which reacts with any human antibody and thus gets stuck to the bead. The beads are again washed to remove any free secondary antibody. Now, we have the beads in the tube with the antigen of the pathogen plus its primary antibody plus the secondary antibody with the linked enzyme, laid one over the other. Now in the third and final step, an appropriate amount of a substrate upon which the enzyme works is added, yielding a visible colour. The colour will be proportional to the amount of primary antibody present in the patient's serum, and the reported results are considered quantitative in nature.

Radioimmunoassay

RIAs represent some of the earliest additions to the modern generation of immunoassays. They can be divided into either solid phase RIA Fig. 31.14 or liquid phase RIA (Fig. 31.15). The illustrations provided will give you an idea of this sensitive analytical technique. The methodology requires expensive equipment for the measurement of radioactivity. This limits their popularity in developing countries.

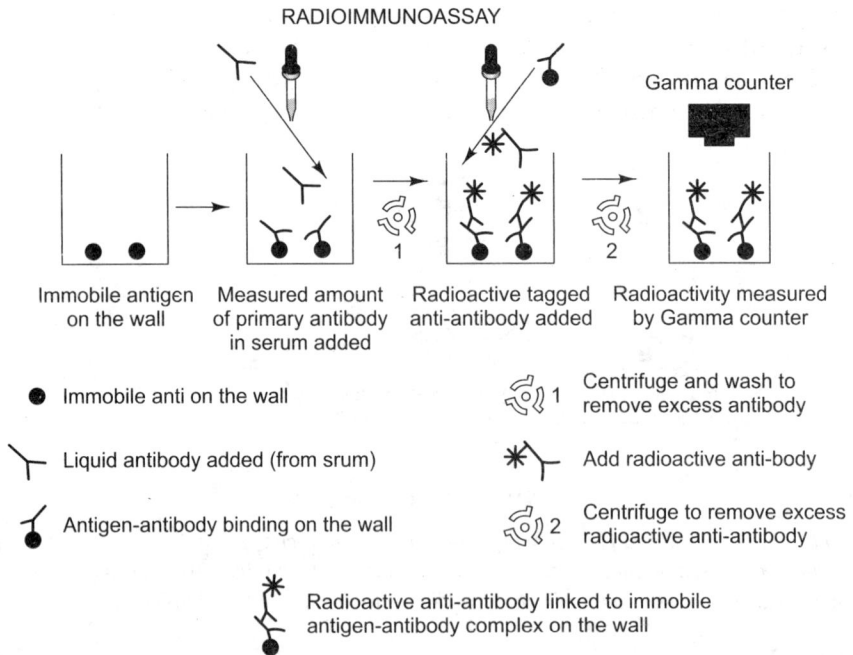

Fig. 31.14 Solid phase radioimmunoassay.
Plastic tubes (or beads) are coated with non-radioactive antigen (or antibody), which reacts with the corresponding antibody (or antigen, Hepatitis virus HAA) present in patient's serum. The antibody (or antigen) gets fixed and the excess antibody (or antigen) is washed away by the buffer. In subsequent steps, radioactive anti-antibody (or antibody) is added which sticks to the antibody (or antigen, HAA) and the excess is washed away. The radioactive tubes (or beads) are then subjected to the counting of radioactivity. In case of absence of antigen (normal serum), radioactive antibody does not stick and the tubes (or beads) stay non-radioactive.

Fluorescent antibody technique

In FA tests, a fluorescent dye is conjugated to the antibody. These dyes fluoresce when excited by a beam of UV light, and epifluorescence microscopes must be used to read and interpret the reactions (Fig. 31.16). An FA test can be direct or indirect. In the case of a direct test, there is no secondary antibody (anti-antibody) used (like tagged human globulin) to react with patient's antibody. The method allows the laboratory to detect antibody in a patient's serum or antigen in a patient specimen. FA tests are used in microbiology and parasitology. It is also used to detect auto-antibodies present in autoimmune diseases such as lupus.

The FA technique is successfully used in the diagnosis of syphilis. Syphilis is the venereal disease caused by *Treponema pallidum*, a spirochete or spiral bacterium. Because of the difficulty of growing *Treponema* in culture, the screening method of choice has been the detection of serum antibody. Since several non-syphilitic conditions can cause biologically false positive (BFP) reactions using other tests, including tuberculosis, hepatitis, pneumonia, pregnancy and rheumatoid arthritis, the fluorescent treponemal antibody test is considered both specific and confirmatory of a diagnosis of syphilis. A prepared slide of the laboratory strain of *Treponema* is incubated with a patient's serum, if the patient is suspected to have circulating antibodies associated with *T. pallidum* infection (syphilis). After incubation, the slide is gently washed to remove unbound non-specific antibody, and the specimen is then incubated with fluorescently labelled antihuman globulin. The slide is washed again and then examined under a fluorescent microscope. The presence of fluorescent-stained spirochetes indicates that the patient's serum is positive for antitreponemal antibodies. The method is also applied in the diagnosis of infection by *Mycobacterium* or *Cryptosporidium*.

A newer method called a *T. pallidum* microhaemagglutination assay (MHA-TP) is more suitable for underdeveloped countries, as it does not require the expensive fluorescent microscope. The method is discussed in Chapter 23 in Vol. II.

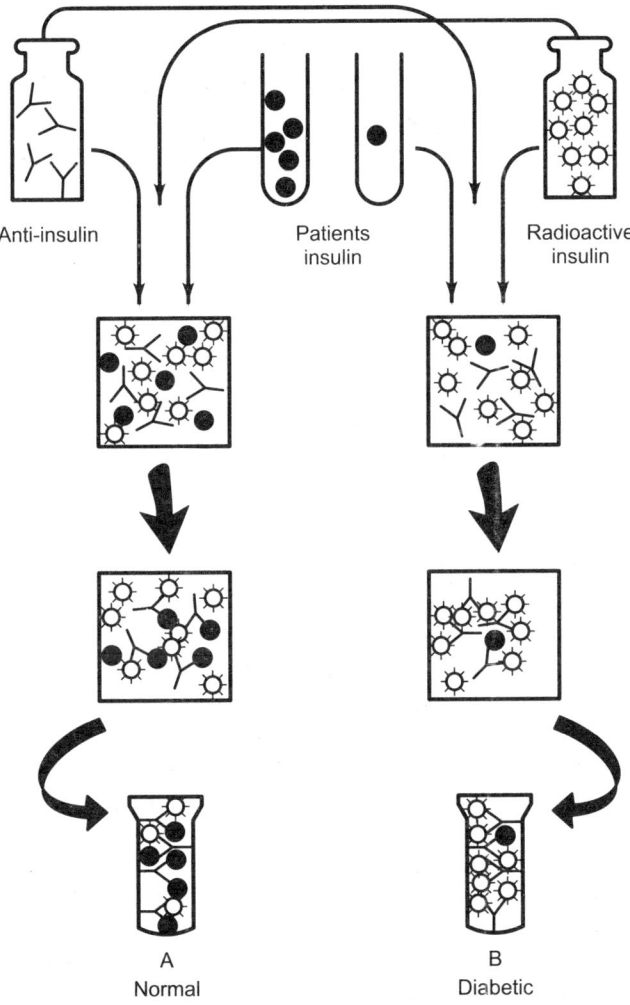

Fig. 31.15 *Liquid phase radioimmunoassay. In a liquid phase radioimmunoassay system, a competition is set up between the antibody (e.g. anti-insulin) and two kinds of the same antigen—radioactive (commercially available) and non-radioactive, which comes from the patient. At the end, the binding of the radioactive antigen is inversely proportional to the amount of antigen present in the serum. The method is applicable in the diagnosis of diabetic patient. The serum of a normal person has a higher concentration of insulin and thus less radioactive insulin is attached to the antibody (series A), than in the diabetic patient (series B).*

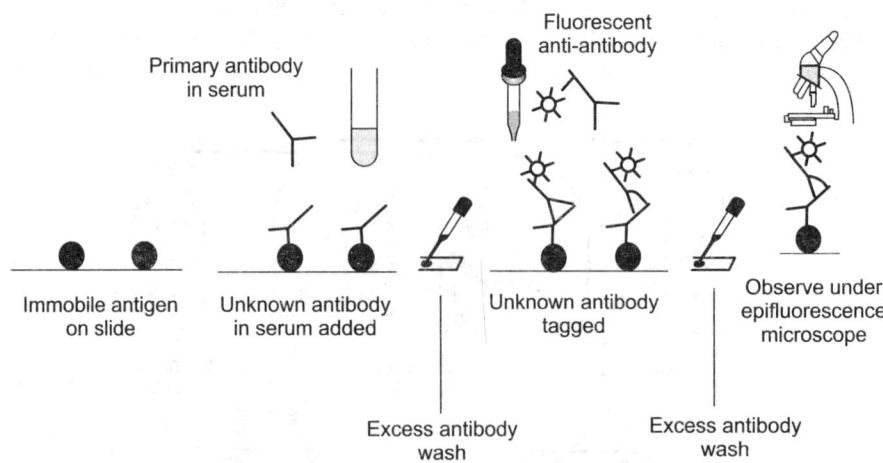

Fig. 31.16 *Antigen (e.g. Treponema sp.) from laboratory culture is laid on the slide. This is reacted with its corresponding antibody, suspected to be present in the serum. The excess antibody is washed away after a while and then overlaid by fluorescent anti-antibody (anti-human globulin). This is followed by a second wash in order to remove the excess fluorescent anti-antibody. The slide is then observed under an epifluorescence microscope. If the patient's serum has the antibody against the antigen of interest, the antigens will glow and test will be reported as positive.*

Electrochemical Technology

Blood gases and pH are determined electrochemically. This is further discussed in Chapter 33 in this volume. Determinations of pH and PCO_2 are done by the potentiometric method. The blood analyser is convenient to use; it is accurate but expensive under conditions of developing countries.

In recent years, electrochemical principles are applied in wider range. This developing new technology has suddenly captured the market and has proved to be of great value for POC service, which may take place at home or in the physician's office. Several hand-held analysers such as glucose meters are based on electrochemical technology. Other terms used for this technology include amperometry and coulometry. Patient samples are applied to disposable biosensors, strips that look similar to other reagent strips. These biosensors, in addition to containing reagent for the chemical reactions, also contain an electrode called electrochemical sensor. When the sample interacts with the reagents in the biosensor strip, the current (electrons) generated is detected by the meter and converted into glucose units.

In the case of haemoglobin A1c (also termed glycated haemoglobin or GHb) determination, which is crucial for diabetic patients, the reports are available within 5 min using a table-top HbA1c analyser. The technology employed by the manufacturer is '**affinity chromatography**' and requires only 10 µL of blood.

Affinity chromatography is almost exclusively used for the purification of biological molecules such as proteins (haemoglobin A1c) and other macromolecules. Biotech research has used affinity chromatography because of its ability to separate one desired species from a host of other biological molecules. It operates on the principle that ligands, attached to a matrix made up of an inert substance, bind to the desired molecule within the solution to be analysed (Fig. 31.17a). Ideally, the ligand will interact only with the desired molecule and form a permanent bond. All other compounds (impurities) in the solution will be eluted (Fig. 31.17b), leaving the desired product in the column. The desired molecule is then removed from the column by using a wash (typically changing the pH) that lowers the dissociation constant and allows recovery of a nearly pure sample (Fig. 31.17c).

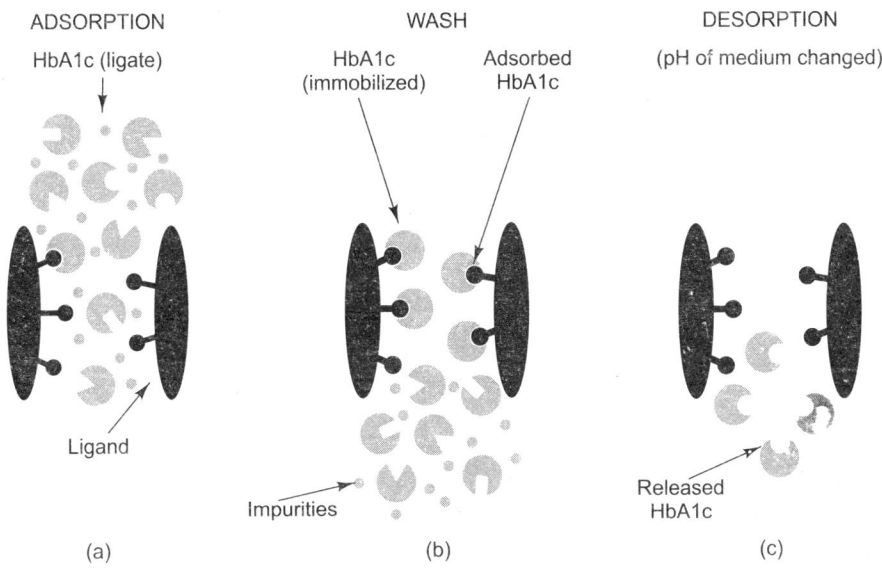

Fig. 31.17 *Determination of haemoglobin A1c by affinity chromatography. Blood specimen with HbA1c ligate is laid on the ligand (a) that results in the adsorption of the HbA1c on the ligand due to its nature of selective affinity. In the following step (b), the washing process removes the impurities but not the ligate. The ligate (HbA1c) is then finally released by desorption for its measurement following change in the pH of the medium.*

Electrophoresis

Electrophoresis is a method of separating a mixture of organic compounds. The technique of electrophoresis is used in separating haemoglobins, proteins (haemoglobin, serum proteins, lipoproteins and isoenzymes) and diagnostic enzymes. It has proved to be most useful in the diagnosis of haemoglobinopathies. The method allows various components of haemoglobins, as well as abnormal haemoglobins, to get separated and quantitative measures of each can be presented to the physician.

Principle: Electrophoresis is the migration of charged particles (e.g. proteins) in an electrical field. The protein has both amino as well as carboxyl groups that can potentially carry either a net (+) or a (−) charge, depending on whether the pH of the medium is acidic or alkaline. During electrophoresis the pH of the buffer (barbital) is kept at 8.4.

Components: Components of electrophoresis equipment are shown in Fig. 31.18. The buffer (sodium barbital) flows through the support medium when the electrodes are connected. This enables the mixture of the organic compounds on the spot to get separated based on charge. The medium is then removed after a specified time, stained and read under a photo sensor. An electrophoretogram (Fig. 31.19) shows the migration rate and can be used for diagnostic purpose.

In the case of a serum protein study, the serum specimen, which is a mixture of various proteins, is placed as a spot on a support medium. The medium is wetted with the buffer used for the free flow of the electric current. As the electric current passes through the sample, different proteins (albumin, globulins—$alpha_1$, $alpha_2$, beta and gamma) migrate at different rates based on charge. Albumin has the highest rate of migration and gamma globulin is the slowest. The location of each separated protein-spot is determined by staining with a protein-staining dye (Ponceau S). Photometric measurements (Fig. 31.19) can also track the migration of the proteins on an electrophoretogram. Figure 31.20 shows several patterns associated with normal and abnormal clinical conditions.

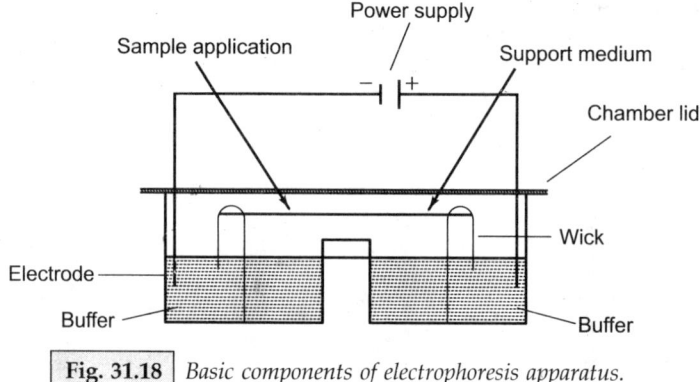

Fig. 31.18 *Basic components of electrophoresis apparatus.*

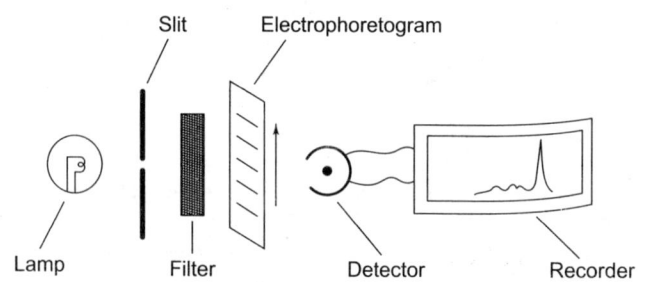

Fig. 31.19 *Reading of electrophoretogram through transparent support medium.*

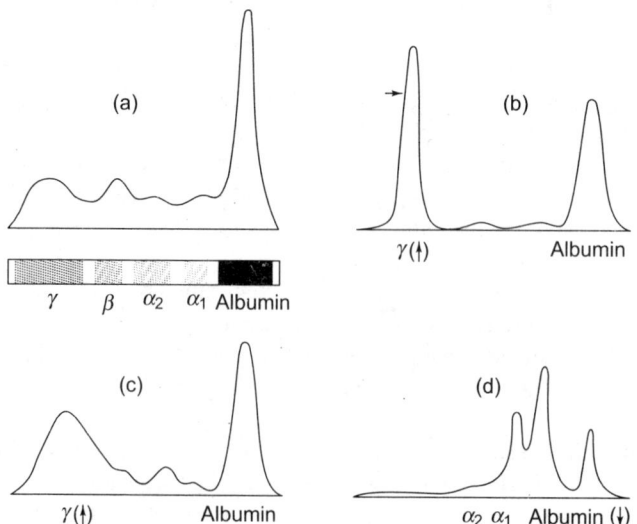

Fig. 31.20 *Separation of serum proteins by electrophoresis.*
Serum electrophoretogram of normal subject (a), of patient with multiple myeloma showing monoclonal peak of Bence Jones protein (b), of patient with chronic infection and increased gamma globulin (c) and of patient with nephrotic syndrome showing fall of albumin (d).

Electrophoresis of haemoglobin is done with the goal of identifying abnormal haemoglobin. The migration rate of abnormal haemoglobins varies from the normal haemoglobin (HbA), and thus they are identified based on their location. Staining is not necessary for locating haemoglobin spots due to the inherent colour of these proteins.

Review Questions

1. What are the basic steps of analytical chemistry?
2. Define the following: Standard solution, a control serum, reagent blank and water blank.
3. What is Beer's law? Discuss its significance to analytical chemistry.
4. What is the principle of colorimetry? How does it differ from spectrophotometry?
5. How does absorption photometry differ from reflectance photometry?
6. State the basic difference between a colorimeter and a spectrophotometer.
7. What is the basis of solid phase technology? What is its future in developing counties?
8. Discuss the principle of electrophoresis and its application in the separation of haemoglobin and serum proteins.
9. List the components of an electrophoresis apparatus and state the function of each component.
10. Which of the following techniques is most suitable for developing countries: enzyme immunoassay, radioimmunoassay or fluorescent immunoassay?
11. Which instrument will detect the immunologic reaction in an Enzyme Immunoassay?
12. What is the basic difference between nephelometry and turbidometry?
13. What is the principle of the latex agglutination test?
14. How does the immunofluorescent assay confirm a diagnosis of syphilis.
15. What is biologically false-positive report?
16. What is the principle of affinity chromatography? Give an example of its application.
17. How is glucose determined by hand-held glucometers?
18. What is the significance of an HbA1c determination?
19. What is the difference between the terms ligate and ligand?

32

Automation in Clinical Biochemistry

◆

Kanai L. Mukherjee, Dipto Chakravarty and Aurin Chakravarty

Chapter Outline

- ◆ Classification of Automated Systems
  - Continuous flow analysis
  - Discrete analysis
  - Centrifugal analysis
- ◆ Steps of Automation
  - Sample handling and sample measurement
  - Sample handling
  - Overcoming interference
  - Transport and delivery of specimen and reagent
  - Reagent handling
  - Reaction conditions
  - Reaction measurement
  - Calculation of results
  - Quality control and preventing maintenance
  - Automated 'stat' testing
- ◆ Computers in the Clinical Laboratory
  - Computer application in clinical laboratories
  - Challenges of computerization
  - Glossary of terms
  - Operation of a computer
    - ❏ Hardware
      - ○ Central processing unit (CPU)
      - ○ Input/Output (I/O)

- Automation in Clinical Biochemistry 873

  - o *Memory/storage unit*
  - ❑ *Software*
  - • *Computerization of clinical laboratory instruments*
    - ❑ *Machine failure*
    - ❑ *Computer housing*
    - ❑ *Conclusion*
  - ◆ *Automated Analysers in Developing Countries*
    - ❑ *Auto Analyzer*
    - ❑ *Clinical Corona*
    - ❑ *Auto Pacer*
    - ❑ *SEAC (Ames)*
  - ◆ *Point-of-care-testing (POCT): A New Approach*
  - ◆ *Time Saving Devices and Kits*
  - ◆ *Automation in Developing Countries*
  - ◆ *Review Questions*

In clinical biochemistry, automation is the mechanization (and computerization) of the steps in a procedure. In this chapter, the reasons for automation and the ways to achieve it are considered. Examples from the major instrument categories often seen in developing countries are examined.

Contrary to common belief, automation is not intended merely to save labour, which may not be a limiting factor for the developing countries, but it allows reliable **quality control** (QC) measures to be imposed strongly. Other advantages include increased accuracy, less discrepancy in results, better QC, reduced subjective errors and the use of smaller quantities of samples and reagents which may ultimately prove to be economical. More and more laboratories in the developing countries are thinking in terms of at least semi-automation because of poor quality of technicians, frequent labour problems, reduction of cost per test and increased reliability. The problems that the developing countries are facing include the repair and maintenance of equipment, and difficulty in obtaining spare parts. Alternate manual methods must be available in order to save the laboratory from complete breakdown.

CLASSIFICATION OF AUTOMATED SYSTEMS

Automated systems are seen only in the urban settings of both advanced as well as in the developing countries. They can be grouped under three basic categories.

Continuous Flow Analysis

This is the first automated system introduced into the market in the 1960s by Technicon (USA) which has since been followed by other systems. In this system, liquids such as specimen, reagents and diluents are pumped through a continuous tubing system leading to continuous flow. Samples are introduced in a sequential manner, following each other through the same network. A series of air bubbles at regular intervals serve as separating and cleaning media. The system is most profitable for larger laboratories. The commonly used models SMA 6/60 and 12/60 process 60 specimens per hour and, respectively, report the results of 6 and 12 diagnostic tests simultaneously. This automated system suffers from the disadvantage that the physician may not be interested in all the tests reported by the instrument. Conversely, he may be interested in some other tests which the instrument does not report.

Discrete Analysis

In this system each sample is separated along with the accompanying reagent. This can be used both for special tests as well as for routine tests. It is ideal for smaller laboratories. Some of the popular ones that fall in this category are Clinicon (Boehringer Mannheim) and Auto Pacer (Miles of India Ltd.).

Centrifugal Analysis

This is the most recent introduction in the markets of developed countries that can be broadly classified under the discrete system. After placing the specimens and the corresponding reagents in their places on the special centrifuge head, the machine is run and the force generated by centrifugation transfers the reagents and the specimen to a cuvette for chemical reaction. Optical measurements are made while the cuvette is in motion (2500 rpm). The method is most useful in performing enzyme assays.

In the following sections, we will try to present the basic principles of these technologies without going into many details.

STEPS OF AUTOMATION IN BIOCHEMICAL ANALYSES

The steps of biochemical analyses can be broadly divided under the following headings—sample handling, sampling processing, reagent handling, analytical procedures (e.g. mixing, heating, etc.), reaction analysis (e.g. reading the absorbance) and calculation. The approach of various automated systems to expedite these steps is discussed here. The goal of this description is to give an idea that automation does not replace our classical approach but it only makes adjustments to speed up the manual process.

Sample Handling and Sample Measurement

Very little automation is applied in this step. By and large, the specimens are manually labelled, centrifuged and divided into aliquots if tests for more than one work station have been requested. This manual processing of the specimen is also important from the point of view of rejecting those specimens which are not acceptable for the analysis (e.g. haemolysed or lipaemic specimens, presence of debris), and review the request form received with the specimen. Extreme care is needed in this step to avoid mislabelling of patient samples or their aliquots.

In automated systems the instrument must be fed with the specimen in an **identifiable manner**. Therefore, the sample-holding containers must be placed in the same order and the technician must write down clearly the order of the arrangement and should never rely on his memory. One should anticipate the problem involved when there is a mix up. Some laboratories prefer to number the sample cups so that if they are misplaced, they can be put into the proper slot. In most automated systems, the samples are held in small cups which are placed on a circular tray. The slots are sequentially numbered. One can use an **automatic pipetter** for taking aliquots of specimens into the sample cups. Use a fresh tip for each sample which may be disposed of or recovered after thorough cleaning and drying. In case of continuous flow analysis, the requisite amount of specimen is picked up by the sampler while in others an aliquot of the specimen may have to be manually placed. Probes used in the automated systems for picking up specimen must be thoroughly washed, preferably with a diluent, before the following specimen is drawn. One convenient way to avoid **carry over effect** is to dispense the specimen first and then the diluent.

While handling the sample one must avoid the exposure of the aliquot to the air for a prolonged period. This will increase the concentration of sample constituents due to evaporation and aliquots taken after evaporation will lead to false high results. Decay of the constituents should also be considered.

Overcoming Interference

Protein causes major interference in many analyses. In the continuous flow system, use of a **dialyser** eliminates the protein in order to facilitate the determination of other components. The dialyser is, however not used for total protein determination. In other systems, there is no such step as protein removal. They either use such a method as will be least interfered with by protein; or they use a more sensitive method, or they add appropriate chemicals to remove the protein. Some discrete analysers read absorbance with two wavelengths (bichromatic) which also help to reduce the effect of protein.

Transport and Delivery of Specimen and Reagent

The volume of reagent required for the determination of a given analyte is related directly to the volume of sample used. Most chemical reactions rely on the combination of reagents and sample in exact proportions to yield accurate results. For most instruments, the manufacturer has predetermined these proportions. However, some manufacturer allows the instrument users to develop and use their own test applications.

In unit test systems, the volume of reagent has been pre-measured. The '**dose**' of reagent, already in the reaction vessel, needs only to be delivered to the area where the sample will be added. This is usually done mechanically by pushing the reaction container to the sampling station or loading zone.

In continuous flow systems, **peristaltic pumps** and plastic tubing transport the specimen and reagent through the system. The volume of reagent is determined by the inside diameter of the rubbing, just as the volume of sample is determined. As the samples flow continuously through the tubing, reagents are added at different points, reaction conditions are provided around the tubing, and timing is determined by the distance of the coil to travel through the reaction chamber.

Positive displacement syringes are another method to deliver specific volumes of reagent to a reaction chamber. These syringes operate in the same manner as the positive displacement syringes used for sample aspiration and delivery. The speed of the driving motor should be controlled as closely as possible to prevent sudden changes in velocity and the accuracy should be verified.

Reagent Handling

Most chemical reactions require the combining of the reagent and sample in exact amounts. This is called proportioning. In continuous flow analysis, the diameter of the tube regulates the volume of the reagent fluid picked up; for the amount of specimen, the dwelling time of the probe inside the specimen container determines the amount of specimen picked up. The rate of flow for all fluids is the same. A single peristaltic pump is used for drawing the fluids. For the discrete system, a single probe may measure the volumes of specimens and reagents but the dwelling time in them varies. Individual automatic dispensers are also used in some discrete systems where syringes and volumetric overflow devices are used to dispense requisite quantities of sample and reagent into test tubes or containers. A single-reagent assay is ideal for automated biochemical analyses. This, however, is not possible and single-reagent assay is not as accurate.

Reagents can be dispensed directly from bulk containers supplied by the manufacturer, or reconstituted in the laboratory. Reagents prepared by the manufacturer are expensive and under the conditions of most developing countries with transportation difficulties and cold storage problems, the preparation of reagents in the laboratory becomes a necessity. Hence those manufacturers, who are able to supply dry reagents or provide the necessary formula for the preparation of reagents within the laboratory, will be most successful in marketing their goods in the developing countries.

Specimen carry-over is a common problem in continuous flow analysis. Thus, if a low-concentration specimen follows a high-concentration specimen, the, former will have carry-over effects due to contamination. Either in such a case the specimen should be re-run or water blank introduced to flush out the system. Alternatively, increase the wash time between specimens.

Reaction Conditions

Mixing of reagents with the specimen is a vital component of biochemical analysis. This is accomplished in several ways in the automated systems. In the continuous flow, it is done through glass coils where the liquid rotates and the liquids (specimen and reagents) fall through one another during their rise and fall through the loop. In the discrete systems, other methods are adopted—vibration, slewing action, centrifugal rotation (in centrifugal analysers), pressing and releasing of plastic bags which receive the fluids and ultrasonic waves.

Automated incubation is merely a **delay station** where the test mixture is allowed to react. The chamber where the incubation is held is heated to the desired temperature by the use of a heating block, air, water bath or oil bath. Time is a definite limitation. To sustain the advantage of speedy multiple analyses, the reaction is not taken to completion, as is required in the manual procedures. Rather, the rate of the reaction can be measured and the values after the completion of the reaction are extrapolated. The instrument may also delay the measurement for a pre-determined length of time or present the reaction mixtures for measurement at constant intervals of time. In case of continuous flow analysis, all measurements are made against a standard and as the procedures are precisely timed, the result of the standard is highly reproducible even if the measurement is made much before the completion of the reaction. In the discrete system, there are a number of delay stations before the readings are taken.

Dry slide methods accomplish mixing of the sample with premixed, pre-measured reagents through diffusion. As the sample comes into contact with the top layer of the slide, it is drawn by capillary action into the porous layer. As the reagents hydrate, components of interest diffuse into the reagent layers.

Discrete system mix reaction components by means of stirring paddles of sticks, motion of the reaction vessel, forceful addition of reagents and agitation by air bubbles or ultrasonic waves. Some system use magnetic stir bars.

Mention should be made of the use of **ion-selective electrodes** for the measurement of sodium, potassium, chloride and occasionally carbon dioxide. The reagent handling systems and reaction conditions for ion-selective electrodes are typically separate from those previous described with colorimetry or enzymatic measurement. Most ion-selective electrodes are of the flow-through variety in which the sample and reference solutions are moved via peristaltic pumps through chambers containing fixed indicator and reference electrodes. The specimen must remain in contact with the electrodes long enough to reach steady state. The electrodes are designed to minimize response time so that a steady state can be reached rapidly, maximizing the throughput of the system.

Reaction Measurement

After the reaction is completed, there must be a sensing device to measure the change like development of colour. Traditionally, **absorbance photometry** has been used for the measurement of analytes. This method has three basic components—light source, spectral isolation and a detector. **Light** sources commonly include tungsten, quartz-halogen, deuterium, mercury and xenon lamps. Each has advantages and disadvantages. Interference filters, monochromators, such as diffraction gratings help in **spectral isolation**. Diffraction gratings provide a continuous spectrum and therefore a great choice of wavelengths for use. A diffraction grating also allows the use of two or more wavelengths (bichromatics) at the same time for correction purposes, to eliminate the absorbance contribution of interfering substances. Photomultiplier tubes (PMTs) are the most prevalent detectors in automated systems. They are sensitive and give a very rapid response.

In recent years, methods other than absorbance photometry have been developed for the measurement of analytes. Reflectance photometry is one of them. In reflectance photometry, diffuse, reflected light rather than absorbed light is measured. This is used in many equipments that employ '**dry chemistry**'. One draw back to reflectance photometry is that intensities are not linear with concentration of the analytes of interest; they do not follow Beer's Law. To correct for this deviation, mathematical algorithms are used to linearize the relationship between the intensity and reflected light and the analyte concentration. Other photometric methods include turbidometry, nephelometry and fluorometry. Many of these techniques are used in automated immunoassays.

The **sensing** can be done on the original site where the reaction occurred (internal) or taken into another vessel (external) to make the measurements. In the continuous flow analysis, the reagent stream under analysis flows continuously through the flow cell which acts like a cuvette. The air bubbles are removed by the de-bubbler before the reacted solution enters the flow cell for photometric measurements. The sensing device converts the optical response into electrical impulses which are then sent to the read out device. The read out device can be the strip chart on which the results are traced or on the digital display.

Chemical reactions can be monitored either at one time point or at many. Commonly, **single-point** monitoring is used for **end-point** (or midpoint) analysis in which the reaction has gone to completion or the instrument extrapolates the value, as mentioned earlier. Multiple-point monitoring is done in case of kinetic studies (enzyme activity).

Calculation of Results

In the automated system the results are automatically computed from the response of the sensor and finally printed out in appropriate units. The printing can be done directly on the patient's request slip (or reporting slip) or on the laboratory form. In order to avoid transcription errors, it is advisable that multiple copies of the print out should be made so that different copies of the same report can be routed to different destinations—financial office, physician, patient's record, laboratory record and others.

Quality Control and Preventing Maintenance

Automated systems are not free from errors. In fact, they frequently render a false sense of security among the users and the results may be far from reliable. The system must be frequently subjected to QC procedures using control sera. Control runs should be done in the beginning of each day and the results plotted on the QC chart (Chapter 7 in Vol. I).

Preventive maintenance is done to ensure the analyser continues to function properly. Keeping an analyser clean may be the most important maintenance procedure, regardless of the instrument. Cleaning up spilled specimens and reagents will help prevent future malfunctions. Other maintenance procedures include discarding waste, cleaning water baths, cleaning reaction vessels (if reusable), replacing reagents, replacing worn or damaged parts (e.g. filters, rubbing syringes, probes and lamps), and readjusting components to ensure proper functioning.

Automated 'Stat' Testing

The word 'stat' is an abbreviation of the Latin word **statin**, meaning immediately. Many clinical conditions require **immediate** reporting of results. If the automated system cannot be adapted towards such a condition of changing the priorities, it will be a handicap. In some systems, such as the continuous flow analysis, the interruption in the processing of the current samples and the time required to change to the proper reagents may not be acceptable or practical. In such cases discrete analysers are handy. The other requirement for automated stat procedures is to have a short dwell time. The machine may not have a high **throughput**. Throughput is an expression that indicates the maximum number of individual samples or test analyses that can be practically performed per hour by an assay system with the required dwell time taken into account.

COMPUTERS IN THE CLINICAL LABORATORY

Computing and use of computers has become pervasive in our society. With commoditization of personal computers, and availability of broad spectrum of software applications, computers are used in every scientific field, including the field of laboratory medicine. The era of computerization has effectively driven high levels of QC, while increasing the laboratory output, and expediting the effectiveness of diagnosis.

Computer Application in Clinical Laboratories

Computer application in the clinical laboratory can be classified into five groups:
1. Specimen handling: Identification and recording.
2. Operation of instruments: Automatic and semiautomatic.
3. Storage of information: Results of laboratory findings.
4. Communication: Facilitates information transfers between laboratories and the physician.
5. Robotics: Robot-driven automation (commonly referred to as *robotics*), further streamlines the processes in clinical laboratories. Robotics is applied in two ways: to reduce the risk of humans in handling contaminated samples, as well as to achieve higher level of precision.

Computer systems have many definite advantages over other laboratory management systems. Not only they are capable of processing vast amounts of data with higher accuracy; they are also able to store and retrieve information in real-time, thus making the end to end performance evaluation (QC) of laboratory instruments with new degrees of efficiency.

Computers have become a pervasive part of the human society. The usage and applications of computers and computer-assisted systems have proliferated across the advanced nations as well as third world countries. Given the widespread application of computers, it is desirable to understand WHAT types of computers exist and HOW basics of computers work.

A **computer** in its simplest term is expressed as a machine that manipulates data according to a list of **instructions**. The ability to store and execute instructions called **programs** makes computers extremely versatile and distinguishes them from calculators. The heart of a computer is its central processing unit (CPU), which is essentially a sophisticated integrated circuit which enables it to carry out arithmetic functions, logic functions and to move data in and out of memory. Memories are of two types: one is referred to as random-access-memory or RAM, which is programmable and erasable, and the other is called read-only-memory or ROM, which normally cannot be modified. This part of the memory allows the computer, in conjunction with the CPU, to function independently of human input, a feature which allows for almost complete automation in the laboratory, which is the focus of this chapter.

The aforementioned parts of the computer, along with a variety of input devices (such as keyboard, mouse, scanner or a tablet) have become a very useful tool in the laboratory. Although it may not be obvious at times, several automated laboratory instruments have incorporated these devices into their designs in a pervasive way. Add to it, a variety of output devices (such as screen, printer, plotter or speaker), which has made data retrieval very simple. Via this modernization of technology, every laboratory has benefited in terms of effectiveness and efficiency.

Computers come in many different sizes and complexity depending on their use.
1. **Supercomputers** and mainframes are the most powerful machines, and tend to have no use in the average clinical laboratory setting. These machines are equivalent of multiple high performance computers working in parallel as a single system.
2. **Servers** are computers that have been optimized to provide services to other computers over a network. Servers usually have powerful processors, lots of memory and large hard drives. This class of machines used to be referred to as mini-computers.
3. **Workstations** are high-end desktop computers that typically have powerful processor, and enhanced capabilities for performing a special group of task, such as 3D Graphics or game development.
4. **Desktops** or personal computers are the most common and widely used, and have proliferated in office and laboratories due to their small portable size and versatility. The personal computer defines

a computer designed for general use by a single person. While a Mac is a PC, most people relate the term with systems that run the Windows operating system. PCs were first known as microcomputers because they were a complete computer but built on a smaller scale than the huge systems in use by most businesses. A PC that is not designed for portability is a desktop computer. The expectations with desktop systems are that you will set the computer up in a permanent location.

5. **Laptops** or Notebooks are portable computers that integrate the display, keyboard, a pointing device or trackball, processor, memory and hard drive all in a battery-operated package slightly larger than an average hardcover book.
6. **Handhelds** are palm-top computers (commonly called Personal Digital Assistants or PDAs) are tightly integrated computers that often use flash memory instead of a hard drive for storage. These computers usually do not have keyboards but rely on touch-screen technology for user input. PDAs are typically smaller than a paperback book, very lightweight with a reasonable battery life.
7. **Wearables** are ultraportable computers that can be integrated into watches, cell phones, visors and clothing. This class of computers support common consumer applications such as email, camera, database, multimedia, calendar and phonebook.

Challenges of Computerization

Automation and computerization are enablers for efficiency and effectiveness. However, the steps of computerization in the laboratory are not necessarily a panacea. As with all machineries, the computer is subject to upkeep and breakdown. Environmental conditions can adversely affect the computer and its peripheral equipment. Excessive heat, humidity, dust, magnetic fields, smoke and transient loss or changes (even minor) in electrical line currents, can cause adverse results, such as data loss or data corruption. Therefore, wherever computers are deployed, it is imperative that:

- Electrical voltage stabilization is provided, with preferably uninterrupted power supply (UPS) backup units.
- Backup copies of all data (raw or otherwise) are kept in an off-line storage so that the information is intact and the data can be re-created in the event of a problem.
- Automated procedures can be bypassed manually or alternative procedures be made available in the laboratory, particularly those procedures which are vital in the emergency situation. In cases where electricity is frequently interrupted, supplemental units such as voltage stabilizer, battery backup (UPS unit) or inverter is essential, depending on the extent of power fluctuation and/or the duration of power loss. A typical UPS unit usually keeps the computer running until data gets saved to the desk and the computer has had a chance to shut itself down gracefully.
- In developing countries, a fully redundant computer system that can function as a backup is desirable due to the frequent scarcity of technical labour to expedite the repair of the primary computer in the event of a failure.

In the following section, an attempt has been made to provide a primer to orient the reader's general understanding of computers. The concepts include hardware, software, interfacing, storage, input, output and computer compatibility.

Glossary of Terms

Before beginning the discussion of the computer, familiarization with some of the terms commonly used in computer technology is necessary:

Address: The physical location of a piece of information within the computer's memory. **Algorithm**: The series of operations required to do a simple task. For example, algorithm might be set up to calculate the mean from a list of numbers.

Binary code: It is a numeration system having a base of 2. It has only 0's and 1's (or 'ON' and 'OFF' switches), which are expressed in powers of the number 2. The word 'bit' evolved from binary digit which happens to be the computer's smallest unit of data representation. A bit is like a toggle switch, which can have only two possible states, either 'on' or 'off'.

Booting: The process of starting a program of the computer after it has been turned off. It is derived from the phrase 'pulling oneself up by one's bootstraps'.

Browser: An 'easy to use' standard user interface which is the most popular way to interact (or browse) with the interconnected computers on the Internet.

Bug: An error or problem in the code of a program. It can be a logical or a typographical error.

Byte: A set of 8 bits makes a 'byte' that represents a character to the digital computer (e.g. one alphabetical or numerical character is represented by a byte).

Code: The set of instructions written to perform a task in the computer. A code may be written in any language compatible with the computer.

CD: Compact Disc or CD is a low-cost analogue optical storage medium that has essentially replaced the floppy disk. There is a variety of CD-s available, depending on user's need. Some common variations of CD (also called CD-ROM) are, write-once audio and data storage CD-R, rewritable media CD-RW, Super Audio CD (SACD), Video Compact Discs (VCD), PhotoCD, PictureCD and Enhanced CD. Of these media types, CD-ROMs and CD-Rs remain widely used technologies in the computer industry.

Database: This is the file or series of files in which all the data of a project are stored. From the data base other files can be made to suit various applications and produce various reports.

Directory: The index of file names and locations in a data-storage device such as a disk; it corresponds to the contents of a book.

Disk: An internal or external device that stores data.

DSL: It is a data communications technology that enables faster data transmission over copper telephone lines than a conventional voiceband modem can provide. It does this by utilizing frequencies that are not used by a voice telephone call. The acronym DSL or xDSL, stands for Digital Subscriber Line.

DVD: Digital Video Disc or DVD is a low-cost digital optical storage medium that has essentially replaced the floppy disk and CD-s. There is a variety of DVD-s available, depending on user's need. Variations of the term DVD often describe the way data is stored on the discs: DVD-ROM (Read Only Memory), has data that can only be read and not written, DVD-R and DVD+R can record data only once and then function as a DVD-ROM. DVD-RW, DVD+RW and DVD-RAM can both record and erase data multiple times.

File: A set of data blocks, which corresponds to a chapter in a book. In a laboratory computer there might be a file of all the tests offered by the laboratory along with their names, costs and reference ranges.

Disk: A device that stress the computer data. It may be internal or external to the computer. Also, it may be removable or fixed, depending on how it is hooked up. Popular storage devices are USB drives, Media Cards and portable drives, which have replaced the floppy drives in the last decade.

Hardware: This is a general term for the physical equipment used in a computer system. Hardware includes the CPU, the monitor, keyboard, mouse, printer, etc.

HTML: HTML or HyperText Markup Language, is the predominant mark up language for web pages. It provides a means to describe the structure of text-based information in a document and to supplement that text with interactive forms and embedded images. HTML is written in the form of tags, surrounded by angle brackets.

Instruction: Commands given to the computer that specify a set of operations that the computer is to do.

Interface: The connection between different components of a computer system or between different computers.

Internet: A global network of interconnected computers worldwide, linked via a variety of connections, which may be via modem, cable, ADSL or satellite link.

I/O: Acronym for Input/Output

Magnetic tape: A data storage medium which closely resembles the tape used to record music. These devices used to be used as low-cost, high-capacity storage medium for data, but have been phased out given the advent of new modern technology.

Memory: The part of a computer system which stores data and programs for use by the computer.

Microcomputer: A computer who's CPU is a microprocessor. It is usually a desk top or portable machine having a substantial amount of memory, and a limited number of I/O ports or peripherals.

Microchip: A semiconductor device with the property to hold transient or permanent data. It has extensive use in electronic industries. Integrated electronic circuits are embedded on silicon wafers to construct these microchips.

Microprocessor: A processing unit built in a single silicon chip. They are used to control and execute tasks involved in the operation of electrical equipment.

Modem: An acronym for modulator-demodulator. It is a device used for communication facilitation connecting two computers or computer systems through a telephone line. Modems have become less common, given the advent of the Internet and 'on-line' systems.

Program: A set of step by step instructions designed to perform designated tasks on a computer.

RAM (random-access memory): Memory to which one can both read and write, changing the contents many times during processing. RAM is used to store data temporarily in the sense that these data are retained only as long as the power is on (refer ROM).

Random access: The ability to have access to a piece of information from an array without having to look at all the elements from the beginning. An example of random access is the ability to play a particular selection on a phonograph record without having to play all the record up to that point.

ROM (read only memory): Storage whose contents cannot be changed by stored program instructions; it generally contains non-alterable programs and built-in functions of the computer (see RAM).

Software: The generic name for the programs, routines and the operational procedures for computers.

Monitor: The most common display device for computers. It usually consists of a keyboard and mouse that helps interact with the computer.

USB: Universal Serial Bus is a serial bus and I/O standard to connect devices to a host computer. It was designed to allow several peripherals to be connected using a single standardized interface socket and to improve plug and play capabilities of multifarious computer peripherals such as mouse, keyboards, PDAs, gamepads, joysticks, scanners, digital cameras, printers, flash drives and external hard drives.

Word: Group of bits which the computer processes at a time. The size of a word ranges from 8-64 bits and is defined by the hardware and software used in any particular system.

World Wide Web: A 'web' or network of networks, which links millions of computers together, and allows the user to interact with the information via an 'easy to use' standardized universal user interface, called the 'browser'.

XML: XML or eXtensible Markup Language is a general-purpose specification for creating custom mark up languages, and its most common purpose is to aid information systems in sharing structured data, primarily over the Internet

Operation of a Computer

A computer is made operational by combinations of two major components the hardware and the software.

Hardware

The hardware is the physical structure of the computer which has three major components CPU, Input/Output and Memory, as outlined in form of a conceptual view of the computer in Fig. 32.1.

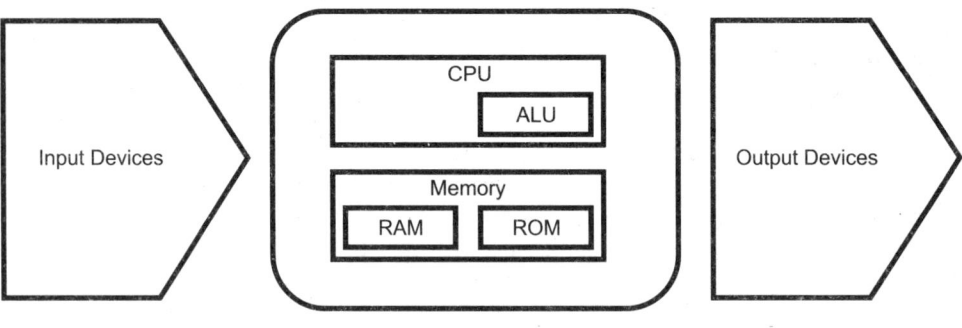

Fig. 32.1 *Conceptual view of primary parts of a computer.*

Central Processing Unit This unit coordinates and directs all the operations of a computer system. The CPU has two components, the arithmetic-logic unit (ALU) that performs numerical computations, and the control unit (CU) that regulates the timing and coordination of machine activities.

Physically, the CPU is a unit of electronic circuitry (integrated circuit). Miniaturization of technology has made large-scale integrated circuits fit in tiny footprint, thus shrinking the size of the CPU. A computer can have a single or multiple CPUs, which functions as a cluster, and supervises the operations within the computer. The other components such as ROM and RAM are under the control and governance of the CPU.

When a software program is executed, it is the CPU that orchestrates its execution by performing the operations specified by the encoded instructions (Fig. 32.2). When a mathematical calculation is involved the ALU is activated; if storage of data in memory or secondary storage is required, the CPU sets up and supervises the storage of data. If a printout of data is called for by the programs, the printer is activated and the data from the memory is passed through the CPU and transmitted to the printer. The connectors which indirectly link the CPU with its peripherals are referred to as the **interface cards**. In summary, the CPU is the brain and '**command centre**' of the computer.

Input/Output (I/O) This interface unit transfers information into and out of the computer. It may include a monitor, keyboard, mouse, scanner, printer, bar-code reader, speaker or a laboratory instrument. Some of the common components of the computer are shown in Fig. 32.2.

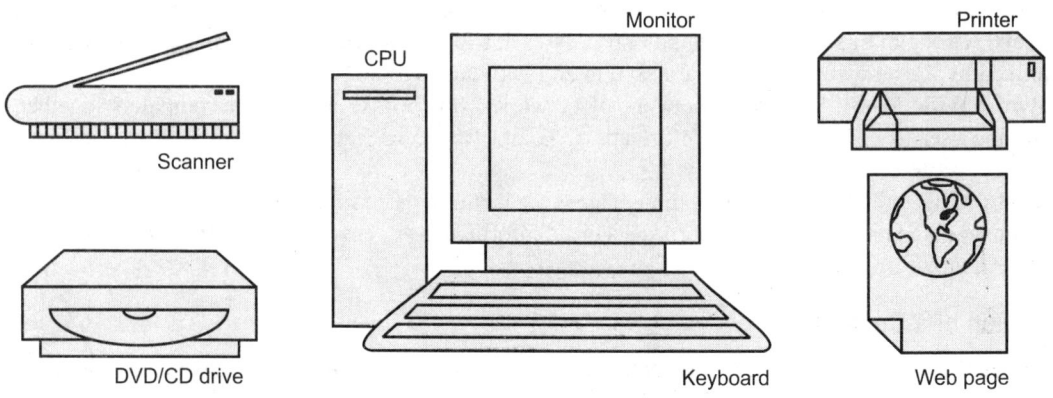

Fig. 32.2 *Components and primary parts of a computer.*

Memory/Storage Unit The memory unit stores data for use by the computer. There are two kinds of storage units—the primary storage unit and the secondary storage unit. The primary storage unit is built into the computer system. Part of primary storage contains permanent information which never gets erased or altered. This is called ROM. It contains pre-defined tasks or perhaps a built in computer language. The other part is called RAM. This is designed to contain temporary information and is addressable and erasable. It may contain the user's computer program, program data and its computed results.

Secondary storage units (also called external memory) can be thought of as being '**accessory**'. Its usage is not indispensable for a computer. Disk drives, tape drives or removable media are some of the most widely used secondary storage units. Their purpose is to expand the memory and to store data for later usage, accessing the data as needed by the program.

Conceptually, the memory is a large array of electronic circuits. Each individual circuit may be switched '**on**' (coded as 1) or '**off**' (coded as 0). As long as there is an electric current, the condition of being on or off codes the memory with bits of data. The ability to manipulate data in the form of an on/off code is the fundamental task of the digital computer's CPU. The on/off property of microchips makes them binary machines. As a result, many coding attributes are in powers of 2. The simplest memory element, the on/off (I/O) condition, is termed a bit and groups of 8 bits are called bytes. Memory is generally expressed in terms of megabytes (MB), which is approximately a million bytes. A single character, like the letter '*A*', takes up 1 byte (or 8 bits) of memory. It follows that in one line of 80 characters, 80 bytes will be required. (*Note*: each space should also be considered as a character.)

The discussion of computer memory would be incomplete without mentioning two terms—the address and the content. In order to logically store data in the computer's memory, data must be placed in an orderly way into locations within the computer's memory array. The location of the data within the array is called the address and the information stored at the address is referred to as content. The content may be determined by addressing the memory location. A **programmer** prepares the program (software) using a suitable computer or programming language. On booting up the program, the stored codes get converted by a translating unit into binary language. It then gets loaded into the RAM and the program is ready for execution. Pre-written programs, which are saved on disk, card or tape, can be re-loaded time and again into RAM.

The laboratory technician need not know anything about the 'program' or computer to accomplish his goals. He only needs to be familiar with the program's purpose and the user's commands.

Software

The programs and routines involved with the operational procedures are broadly referred to as software. The computer does not understand the human language. Hence, the instructions must be interpreted into a language that the computer understands. To facilitate programming, various computer languages have been developed which resemble the English language. The process of programming is relatively complex and requires a set of specific skills; rules must be followed, and the computer must be instructed every step which is to be performed in order. There are a variety of programming languages, and programmers usually select the language best suited for the application. The program code written is translated into machine language (binary code) before execution.

The programming task can be simplified through the use of a flowchart, which is a symbolic presentation of the steps required to solve the problem. Typically, the programmer and laboratory technician collaborate closely in order to achieve the desired results.

Computerization of Clinical Laboratory Instruments

Computer applications in laboratory instrumentation are relatively new. The development of, the microprocessor has revolutionized the very concept of analytical chemistry and instrumentation (Fig. 32.6). In, automated systems, the computer controls each step, including identification of specimen, aspiration of specimen and reagents, reading of results after periodic time intervals, standardization, collection of data, tallying of information, comparing and writing to data bases, calculation, and output of results. One of the major roles of laboratory computers is to regulate the QC of data. **Quality control** is a natural application for the CPU because of the ease with which large amounts of data can be collected and compared, calculated, interpreted or standardized. In some cases the computer can be interfaced directly to a laboratory instrument so that the QC data and patient's results may be easily collected and stored in a data base for later use. In less sophisticated programs, the computer can simply compare the patient's laboratory values to standards with the acceptable range supplied by the user. If the result is outside this range, it can be identified automatically with an asterisk or other mark so that the user may choose to reject the run, collect another sample or notify the physician of the results.

Storage of laboratory information and the easy access to the stored data have proved to be most helpful in modern laboratory operations, particularly with increased number of tests available. This has reduced the time and space needed for filing of papers and in addition, has made it much easier to provide the previous history of the patient's laboratory findings.

Machine failure

The computer is a blessing for the modern era as long it is working. Its failure is always possible and this can paralyse the entire system, if contingency planning is not in place. This may occur because of failure of electronic components or occasional abuse and misuse by the users. The components most likely to fail are those that involve mechanical parts, such as are found in disk drives and printers. If an electronic component does fail, the usual way to approach repair is to replace the computer circuit boards that might be involved. It is a good idea to keep spare parts or backup computers, if at all possible. It is equally wise to identify a source of technical assistance in the event that mechanical or electronic problems cannot be serviced promptly by the user.

Computer housing

Computer equipment must be kept at a cool temperature (24 °C) and at low humidity. The level of humidity should be low enough so that it is non-condensing but high enough so that static electricity is not a problem. These environmental problems are likely to appear in the form of a memory error or a disk read error.

Conclusion

Computerization is an integral part of laboratory automation and operation. As the numbers of laboratory tests, patients and diagnostic techniques increase, it becomes imperative that data be processed and managed more efficiently and effectively.

Despite the drawbacks noted in this chapter regarding computerization (including computer failure), careful and thoughtful selection of the computer system together with the identification of specific purposes for utilization of such a system will resolve most, if not all of the potential problems before they occur. A common obstacle that must be quickly overcome is fear and apprehension of computers-assisted technology. As explained in this chapter, the user of the computer need not have any prior knowledge of computers to get high-quality results, as long as the individual follows instructions.

The following can serve as guidelines in taking the efforts out of the process of computerization):
- Identify tasks that are best suited for the computer in the laboratory.
- Evaluate pre-packaged software available for performing these functions.
- Investigate available computer models that can run the packaged software per its specifications, keeping in mind that expandability and flexibility in the system are important (both in terms of data storage and future applications).
- Prepare laboratory personnel for the new technology, and reducing anxiety or 'technophobia'. The staff should be assured of the productivity gains to be achieved with the new machinery.
- Arrange for appropriate end-user technical training, diagnostic training as well as repair assistance procedures.

- Setup backup procedures (preferably in manual form) for anticipated problems (lost data, machinery failure, power failure, etc.) well in advance.
- Create backups often, and make it a part of the prescriptive steps so that backup copies of data files are always available.
- Assign a resource to champion the computer operations and function as the laboratory's on-site staff to run initial set of diagnostics in the event of a malfunction.
- Periodically repeat the aforementioned tasks of computerization upkeep, revise the operational guidelines and retrain the staff on any new extensions or software, as needed to ensure a smooth and uninterrupted operation in the laboratory.

AUTOMATED ANALYSERS IN DEVELOPING COUNTRIES

Historical Background

The first automated system was introduced into the market by Technicon under the name of AutoAnalyzer. The company is now owned by Bayer. It is a continuous flow system where the specimens flow in a continuous stream while separated by air bubbles. At the final stage, the air bubbles are released and colour of the mixture is measured by absorption photometry. Acid, phosphatases and bicarbonate—any of these can be chosen according to the need of the laboratory.

Centrifugal fast analyser is the next generation of automation and has many unique features. It is a discrete system where reagents and specimens are placed in the innermost discrete compartments in a rotor using positive displacement syringes. The reagents and samples get mixed and delivered to outer compartment by centrifugal force. The outer chamber provides appropriate reaction conditions and read the change in optical density at quick sequence each time the cuvette passes over the optical device during rotation. The instrument is very useful for the determinations in rate reactions.

The dry slide technology has become quite popular not only in large laboratories but also serve the needs of POC in the physician's office. The colour reactions in dry slide technology are read through reflectance photometry.

Dade Behring (formerly Dupont) is marketing a different kind of discrete analyser. All the reagents are put in different pouches of a plastic bag where they are mixed with the specimen and the mixture undergo the required chemical reaction conditions. Finally, the optical absorption of the reaction fluid is read at specific wavelength through the plastic bag. A bar code marked at the top of the bag prompts the machine to respond to specific test.

We will focus here on three automated analysers which are commonly seen in various laboratories of India and other developing countries—AutoAnalyzer (Bayer), Clinical Corona (Boehringer Mannheim) and Auto Pacer (Miles of India Ltd.). We will focus here the operation of these analysers

AutoAnalyser

This is grouped under the 'continuous flow' where the specimens move in a stream, separated by air bubbles. In discrete system all specimens are independent of each other and one can have multiple choice of tests and they can have random access. Three unique approaches of the discrete system include centrifugal fast analysers, dry slide technology and compartmental pre-packaged reagents that move on a belt, meeting all the reaction conditions and ultimately subjected to optical measurements before packages are disposed off. Bulk reagents are available and spare parts are becoming easier to obtain through the Internet.

Components of AutoAnalyser

The five major components of the AutoAnalyser is shown in Fig. 32.3.

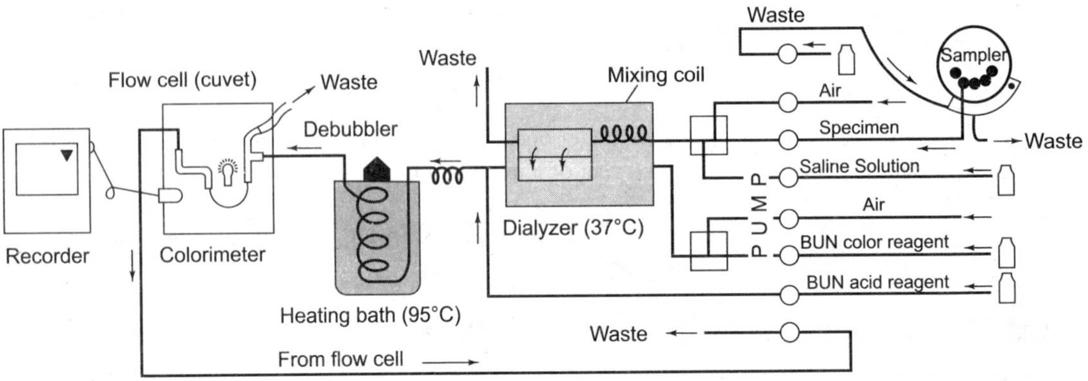

Fig. 32.3 *Continuous flow automated system. Components and working of AutoAnalyser for the analysis of blood urea nitrogen (BUN) by diacetyl monoxlme method.*

Sampler and Cam The sampler is a circular platform that holds the cups containing the standards and specimens for analysis. As the sampler rotates, it brings each cup in turn under the sampling probe, which aspirates for a FT, decides sample volume, and alternates with the wash cycle. The dwell time in the specimen and the sample-to-wash ratio are governed by the cam. An appropriate cam is selected to determine the rate of analysis. The most common sample-to-wash ratio is 2 : 1.

Pumps and Manifolds The pump is the heart of the AutoAnalyzer, and the manifolds are the arteries. The proportionating pump has a peristaltic action that moves the fluids inside the tube in one direction at a constant speed, rendering a uniform rate of delivery throughout the system. The advancing movement accomplishes sample aspiration reagent pickup, mixing, and all other actions. The diameter of the manifold tube determines the volume of the fluid. Before the sample stream enters the dialyser, **air bubbles** are introduced in both specimen and reagent streams. The air bubbles help in cleaning the manifold tubing and avoid carry-over effects. In an enzyme study, substrate and the serum specimen (containing enzymes) are first mixed in an incubation chamber kept at 37 °C for a certain period. The extended coil determines the time delay. After incubation, the specimen stream with products of the substrate enters the upper chamber of the dialyser.

Dialyser The dialyser is a double compartment separated by a semi-permeable membrane. A diluted sample stream ('**donor stream**') circulates on one side of the membrane while the recipient stream (generally one of the reagents or saline solution) circulates through the other side. The membrane allows part of the sample constituents of low-molecular mass (the analyte) to pass through while it holds back, the compounds with high-molecular mass (protein) that flow into the waste. The amount of solute that passes through the membrane is influenced by the instrumental factors, which are kept constant and the variable concentrations gradient, which is the basis of flow analysis. Although only a fraction of the total amount of the analyte present in a unit volume of specimen passes through the membrane, the ratio of diffusion remains constant. The AutoAnalyzer operates on the accurate measurement of the sample-standard ratio. It is not important to have the total amount of compound to be taken for analysis, nor is it necessary to take the chemical reaction to completion. As long as a photometric measurement is possible at the final step, there is no loss of accuracy.

Reaction Chamber or Heating Bath This provides elevated temperature and a time delay which are required for the development of a coloured reaction product. The temperature is usually maintained at about 95 °C, and occasionally at 37 °C, depending on the analysis. The time delay is accomplished by introducing a long glass coil inside the chamber in continuation with the manifold tubing.

Detector and Recorder The basic analytic procedure of the AutoAnalyzer is colorimetry. Thus the colour of the reagent stream, following the chemical reaction, is proportional to the amount of reacting compound. A small amount of coloured reagent is drawn by the continuous flow system into a microcuvette. The air bubbles are discarded by the 'F' tube or **debubbler**. To avoid fluctuation of the light source caused by voltage fluctuation, the colorimeter employs a dual-beam system. Light from a single tungsten filament lamp is split and **collimated** into two beams, one of which acts as a reference (null balance) while the other goes through the cuvette. Initial baseline conditions are achieved by controlling the light intensity of the reference beam through the introduction of a suitable aperture plate. The photocell of the colorimeter reads the light energy that is transmitted through the coloured solution (%T) and converts it to electrical energy. The electrical impulse is finally communicated to the mechanical device of the recorder or directly to the computer.

The recorder chart provides a continuous measurement of the intensity of the light that has passed through the **flow cell** and is received by the **detector** (%T). The response is shown as **peaks** indicating the concentrations of the analytes. The highest concentration is at the centre of the peak with adjoining slopes that indicate a decreasing concentration of the analyte in the wash cycle phase. The peaks obtained from the specimen on the recorder chart are compared against the peaks of the standards. It is therefore important to **calibrate** the AutoAnalyzer prior to the running of specimens. Variation from a smooth shape of the peak frequently indicates many internal problems. For example, a sharp spike in the middle of a peak or between peaks indicates the presence of air bubbles at the time of colour measurement; trailing indicates possible obstruction in continuous flow; and overlapping peaks are indicative of poor wash.

Clinical Corona

The Clinical Corona (or Corona) made by Boehringer Mannheim is a discrete, compact and fully automated clinical batch analyser (Fig. 32.4). It is a bench-top model that requires minimal space. A microcomputer system controls the whole analytical process via its programs. The program to be used in a specific assay is selected by the operator, who enters an analysis code through the keyboard.

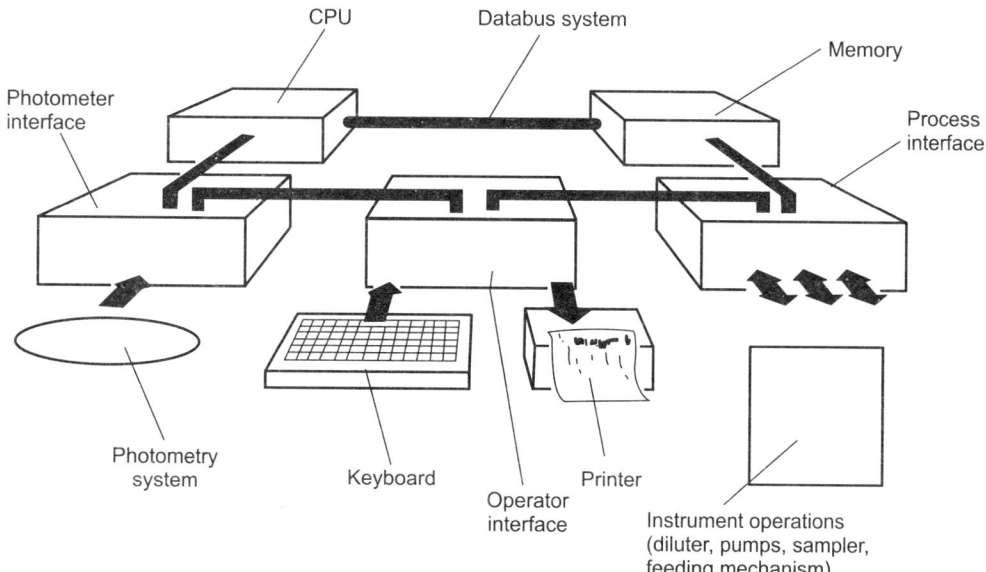

Fig. 32.4 *Use of microprocessor in the operation of laboratory instruments. The communication between different modules in the operation of Clinicon (Boehringer Mannheim, Sweden).*

Corona performs methods for routine biochemistry and is also capable of handling special tests with appropriate reagents. Its throughput (maximum number of tests that can be performed per hour) is 200 samples per hour for end point analysis (single observation) and 140 samples per hour in kinetic mode (multiple; observations) for enzyme assays. The required serum volume for a set of 20 chemistries is as small as 500 µL, and the reagent consumption per test is typically 400 µL (Fig. 32.5).

Substances analysed (kinetic or end point) in the Corona are: Glucose (hexokinase), total protein (biuret), albumin (bromocresol green), bilirubin (dichloro diazophenyl), creatinine (Jaffe), triglyceride (ATP method), urea (UV method), uric acid (UV method), calcium (o-cresolphthalein complexone), cholesterol (p-aminophenazone) and iron (bathophenantrolin). Other tests can be introduced according to the need of the laboratory.

The enzyme assays (kinetic) include—SCOT, SGPT, LD, CK, ALP and GGT.

Components of Corona

Various components of Corona and their functions are described here (Fig 32.5). It is important that the operator understands the function of each component in order to trouble shoot.

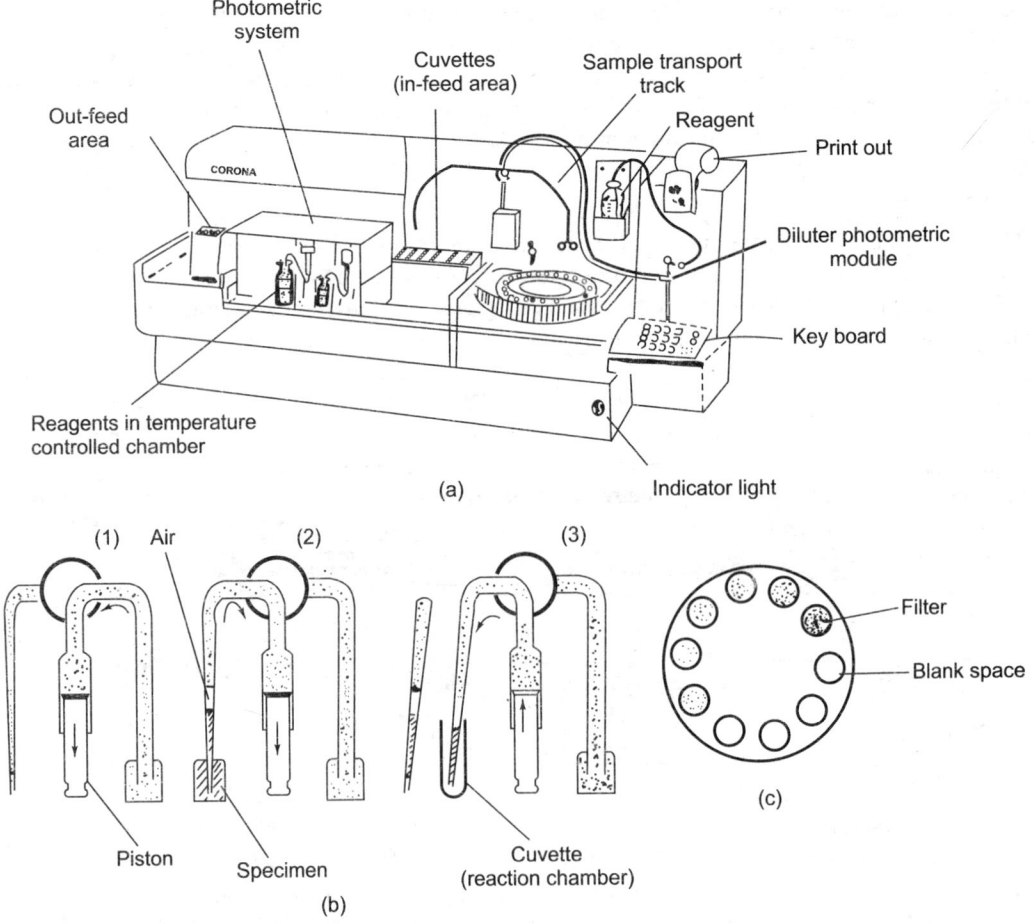

Fig. 32.5 *Discrete automated system—Corona (Boehringer Mannheim, Sweden). (a) Principle components of Corona. (b) Operation of diluter: (1) filling of reagent, (2) aspiration of specimen and (3) transfer and delivery of specimen and reagent. (c) Filter disc used in the photometric system (visible range).*

Sampler The sampler is a 40-position carousel that carries the specimen. Specimens must have clear identification, and the sequence must be noted in a register. Movement of the sampler is controlled by the microcomputer. The slots are numbered and it is possible to run replicates and standards simultaneously by choosing the slots.

Diluter This prepares the specimen for the assay, mixes the reagent and the sample, and delivers it into the reaction chamber. It is fully integrated to function with a single syringe and one valve whose movements are totally controlled by the microcomputer. The diluter has a small dead volume as only one syringe is involved in the whole dilution process. The dilution cycle begins by sucking the reagent into the syringe. The valve is switched on and thereafter the sample is aspirated and separated from the reagent by air. When the pipette has left the sample cup, another segment of air is sucked in and the outside of the pipette is wiped in order to minimize carry-over. The pipette is then transferred to the cuvette into which the sample and reagent are delivered. The volumes of the fluids are regulated by the length of the stroke, and pickup deliveries of the fluids are regulated by the valve. The syringe is capable of delivering 5–1000 μL of the specimen.

Reaction Chamber The main chemical reaction for the test is in the reaction chamber which is temperature controlled and newer chemicals are added. The instrument uses disposable **cuvettes** (which add to the cost of its running) which are placed in racks in the in-feed area of the instrument, and end up in the out-feed area when the analytical process is complete. Just before entering the thermostat the cuvette receives the reagent and sample previously picked up by the diluter from a cup in the sampler. The racks travel through the thermostat and during this travel the reaction mixture is gradually heated to the set temperature. At any point in time during this feeding through the thermostat it is possible to add two additional reagents. These reagents are preheated in order not to upset the temperature of the reaction mixture already in the cuvette. The pipette, tubing and heating block are in one piece which is easy to position and remove from the top of the thermostat. The reagent pumps are controlled by the microcomputer.

Detector The detector is built-in within the reaction chamber. The detector is an optical system which is typical of any photometer. Contents of the cuvettes are well mixed before taking **optical measurements**. Most observations are made in the visible range, using a tungsten lamp but the instrument is capable of working in the ultraviolet range as well. **Radiant energy** from the light source passes through two lenses and the emerging parallel beams of light then enter the interference filter in order to choose the desired wavelength of light to go through the cuvette with the test solution. The parallel beam of light is then focussed by another lens in order to concentrate it at the middle of the cuvette. The light is absorbed by the test solution and the non-absorbed light is focussed by another series of lenses onto a **silicon photodetector**. The electrical signal sent by the photodetector is amplified, converted into logarithmic and digital form, and finally transferred to the microprocessor.

Printer After receiving the signal from the CPU the microprocessor then performs the necessary calculations and transfers the final information to the output printer.

Microcomputer System The microcomputer is the brain of the machine and controls the whole instrument through the CPU. The microprocessor receives instructions from the software (program) which is operated by the user of the machine. The memory of the computer has two components, the user file (comparable with random access memory, RAM) and the master file which is provided by the manufacturer. The operator, by a few commands via the keyboard can make a selection of 16 analyses which are automatically loaded into the user file. These analyses are immediately accessible for routine use. Only one analysis should be run for a batch. For different analyses, different chemicals and reaction conditions will be needed.

There are three assay modes—constant rate (CR), fixed time (FT) and end point (EP). Depending on the chosen mode, the arithmetic-logic unit of the CPU makes the necessary mathematical calculations. CR mode is used for enzymes; the slope is determined by the best fit to measured data. The accuracy is checked and compared to a pre-set value (RMS) to yield a factor. The concentration results are obtained by multiplication by the factor. **Fixed time mode** is used for substrates and immunoglobulins. The primary value is determined by integration of the measured data forming the midpoint ($t/2$) of the reaction rate until the plateaus is reached. The EP mode is applied for routine chemistry—albumin, bilirubin, calcium and others. In the EP mode, the absorbance level is determined by the best fit to measured data, and the concentration result is obtained by comparison with standards.

Before starting the machine load the carousel with specimens, check the identifications of the specimens, place the standards, record the sequence, orime the diluter with the reagent, check the temperature light (it must be on), place the empty cuvettes in position, and enter the analysis code, date and sequence number on the keyboard. Then press the 'start' key provided on the keyboard.

The Corona is programmed to check the QC. If a result does not fulfil a pre-set QC parameter or unit value the result will be accompanied by a text or a symbol which depends on the type of error. Error messages are also given when the standard curve of an assay is unacceptable.

When the analysis code is entered by the user, all the settings are completed. The Clinicon Corona, however, is flexible enough to adapt to newer methods to meet the needs of the individual laboratory. In order to adapt to newer methods, 38 parameters have to be fixed such as temperature, wavelength, concentration unit, etc.

Auto Pacer

The Auto Pacer (Chemetrics Analyser – I) made by Ames, USA (Miles of India Ltd.) is a computerized discrete analyser of modular design. It is a bench top model which is fully automated right from the sample dispensing to the final printout of the results. The technician has to load the machine with samples, provide appropriate reagents, instruct the computer through the computer keyboard and set the parameters as required by the tests. It is capable of doing 26 biochemical tests. Although the analyser is pre-programmed for 26 tests, 37 programs are available and it is open for the addition of new tests as they are developed in future. There are also two open programs available to the user (one kinetic for enzyme study and one EP for routine chemistry). Over and above all these programs, a built-in statistical program for QC, i.e. for calculating standard deviations, coefficients of variation, and means, is also available. It is faster than Clinicon Corona and can handle 300 EP reactions per hour (throughput) and 40 kinetic enzyme assays per hour. The analyser processes the sample in batches and it is possible to interrupt a batch run to do a 'Stat' test. The reagents are available from the manufacturer and can also be prepared in the laboratory.

The program provided by the manufacturer is not totally inaccessible. The user can change the test parameters, if needed, such as the number of data points, range of normal and others. The instrument is also designed for handling enzyme immunoassays, and has proved to be an important tool in drug analysis.

Components of Auto Pacer

The modular design provides the following components (Fig 32.6):

Sampler It is a turntable carrying 60 reaction cups and 60 sample cups per tray. The carousel can be separately loaded with fresh specimens while the tests are in progress with one batch.

Automatic Dispenser This component functions in the automatic dispensing and diluting of sample and reagents. Pump and syringes are housed in this module.

Detector This consists of a spectrophotometer for photometric measurements. The spectrophotometer is of high precision and narrowband (8 nm) that incorporates a digital readout. It works in the entire range of photometric determinations for routine biochemical analyses (335–850 nm).

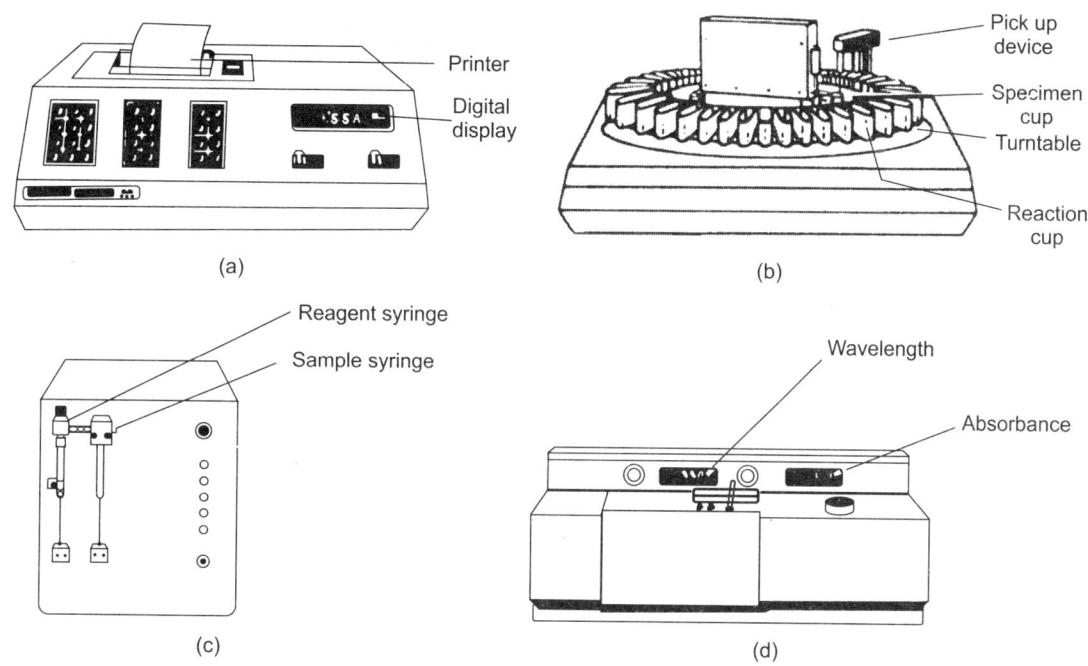

Fig. 32.6 *Various components of auto pacer: (a) digital display and printer, (b) specimen pickup module, (c) specimen and reagent pickup syringes and (d) photometric module.*

Computer This is the brain of the machine. The keyboard is the communication link between the user, the manufacturer's software and the microprocessor. The temperature of the reaction chamber and flow cell is controlled by an internal thermostat (25–37 °C). It is attached to the instrument and is programmed to function according to the test requirement. It has a built-in printer that gives impact paper printouts. If the results are not normal, the printout gives an automatic flag of abnormal, non-linear, invalid or out of range values.

The instrument is capable of performing EP, kinetic or initial rate reactions as the need be. It is designed for continuous batch operation round the clock.

SEAC (Ames)

This is a semi-automated analyser (Ames, USA; Miles of India Ltd.) where the initial preparations are done by the technician and the instrument works like a sophisticated spectrophotometer. The advantage of this machine is that the use of separate cuvettes is avoided, and the conditions of the test can be programmed. Similar products have also been marketed by Boehringer Mannheim and other manufacturers. This instrument is highly effective in measuring enzyme kinetics and is a necessary tool for enzyme-linked immunoassays.

POINT-OF-CARE TESTING: A NEW APPROACH

In recent years there is a growing demand of '**Point-of-care testing (POCT)**' that led to the rapid advancements in technology that will enable the physician to make decision on the bedside. This is making rapid changes in all aspects of health care. One of the major changes in the clinical laboratory has been the implementation and increased use of POCT. This brings the laboratory test to the patient rather than obtaining a specimen from the patient and transporting it to the laboratory for testing. This makes laboratory test results available more rapidly, providing improved patient care. In advanced countries it is applied in numerous situations—nursing homes, physician's office, emergency rooms, intensive care units and for bedside testing in hospital wards. The evolution of small, simple-to-use analysers that require only one drop, or less, of specimen has led to widespread POCT implementation. Handheld portable analysers can measure substances such as glucose, haemoglobin, cholesterol and electrolytes. Most require only a drop of blood, usually obtained by finger stick. Thus in the near future many of the routine clinical laboratory tests will be available in remote villages of developing countries although in the urban setting large automated system will continue to function. The clinical laboratories, however, will have to stay involved in making recommendations and compare the results with the classic procedures.

TIME-SAVING DEVICES AND KITS

The automated systems are 'undoubtedly fast, reliable and prove to be cheaper in the long run. However, the initial investment is high and a breakdown can be disastrous. As most of these automated systems are computerized, unfavourable weather, intermittent electrical supply and lack of technical repairmen make it hard for the laboratories to decide whether to invest in them or not. Modular systems are more advantageous as spare module can be used in case of breakdown, and the defective machine can be sent for repair. Automated system is profitable only when the work load is high.

For smaller laboratories, **kits** have proved to be profitable. Kits must be purchased from reliable companies (Appendix at the end of this volume). The laboratory should purchase such time-saving gadgets as automatic pipetter, diluter, mixer and others to expedite the work. Excessive mechanical work will cause fatigue in the technician and this will result in erroneous results. All technicians must, however, master the manual procedures before they plan for any kind of automation. This reduces the sense of helplessness when the automated system fails.

Final Comments

Automation is a buzzword among clinical laboratories, but it is not a pie in the sky. The future for automation in clinical labs is here. Many clinical laboratory tasks have already been automated, and several manufacturers are offering automated laboratory systems in the marketplace. Automation continues to be the province primarily of hospital laboratories, however, although most large commercial laboratories continue to eschew its usage. Unreliable energy source and instrument breakdown are the main problems of automation in developing countries, other than the high purchase cost and repair. If the laboratory totally relies on automation and neglects the written manual procedures about what to do, when there's a system interruption, which inevitably occurs, it will make a big folly. The laboratory must have a backup plan. The patient has no time to wait until the machine gets fixed.

AUTOMATION IN DEVELOPING COUNTRIES

Technology enables automation, which in turn, drives efficiency laboratories. As automation has become an indispensable part of modern laboratories, its adoption varies by geography. Developing countries tend to take a longer time to adapt the oncoming changes and should select from the large array of automated systems to suit their own conditions. The ideal automated system for the laboratories of developing countries ought to be simple, trouble-free, low-maintenance and reliable. It ought to be able to function with basic chemicals and versatile enough to switch to manual system, if necessary, without sacrificing the accuracy of the results. In developing countries a good backup system must be thought well before the laboratory adopts an automated system. Use of the computers and computer-assisted process control is encouraged and should be leveraged to drive productivity and achieve efficiency.

Review Questions

1. What is the difference between continuous flow atialysis and discrete analysis? Name one instrument in each of these automated systems.
2. Why is it that the centrifugal fast analyser is chosen for enzyme assays?
3. How is the protein interference minimized by the automated systems?
4. Why is it that the discrete system is preferred over the continuous flow system in the laboratories of developing countries?
5. What are the difficulties you anticipate in computerizing a laboratory located in a developing country?
6. Define: CPU, Byte, hardware, software and algorithm.
7. What are the main components of a computer and what are their functions?
8. If you are asked to install a computer in the laboratory where will you place it?
9. List the most important components of an AutoAnalyser and state their functions.
10. Why does the AutoAnalyser introduce air bubbles into the flowing stream of the sample and reagent and how are the air bubbles removed before the detector reads the colour of the solution?
11. What are the functions of the microcomputer system in the Clinical Corona?

33

Routine Biochemical Tests

◆

Shanker Mukherjee

Chapter Outline

- ◆ *Determination of Blood Glucose*
  - *o-toluidine method*
  - *Glucose oxidase method (true glucose)*
  - *Quick screen of blood glucose*
- ◆ *Clinical Significance of Glucose in Circulation*
  - *Diabetes and diabetes management*
    - *HbA1c (glycated haemoglobin)*
- ◆ *Determination of Serum Protein*
  - *Determination of total protein in serum*
    - *Biuret method*
  - *Determination of serum albumin*
- ◆ *Determination of Blood Urea*
  - *Diacetyl monoxime method*
- ◆ *Determination of Creatinine*
  - *Alkaline picrate method*
- ◆ *Determination of Creatinine Clearance*
- ◆ *Determination of Bilirubin*
  - *Jendrassik and Grof method (total, direct and indirect)*
- ◆ *Diagnostic Enzymology*
  - *Routine analysis of diagnostic enzymes*
    - *Alkaline phosphatase*
    - *Transaminases*
      - *ALT and AST*

- Creatinine kinase (CK)
- Lactic dehydrogenase (LD)
- Amylase
* Lipid profile
* Total cholesterol
* Liporoteins—HDL and LDL
* Serum triglycerides
♦ Electrolytes
  * Sodium and potassium
    - Ion selective electrode
  * Calcium
    - Cresolphthalein complexone method
  * Chloride
    - Ion selective electrode
    - Colorimetric method
♦ Acid-base Balance and Blood Gases
  * Determination of blood gases
♦ Review Questions

Chemical constituents in a healthy body are in a delicate balance or equilibrium that is influenced by both internal and external factors. This equilibrium or steady state is referred as **homeostasis**. Under diseased state, this equilibrium is disturbed. The cause of the disturbed state of the body can be diagnosed by analysing various body fluids such as blood, urine and cerebrospinal fluid. In the clinical chemistry laboratory tests are performed with these body fluids for the presence or absence of certain biochemicals (analytes) or for the level or amount of the these substances that indicate the causal agent, may that be infection, metabolic disturbances, toxicity, drug effect or other pathologic states. Physicians use the results of clinical chemistry tests to aid in the diagnosis, treatment, and prevention of disease. Interpretation of test results is based on understanding the physiological and biochemical processes occurring in health and in disease. This has been presented earlier (Chapter 29 in this Volume).

The tests of clinical chemistry can be done through various automated systems or done manually or semi-manually. It is important that the test results are reliable so that the physician can have confidence in basing diagnosis and treatment on test findings. **Reliability** is ensured from the time of specimen collection, handling, storing and performance of the test with appropriate quality assessment measures; so that the results are calculated and reported accurately. Just because the results are coming out of a 'machine' or a 'computer' does not necessarily mean they are all reliable.

'**Routine tests in chemistry**' is defined as the tests that are commonly asked for (80% of the physician's request). A list of these frequently requested tests is given in Table 33.1.

Complete automation is still a dream in the world of struggling economy, unreliable power supply and available health facilities for all. This has been elaborated in Chapter 32 in this volume. Those laboratories which can afford automation should have the manual system as a standby. In this chapter, we will present some of the important biochemical tests which are considered to be routine. All the chosen procedures are followed manually in various laboratories across the developing countries. Many of the test procedures described in this book may not meet the standards of the advanced countries but they fit into the conditions existing in these areas. Most of these methods are approved by WHO. The limitations of each procedure have been stated and if the laboratory can, it must try to switch to more modern methods. Along with the currently existing methods, newer methods have been proposed which, according to the authors, can be adopted in the progressive laboratories of developing countries.

Table 33.1 Routine diagnostic tests in clinical chemistry and their normal range

Tests	Reference values (Normal range)*	
	Conventional Units	SI Units
Glucose	70–110 mg/dL	3.9–6.2 mmol/L
Total protein	6.0–8.0 g/dL	60–80 g/L
Albumin	3.5–5.0 g/dL	35–50 g/L
Urea (BUN)	15.0–38.5 mg/dL	2.9–6.4 mmol/L
Creatinine	0.9–1.5 mg/dL	62–125 µmol/L
Total bilirubin	0.1–1.2 mg/dL	2–21 µmol/L
Direct bilirubin	0.0–0.3 mg/dL	0–6 µmol/L
Indirect bilirubin	0.1–0.9 mg/dL	2–15 µmol/L
ALT/SGPT	3–30 U/L	3–30 U/L
AST/SGOT	10–37 U/L	10–37 U/L
Gamma glutamyl transferase (GGT)	3–40 U/L	3–40 U/L
Alkaline phosphatase (AP)	20–130 U/L	20–130 U/L
Lactate dehydrogenase (LD)	110–230 U/L	110–230 U/L
Amylase	60–180 Somogyi unit (SU)/dL	95–290 IU/L
Creatinine kinase (CK)	30–170 U/L	30–170 U/L
Cholesterol	140–250 mg/dL Desirable level <200 mg/dL	3.64–6.50 mmol/L
Triglyceride	10–190 mg/dL Desirable <150 mg/dL	0.11–2.15 mmol/L
Calcium	8.7–10.5 mg/dL	2.18–2.63 mmol/L
Sodium	135–148 mEq/L	135–148 mmol/L
Potassium	3.5–5.4 mEq/L	3.5–5.4 mmol/L
Chloride	98–106 mEq/L	98–106 mmol/L
Uric acid	3.5–7.5 mg/dL	0.21–0.44 mmol/L

* The normal values quoted here are for adult males. These may differ from laboratory to laboratory due to variation in population and methodology used. Hence they may not be identical with the values quoted in the text describing the methodology.

The current advancement in '**Point-of-Care**' approach with the use of dry chemistry (Chapter 3 in Vol. I) brings hope to affordable fast chemical analysis on the bed side of the patient or in the physician's office without referring to the laboratory for 'wet chemistry'. In another decade more of these routine chemical tests will be coming into the market for performing them at home. (Tests such as blood sugar and pregnancy testing, etc. are already done at home.)

DETERMINATION OF BLOOD GLUCOSE

A request for serum glucose analysis is made in case of suspected **diabetes mellitus**. Increased serum glucose level (hyperglycaemia) with associated glucosuria is diagnostic for diabetes mellitus. An increased level of glucose is also noted with increased endocrine activity (such as glucagons secreting tumour of Pancreas), or pregnancy. A decreased level of serum glucose (hypoglycaemia) is often associated with starvation, hyperinsulinism as in insulin producing tumour of the pancreas, and decreased activity of certain endocrine glands. In case of suspected brain tumour or meningitis, CSF specimen is submitted for glucose assay, which shows a decline.

Normal values

The normal level of serum glucose, determined by *o*-toluidine method, as reducing substance, is 70–110 mg/dL. It is essentially the same as those for the glucose oxidase method which is 65–95 mg/dL. In patients with uraemia, however, higher values are obtained by the *o*-toluidine method. The concentration of serum is about 15% higher than in whole blood.

O–Toluidine Method

The *o*-toluidine method is superior to the older method of Folin-Wu. *o*-Toluidine method reports glucose as 'reducing substance' and not as 'true glucose' because the colour reaction can occur with substances other than glucose although the results are close. If the physician asks specifically for '**True glucose**' enzymatic method has to be followed. The procedure is based on a condensation reaction instead of the reducing action involving the same organic group present in glucose-aldehyde.

The method described here (*o*-toluidine) is recommended by WHO (Manual of Basic Techniques for a Health Laboratory, 2003). The *o*-toluidine method of glucose determination is discontinued in most western laboratories due to its carcinogenic effects, and replaced by the enzymatic method described later. The latter is available as commercial kits, or the reagents can be made in the laboratory. The *o*-toluidine method, however, is cheaper.

Principle

The proteins are first precipitated by trichloroacetic acid (TCA). The aldehyde group of glucose in the filtrate condenses with *o*-toluidine in glacial acetic acid (colourless) on heating, giving an emerald blue-green colour which is measured photometrically. The intensity of colour is proportional to the glucose concentration. The presence of thiourea stabilizes the o-toluidine reaction. The reaction is not specific for glucose but there are much fewer substances (e.g. aldohexoses such as fructose and galactose) that can affect the colour. This method is discouraged because of the carcinogenic effect of *o*-toluidine. It is still popular because of its simplicity, accuracy and rapidity. The chemical *o*-toluidine must be handled carefully; it should not touch the skin and the acetic acid fumes should not be inhaled.

Materials and supplies

- Conical centrifuge tubes and large test tubes (to hold 20 mL).
- Test tube racks.
- Blood (Sahli) pipettes.
- Pipettes, 0.5 mL, 5.0 mL.
- Water-bath at 100°C.
- Whole blood (capillary and venous), plasma or serum, taken from a fasting patient. The use of fluoride oxalate as the anticoagulant is recommended as this prevents the glucose from being destroyed in the blood by oxidation.
- Control serum. *Note:* A control serum should be used with each batch of tests. If the result of the test with the control serum is correct, it can be assumed that the patient's results will also be correct.

Reagents

- *TCA (3%, 30 g/L)*

TCA (CCl_3COOH)	15 g
Distilled water	q.s. 500 mL

Weigh the acid out quickly, since it is highly deliquescent. Transfer to a beaker. Add distilled water to dissolve the chemical. Transfer to a 500-mL flask and make up to volume to 500 mL with distilled water. Label the flask (3% TCA) with date. Keep in the refrigerator.
Warning: TCA is highly corrosive.

- *o-toluidine reagent*

Thiourea	0.75 g
Glacial acetic acid (CH_3COOH)	470 mL
o-toluidine	30 mL

Dissolve the thiourea in the glacial acetic acid. (If it is difficult to dissolve, stand the flask in a bowl of hot water.) Add the *o*-tolouidine and mix well. Transfer the reagent to a brown bottle. Label the bottle and write the date. Keep at room temperature. Allow to stand for at least 24 h before use. This reagent may be used for months but older reagents tend to give increased absorbance values with glucose. *o*-Toluidine reagent should be dispensed only with an automatic dispenser (set at 3.5 mL). Glacial acetic acid is highly corrosive. Contact with the skin should be avoided.

- *Benzoic acid solution (1 g/L)*

Benzoic acid	1 g
Distilled water	q.s. 1000 ml

Measure 1000 mL of distilled water and heat to just below boiling. Add the benzoic acid and mix well until it is dissolved. Allow to cool. Transfer the solution to a 1000-mL glass-stoppered bottle. Label the bottle and write the date.

- *Glucose stock reference solution (100 mmol/L)*

Glucose, pure, anhydrous	9 g
Benzoic acid solution (0.1% or 1 g/L)	q.s. 500 mL

Label the flask ('Glucose stock reference solution') and write the date.

The general method of preparing stock reference solution is shown in Fig. 33.1.

- *Glucose working reference solutions (2.5, 5, 10, 20 and 25 mmol/L)*

Allow the glucose stock reference solution to reach room temperature. Carefully pipette 2.5, 5, 10, 20 and 25 mL of the stock reference solution into each of five 100-mL volumetric flasks. Make up to the mark with the benzoic acid solution and mix well. Label the flasks as described earlier and write the date. Store the working reference solutions in a refrigerator. Renew monthly.

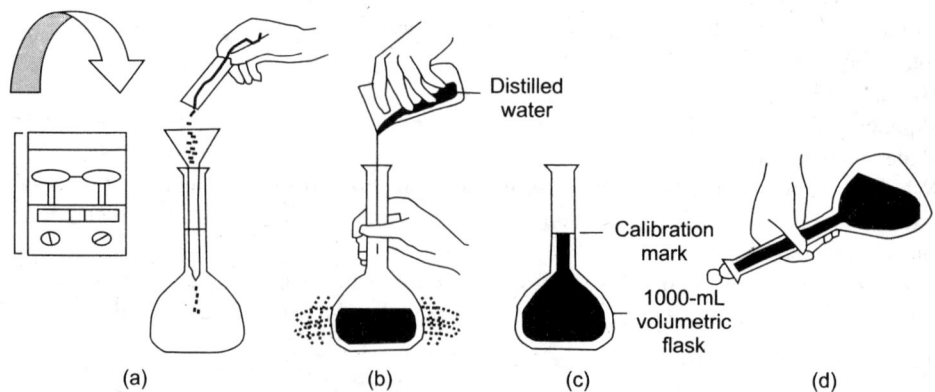

Fig. 33.1 *Preparation of stock solution: (a) Weigh the standard on an analytical balance on a pre-weighed paper and transfer the standard into a volumetric flask. (b) Pour distilled water to dissolve by swirling. (c) Bring to the mark (q.s.) of the volumetric flask. (d) Finally, mix by inversion.*

Procedure

1. Pipette 1.8 mL of TCA solution into each of three centrifuge tubes.
   Note: TCA is corrosive. Use it with care.
2. With a 0.2-mL blood pipette (Sahli), deliver 0.2 mL of the blood specimen to the bottom of the first centrifuge tube i.e. under the TCA solution. The TCA solution will become cloudy where it makes contact with the blood specimen.
   Note: Always use safety devices for pipetting. Do not pipette by mouth.
3. Raise the pipette and draw clear TCA solution into it in order to wash out all traces of the blood specimen.
4. Expel the TCA solution from the pipette into the centrifuge tube.
5. Mix well (the entire solution will become cloudy) and allow to stand for 5 min.
6. Using a clean 0.2 mL blood pipette, deliver 0.2 mL of distilled water and 0.2 mL of glucose working reference solution (e.g. 10 mmol/L) to the second and third centrifuge tubes, respectively, as described in step 2. These tubes will be used to prepare the reagent blank and the glucose working reference standard, respectively.
7. Centrifuge the three tubes at 3000 g for 5 min. (*Note:* you can skip this step for the blank or the standard). The precipitated proteins in the tube containing the blood specimen will sediment and a clear supernatant fluid will be obtained.
8. Take three (or more if needed) large test tubes and label them as B for blank, R for reference and P for patient *Note:* With more specimens, carefully number them as P_1, P_2, etc.
9. Pipette into each tube as follows:
   - *Blank (B)*: 0.5 mL of fluid from the second centrifuge tube and 3.5 mL of *o*-toluidine reagent.
   - *Reference (R)*: 0.5 mL of fluid from the third centrifuge tube and 3.5 mL of *o*-toluidine reagent.
   - *Patient (P)*: 0.5 mL of supernatant fluid from the first centrifuge tube and 3.5 mL of *o*-toluidine reagent.
   Note: *o*-toluidine reagent is corrosive.
10. Mix the content of each tube. Place all the tubes in the boiling water-bath at 100°C for exactly 12 min.
11. Remove the tubes and allow them to cool in a beaker of cold water for 5 min.
12. Measure the intensity of the colour produced at a wavelength of 630 nm (orange-red).
    (a) Set the wavelength (630 nm).
    (b) Fill the cuvette with the blank solution and place in the colorimeter.
    (c) Adjust the reading of the colorimeter to zero.
    (d) Pour solution B out of the cuvette, rinse with a small amount of solution R (reference), pour this out and fill the cuvette with solution R, place the cuvette in the colorimeter and take the absorbance reading (A_R).
    (e) Pour solution R out of the cuvette, rinse the cuvette with a small amount of solution P (patient), pour this out, and fill the cuvette with solution P; place the cuvette in the colorimeter and take the absorbance reading (A_P)

Calibration of the Colorimeter Before taking the readings prepare a calibration graph using different concentrations (2.5, 5, 10, 20 and 25 mmol/L) of the glucose working reference solution. Set up six test tubes labelled 1–6. Tube #1 is the blank (B) and others in the increasing order of glucose working standards (S_1–S_5).

1. Put 0.5 mL of water in the tube #1 (Blank) and 0.5 mL of the working standard solutions in the rest five test tubes (S_1–S_5: 2.5, 5, 10, 20 and 25).
2. Add 3.5 mL of *o*-toluidine reagent in each.
3. Then follow steps 10–12 and note the absorbance readings for each standard, against the blank.
4. Prepare a graph in the way described in Chapter 4 in Vol. I for haemoglobin. The graph should be linear up to the highest concentration and should pass through the origin. Prepare a new graph whenever the *o*-toluidine reagent is renewed, to confirm the linearity.

Calculation and reporting
Calculate the concentration of glucose in the blood specimen using the following formula:

$$\text{Concentration of glucose in Patient's blood (mmol/L)} = \left(\frac{A_P}{A_R}\right) \times C,$$

where A_P is absorbance reading of patient specimen, A_R is Absorbance reading of the glucose working reference solution and C is concentration of the glucose working reference solution (we chose 10 mmol/L).

Note:
- If a control serum is included, make the calculation for that serum in exactly the same way, substituting AC (absorbance of the control solution) for AP in the formula.
- The calculation is for SI units. Use the following formula in order to convert the SI unit to the traditional unit (mg/dL):

$$\text{Concentration of glucose (mg/dL)} = \text{Concentration of glucose (mmol/L)} \times \frac{1}{0.0555}$$

Normal range
Serum or Plasma: 3.9–6.4 mmol/L (SI) and 70–115 mg/dL

Additional information
- Lipaemic serum may cause turbidity of the final solution. In this case add 2.0 mL of isopropanol to the 8 mL of final reaction mixture, mix, measure the absorbance, and multiply the answer by 10/8. If turbidity persists after isopropanol treatment, repeat the test on a protein-free filtrate.
- The procedure follows **Beer's Law** over a long range (100–500 mg/dL or higher). The technician must, however, establish the linearity by preparing a calibration curve which is good for the instrument and the chemicals in use. The calibration curve should be made with a minimum of four concentrations of standard—100, 200, 300 and 500 mg/100 mL. It is not necessary to prepare the standard curve every day, but this is recommended when there is a change in the photometer (e.g. a new bulb is installed), or a new batch of *o*-toluidine reagent is made.
- If the reading of the test solution is more than 0.8, dilute the final reaction mixture with acetic acid. For five-fold dilution: 1 mL reaction mixture + 4 mL acetic acid; for 10-fold dilution: 1 mL of reaction mixture + 9 mL acetic acid. The final result must be multiplied by the dilution factor of 5 or 10, respectively.

Glucose Oxidase Method
Glucose oxidase method is one of the three enzymatic methods used to report the '**True glucose**' value. These enzyme tests are simple, quick, and specific for glucose and have been adapted for use in many types of glucose analysers both large and small. In general, tests that use hexokinase or glucose dehydrogenase are more specific and have less interference than that using glucose oxidase.

Principle
The glucose oxidase method of analysis is a three-step reaction.

$$\text{Glucose} + H_2O + O_2 \xrightarrow{\text{Glucose oxidase}} \text{Gluconic acid} + H_2O_2$$

$$H_2O_2 \xrightarrow{\text{Peroxidase}} H_2O + O \text{ (active oxygen)}$$

$$\text{Phenol} + O + \text{Chromogen} \longrightarrow \text{Colour formation}$$

In the first step glucose is converted to gluconic acid in the presence of glucose oxidase and oxygen. The amount of peroxide (H_2O_2) produced is proportional to the amount of glucose (substrate) present in the specimen. In the second step, the hydrogen peroxide reacts with the enzyme peroxidase releasing water and active oxygen. In the third step, the active oxygen is accepted by an oxygen acceptor (phenol) and then transferred to a chromogenic substance, aminoantipyrine, a compound that yields a strong red coloured solution. The intensity of the colour is proportional to the amount of available hydrogen peroxide and thus the glucose substrate in the initial phase. The intensity of colour complex is measured colorimetrically at 515 nm (or, 500–530 nm, if a filter is used).

Interfering substances: The method is specific for glucose. High concentrations of reducing substances (e.g. ascorbic acid) may interfere by competing with the chromogen for the liberated oxygen and thus causing **false low values** of glucose. Haemoglobin can also interfere by causing a premature decomposition of hydrogen peroxide (see urinalysis for dip-stick screening of haemoglobin) which may give low results. Haemoglobin concentration of less than 600 mg/dL does not interfere with the test. Bilirubin concentration up to 18 mg/dL does not interfere with the test. If the specimen is haemolysed, icteric (jaundiced with yellow-green colour) or lipaemic, use protein-free filtrate. Creatinine, uric acid, and antidiabetic drugs are not known to interfere with the test. Patients with vitamin C therapy (ascorbic acid) may yield low values of glucose.

Specimen

A serum specimen is recommended for this procedure. *Note:* Serum must be separated from the clot within 30 min after collection. Delay in separation of serum from the clot would result in glycolysis and lower glucose values. This is true for all glucose analyses irrespective of the method.

For plasma and whole blood, collect venous blood in tubes or bulbs containing dried sodium fluoride and oxalate. Mix by repeated inversions. Centrifuge the blood to separate the plasma and then transfer the plasma into a clean, dry test tube for the test.

Preparation of protein-free filtrate

Protein-free filtrate is required for whole blood and for specimens which are haemolysed, icteric or lipaemic.
1. Take 0.9 mL of 4% TCA (w/v) in a large-size test tube (19 mm × 150 mm) which helps in mixing.
2. Add 0.1 mL of the test specimen.
3. Mix the contents of the tube.
4. Wait for about 5 min to precipitate the protein.
5. Centrifuge for 5 min (2500 rpm) or until the supernatant is clear.
6. Use 0.1 mL of the clear supernatant for testing.

Reagents

- *Enzyme-chromogen reagent*:
    (a) *Phosphate buffer* (0.1 mole/L, pH 7.0): Take about 800 mL of distilled water in a 1000-mL beaker. Add to this 8.5 g of anhydrous disodium phosphate ($Na.HPO_4$) and 5.3 g of potassium monophosphate (KH_2PO_4). Dissolve the salts by stirring with a glass rod. Check the pH with a pH meter to 7.0 ± 0.1 by the addition of a small amount of 1 N NaOH or 1 N HCl as required. Then quantitatively transfer the solution to a 1000-mL volumetric flask using distilled water for repeated washing of the beaker. Store the buffer in a refrigerator to avoid the growth of microorganisms.
    (b) *Peroxidase reagent*:
    Take 500 mL of phosphate buffer (a) in a 1000-mL beaker. Add 175 mg of 4-aminoantipyrine (also known as 4-aminophenazone) and 2 mL of peroxidase. Both chemicals are available from Sigma Chemical Co., St. Louis, USA. This solution will remain stable for approximately 4 weeks in the refrigerator.

(c) *Glucose oxidase-peroxidase-chromogen reagent*:
  Add 2 mL of stock glucose oxidase solution (1000 units/mL, Sigma type V) to the previously made 500 mL of peroxidase reagent.
  This solution is stable for 1 week in the refrigerator. If the consumption of the laboratory is limited, mix 50 mL of the peroxidase-chromogen reagent with 0.2 mL (200 units) of stock oxidase solution using a 1 mL serological pipette with 0.01 mL graduation. This is good for at least 40 analyses. Daily preparation of the enzyme-chromogen reagent is recommended and the final solution need not be refrigerated.

- *Phenol solution*:
  (a) Take a 1000-mL volumetric flask and add to it about 800 mL of distilled water.
  (b) Transfer 2 g of phenol and 9 g of sodium chloride (NaCl) into the flask and dissolve the ingredients by swirling.
  (c) Finally, make it up to 1000 mL mark with water. Mix by inversion. This solution is stable at room temperature for several months.

- *Glucose standards*:
  The procedure for preparing benzoic acid solution, which will be needed in preparing glucose standard, is given earlier. Benzoic acid works as a preservative for glucose.
  (a) *Stock standard* (1000 mg/dL):
    Dissolve 1.000 g of anhydrous glucose of purest available grade in 80 mL of benzoic acid solution (0.25%) in a 100-mL volumetric flask. Dissolve the sugar and dilute to 100 mL volume. Tightly put stopper and store in a refrigerator. Warm up to room temperature before use.
  (b) *Working standard* (100 mg/dL):
    Dilute 5 mL of the stock standard to 50 mL in a volumetric flask with benzoic acid solution (0.25%) to obtain 100 mg/dL standard.
  (c) *Series of standards*:
    If a series of standards is needed for preparing the calibration curve, dilute 5, 10, 15, 20 and 25 mL of the stock standard to 50 mL volume with benzoic acid solution. These will correspond to 100, 200, 300, 400 and 500 mg/dL standards. This newly prepared series of standards can be stored in a refrigerator in tightly stoppered glass bottles.

Procedure

1. Take three large-size test tubes (19 mm × 150 mm) and mark them as 'T', 'S' and 'B' corresponding to the test specimen, standard and blank. Use more tubes if there is more than one specimen and mark them as T_1, T_2, etc. Large-size test tubes help to shake and mix the reagents.
2. Pipette 2 mL of the glucose oxidase reagent into the three test tubes—T, S and B.
3. Pipette 0.5 mL of 10-fold diluted serum/plasma or standard (100 mg/dL) into the test tubes marked 'T' and 'S', respectively,
   Dilution procedure: Mix separately 0.1 mL of serum/plasma or standard with 0.9 mL of distilled water.
   Alternatively: Use 50 µL of undiluted serum, plasma or standard. This is not recommended for samples showing haemolysis or high bilirubin concentration. It may yield erroneous results.
4. Add 0.5 mL (or 50 µL for undiluted series) of distilled water in the blank ('B').
5. Add 2 mL of phenol reagent to all the tubes. Stopper and shake (to aerate).
6. Place the tubes in a water bath at 37°C for 15 min or at room temperature (25°C ± 5°C) for 30 min.
7. Measure the absorbance (optical density or O.D.) of the test and the standard against the blank at 515 nm (range 500–530 nm). The final colour complex is stable for more than 2 h at room temperature.

8. *Calculation*:

   Glucose concentration (mg/dL) = $(A_t/A_s) \times 100$,

   where A_t is absorbance or optical density of the test solution, A_s is absorbance or optical density of the specimen and 100 is concentration of standard (mg/dL).

   For the conversion into international unit (SI), use the following formula:

   mmol/L = mg/dL divided by 18   [mmol/L = (mg/dL)/10/MW (mg)]

   Note: Molecular weight of glucose ($C_6H_{12}O_6$) = 180 g and 180 mg is the mmol.

Preparation of Calibration Curve

1. Carry out glucose estimation, as described earlier, with the following series of standards (mg/dL): 50, 100, 200, 300, 400 and 500.
2. Draw the calibration curve for every new batch of reagent (Chapter 4 in Vol. I).
3. It is essential to check the graph by using the control serum in order to find out the variation from previous estimations. The calibration curve is linear up to 500 mg/dL of glucose concentration. In specimens with higher glucose concentration, for greater accuracy, it is advisable to dilute the test sample further one to two times with distilled water and repeat the test. The glucose concentration thus obtained should be multiplied by two to obtain the actual glucose level in the test specimen.

   Note: If undiluted standard is to be used (for alternative method), use concentrated standard of 1000 mg/dL.

Additional information

- The glucose oxidase method is not directly applicable to urine specimens, owing to the high concentration of enzyme inhibitors present.
- Rubber tubing, used for dispensing deproteinizing solutions or distilled water, has been found to interfere with adequate colour development; therefore, rubber tubing connections on dispensers or automatic sampling and diluting devices should be kept to a minimum and should be suspected if standards yield unexpectedly low colour values.
- Because of high dilutions prior to the analysis, common drugs do not have any appreciable effect.
- Anticoagulants have not been found to affect the result seriously (although they are discouraged). Sodium fluoride (2.5 mg/mL blood) with oxalate may be used as a preservative, but not thymol which inhibits the reaction. Contrary to this statement many technicians believe that fluoride inhibits glucose oxidase reaction.

Quick Screen of Blood Glucose

Using test strip

For quick screening of blood glucose in case of diabetic patients, plastic reagent strip with glucose testing spot is convenient (Dextrostix, Ames, Miles of India Ltd., Baroda) Hyperglycaemia can be easily recognized. The procedure is described here:

1. Perform skin puncture and squeeze out a large drop of blood.
2. Touch the test spot on the drop of blood and see that the entire surface of the spot is covered.
3. Begin timing immediately by exactly 60 sec (or according to the manufacturer's instructions). Simultaneously hold dry surgical gauze over the puncture site.
4. After 60 sec, rinse the spot on the strip, blot off the excess water and read the glucose concentration by comparing the colour of the spot with the colour chart. Use the spot reader for glucose, if available.

Using electronic devices

Several hand-held glucose meters are available in the market, which are based on electrochemical technology. This allows the diabetic patients to check their blood sugar at home several times a day without any pain.

Patient samples are applied to disposable biosensors, strips that look similar to other reagents strips. These biosensors, in addition to containing reagents for the chemical reactions, also contain electrodes called electrochemical sensors. When the sample interacts with the reagents in the biosensor strip, the current (electrons) generated is detected by the meter and converted into glucose unit.

Clinical Significance of Glucose in Circulation

Glucose, the major and simplest carbohydrate in blood, is used as the primary energy source by the body cells. Glucose level of blood is controlled by hormonal mechanism. This is why patients with abnormal glucose level of blood are referred to the endocrinology department for evaluation and treatment.

Two disorders of glucose metabolism are common.
- **Diabetes mellitus**, in which there is, increased blood glucose (**hyperglycaemia**).
- **Deficiency of growth hormone (ACTH)**, in which there is decreased level of blood glucose (**hypoglycaemia**).

The former is caused by insulin deficiency (or its insufficient utilization) and the later is seen in deficiencies of ACTH or growth hormone. *Note:* There is another kind of diabetes, called **diabetes insipidus**. This is unrelated to carbohydrate metabolism. It is caused by the deficiency of antidiuretic hormone (ADH which is made in hypothalamus and secreted by pituitary at the base of the brain) that affects water metabolism of the body. Symptoms of diabetes insipidus include polyuria (increased urination) and increased thirst.

Insulin is a hormone produced by the pancreas, **lowers blood glucose** by increasing cellular uptake of glucose and increasing the rate of glycolysis. Glycolysis is a cellular process that produces energy by the metabolic breakdown of glucose. Insulin also increases the rate of conversion of glucose to glycogen, the short-term storage form of glucose in liver. This has been further elaborated in Chapter 29 in this Volume.

On the other hand, there are several hormones such as growth hormone, epinephrine, cortisol, and glucagons, which act in a variety of ways to **increase blood glucose** concentration. Hence these are sometimes referred as insulin antagonists, because their action is opposite to the action of insulin.

Diabetes and Diabetes Management

Diabetes mellitus, commonly called diabetes, is a chronic disease in which the body either produced insufficient insulin or is unable to use insulin properly. It is a serious disease and uncontrolled diabetes may lead to a number of ailments, heart attack, coma, high blood pressure, blindness, kidney failure and increased infection in case of injury. Early diagnosis is very important because proper management of diabetes can lessen, postpone, or even prevent many of these complications.

There are two common types of diabetes—**type I**, insulin dependent and **type II**, adult onset. In type 1, the person has to take insulin injection as their body does not produce sufficient insulin. It usually appears in children and young adults, often inherited. In type 2 diabetes, the body fails to properly use insulin (insulin resistance) and usually appears later in life.

Diagnostic tests for diabetes and hypoglycaemia involve three major tests—testing for fasting blood glucose, oral glucose tolerance test and determination of haemoglobin A1c. These three tests are diagnostic in the following ways:
- Fasting glucose 126 mg/dL or higher.
- Glucose level of blood does not return below 200 mg/dL level after 2 h following heavy load of oral glucose intake. If sugar level is between 140 and 199 mg/dL, it is called prediabetes. In 3 h sugar level should be normal.
- HbA1c is above 6.0.

Diabetes cannot be cured but can be managed. One can lead a healthy life if the blood sugar is kept under control. Monitoring the blood glucose is the first line of action in **the management of diabetes**. Glucose meter has greatly contributed to home glucose monitoring schedule. Early morning fasting glucose concentration in a normal person is 70–110 mg/dL. If the concentration exceeds 126 mg/dL, it will be the condition of **hyperglycemia** and the person may be suspected of diabetes. The result of glucose tolerance test for a normal person will show the levels of blood glucose as 70–110 mg/dL (0 h, fasting glucose); 90–160 mg/dL (1 h after sugar intake); 140 mg/dL (2 h after sugar intake) and normal level after 3 h.

If the level of blood glucose falls below 40 mg/dL (**hypoglycaemia**), the person may experience weakness, visual disturbance, confusion, hunger, faintness, diaphoresis, palsy and confusion. When the level is high (hyperglycaemia), above 400 mg/dL, one may experience coma, confusion, nausea, intense thirst, dry skin and weak pulse. The signs and symptoms vary with individual.

The patient's ability to keep blood glucose levels within acceptable range can be assessed by periodic measurement of **haemoglobin A1c**, also called **glycated haemoglobin**.

Hb A1c (glycated haemoglobin)

Haemoglobin (Hb) is present in all red blood cells and is the molecule that transports oxygen from the lungs to the tissues. The major haemoglobin is Hb A. After glucose is absorbed form the gastrointestinal tract and enters circulation, it is taken up by cells for energy. Glucose, the major and simplest carbohydrate in blood, is used as the primary energy source by all cells and especially by the red cells which cannot consume any other form of carbohydrate, the energy package of the biological world.

During period of high blood glucose levels, glucose molecules enter red blood cells and bind to haemoglobin, forming HbA1c (glycated haemoglobin). The amount of HbA1c is proportional to the amount of glucose in circulation. Since average life span of red blood cells is approximately 120 days, the level of HbA1c is related to the average amount of glucose it is exposed to in the blood for that period of time. In reality the HbA1c more closely represents levels over the previous 2–4 weeks.

As the **fasting glucose level** gives the patient an idea of the lowest level of glucose on the daily basis, the physician reads the HbA1c value for judging how tightly the patient has controlled the blood glucose level over a period of about a month. Recent studies have shown that HbA1c is the single best test for evaluating the risk of damage to nerves and the small blood vessels of the eyes and kidneys. This damage leads to the complications of diabetes, such as blindness and kidney failure. Clinical trials have shown that reducing the HbA1c level in diabetics and maintaining it below 7% will prevent the development of, or further progress of, complications from diabetes. It is true for both type I and type II diabetes.

The traditional methods of HbA1c determination are HPLC, TLC and electrophoresis. These are available only in reference laboratories. Point of care analysis HbA1c is a recent innovation and has proved to be very helpful to diabetic patients. Results are obtained within few min. Additionally, some home glucose meters calculate the HbA1c from the average of the glucose values in memory.

The commonly available automated system (Afinion Analyzer) for HbA1c, gives you reliable results. This instrument uses **boronate affinity assay** for the determination of the percentage of HbA1c in human whole blood. All reagents are contained in the disposable test cartridge which also has an integrated sampling device taking only 1.5 ìL of whole blood from a finger prick. The blood sample is automatically diluted and mixed with a liquid that releases haemoglobin from the erythrocytes. The haemoglobin precipitates. The sample mixture is transferred to a blue boronic acid conjugate, which binds to glycated haemoglobin. The reaction mixture is soaked through a filter membrane and all precipitated haemoglobin remains on the membrane. All measurements and calculations are performed by the analyser and percentage HbA1c displayed on the screen. The analyser system is easy to use, gives reliable and accurate results. The analysis time is about 3 min and measuring range is 4–15% HbA1c. The system is therefore particularly suitable for use in diabetic clinics.

Laboratory determination of HbA1c may use a latex agglutination reaction in which a monoclonal antibody is used as epitope which recognizes glucose bound to HbA1c. The measurement, however, will require an immunophotometer.

DETERMINATION OF SERUM PROTEIN

Serum protein consists of **albumin** and **globulin**. Serum protein analysis can help diagnose liver disorders, nutritional deficiency of protein, renal failure and lymphoproliferative disorders. Decrease in total protein values is associated with cirrhosis of the liver and other liver disorders, malnutrition, nephrotic syndromes and neoplastlc disease. Increased total protein values may be found in multiple myeloma, and conditions associated with high globulin concentration (autoimmune and lymphoproliferative disorders).

Normal values (adult)
Total protein: 6.0–8.0 g/dL
Albumin fraction: 3.5–5.0 g/dL
Globulin fraction: 2.3–3.5 g/dL.

Determination of Total Protein

Biuret method
This method is still popular, easy to follow and provides accurate results.

Principle Proteins and peptides react with alkaline copper tartrate solution to give a violet coloured complex. The intensity of the final colour complex is measured colorimetrically at 540 nm (range 530–560 nm) and is proportional to the concentration of total protein in the specimen under test. Under carefully controlled conditions this method can prove to be very useful but the reagents must be prepared carefully (alkalinity affects colour development).

The name biuret reaction comes from an analogous reaction that takes place between the cupric ion and the organic compound biuret (an ammonium compound). Kits for this method are commercially available.

Specimen Serum or plasma.
Interfering substances: Haemolysed serum or plasma samples should not be used in this testing procedure. Lipaemia has no effect on the total protein values but grossly turbid serum should not be used. If necessary, treat the serum with isopropanol, discard the solvent and use the serum for protein assay.

Reagents
- *Biuret reagent*
  - *Biuret diluent*: 5 g potassium iodide (KI) in 0.25 N sodium hydroxide (10 g NaOH/L). The sodium hydroxide solution may be prepared in larger quantities as a stock solution (2.50 N) which is diluted 10-fold with distilled water fresh from a still (it should be CO_2 free). Always store the sodium hydroxide reagent in stoppered poly ethylene bottles.
  - *Stock biuret reagent*:
    (a) Dissolve 15 g of finely pulverized uneffloresced copper sulphate ($CuSO_4 \cdot 5H_2O$) in 70–80 mL of water placed in a beaker.
    (b) In a 1000-mL volumetric flask, prepare a solution of 45 g Rochelle salt (potassium sodium tartrate, tetrahydrate) in 600–700 mL of biuret diluent [solution (a)].
    (c) Add slowly the copper sulphate solution (a) into the volumetric flask containing tartrate solution (b). Both solutions must be at room temperature when mixed to prevent reduction of cupric ions by the tartrate.
    (d) Add biuret diluent up to the 1000-mL mark of the volumetric flask. Store in a polyethylene bottle, away from strong, direct light.
    (e) Before use, filter the solution through a qualitative paper to remove any deposited cuprous oxide.

o *Working biuret solution*: Dilute the stock biuret solution five-fold with biuret diluent. For preparing 100 mL of the working biuret solution, take 20 mL of the stock biuret solution in a 100-mL volumetric flask and dilute it to the mark with the biuret diluent. This is good for 10 analyses, including the blank and the standard. Store the working biuret solution in the same way as the stock biuret reagent.

  Note: If a slight precipitate forms on storage the reagent should be filtered before use; the sensitivity does not change.

- *Saline* (NaCl, 0.85% w/v in water): Dissolve 8.5 g of sodium chloride in about 800 mL of water placed in a 1-L volumetric flask. Bring the solution to the 1000-mL mark with water and mix by inversion. Keep the solution in a stoppered glass bottle.
- *Standard protein solution*: It is most convenient to purchase the standard from the supplier (Ethnor Ltd., Span Diagnostics, Bharat Laboratories). The value of the protein concentration is imprinted on the ampoule and is usually in the range of 6–8 g protein/100 mL or dL. If it is given in nitrogen value (mg/mL), multiply the value by 6.25 in order to get the corresponding value of protein in g/dL. (*Note:* Nitrogen concentration × 6.25 = protein concentration).

  Alternatively: Use the control serum with a known concentration of protein determined earlier.

- *Control serum*: Prepare this by pooling leftover normal sera, which are free of haemolysis, significant icterus, turbidity or chyle. Mix the pool, pass it through several layers of glass wool to remove the fine clots. Transfer to 15 × 120 mm test tubes in 1 mL aliquots. Many laboratories use smaller glass vials or penicillin bottles. The container must be about 5-mL. Store the control serum in a frozen state. Before assaying, remove a tube, thaw in a bath at 37°C, and carefully mix. Determine the protein value against a commercial protein control.

  Note: This control serum may be used in other tests as well for quality control. All safety precautions of handling patient's serum specimen should be taken while handling control serum as well.

Procedure

1. Prepare 20-fold dilutions of test specimen (T) and standard (S) by the following steps:
   (a) Set up two test tubes marked as 'T_D' and 'S_D'
       Note: Increase the number of test tubes if there are more than one test specimen (T_{D1}, T_{D2}, etc.).
   (b) Pipette 9.5 mL of saline in each.
   (c) Transfer 0.5 mL of test specimen and standard in the tubes marked as T_D and S_D respectively. Avoid foaming during dilution. (Do the same with other test specimens as well T_{D1}, T_{D2}, etc.)
2. Set up three new test tubes (15-mL), marked as 'T', 'S' and 'B' for test, standard and blank respectively. Continue the same if there are more than one specimen, T_1, T_2, etc.
3. Dispense, with the help of a dispenser, 4.0 mL of working biuret reagent in all the three test tubes.
4. Add 1.0 mL of the diluted serum specimen and standard in the tubes marked T and S (continue the same way with other specimens as well). Add an equivalent amount of water (1.0 mL) in the blank tube (B).
   Alternatively: Pipette 5 mL of working biuret reagent into the above test tubes marked as T, S and B. Directly add 100 μL of undiluted specimen and standard in T and S tubes, respectively and 100 μL of water in tube B. This method is not recommended when the serum or plasma samples show haemolysis or high bilirubin concentration (icteric). This method yields erroneous results under these conditions. The 100 μL automatic pipette should be carefully calibrated or else this method will have increased error. An aliquot of 50 μL can also be used.
5. Mix the contents thoroughly. A large-size test tube helps in mixing which is rather inconvenient in the cuvette.
6. Incubate for 15 min at 37°C in a water bath (preferred) or alternatively, for 30 min at room temperature.

7. Measure the absorbance (or optical density, O.D.) of the test (A_T) and the standard (A_S) against the blank (A_0) at 540 nm (range 530–560 nm). Complete the readings within an hour.
8. Calculations:
   Total protein concentration in test specimen (g/dL) = (A_T/A_S) × 6
9. Preparation of calibration curve:
   (a) Prepare five concentrations of the standard: Arrange five test tubes and label them 1–5.
   (b) Mix 1 : 20 dilution of the standard with the saline in the following way:

Tube No.	1 : 20 dilution of protein standard (6 g/dL)* mL	Saline (mL)	Corresponding protein concentration (g/dL)
1	1.0	2.0	2.0
2	1.5	1.5	3.0
3	2.0	1.0	4.0
4	2.5	0.5	5.0
5	3.0	0.0	6.0

*Make the necessary adjustments if the standard is different.

   (c) Carry out the total protein estimation in tubes labelled 1–5 following the testing procedure outlined earlier, including the dilution (or using the specimen/standard directly).
   (d) Tabulate the absorbance (O.D.) readings.
   (e) Plot a graph with protein concentration in g/dL against the corresponding optical density after adjusting the blank to zero absorbance. The graph will be a straight line passing through the origin (0 reading of the blank).
   (f) The calibration curve should be a straight line and it is linear up to 10 g/dL.

Additional information
- The calibration curve should be redrawn with every new batch of reagent.
- It is preferable to check the calibration graph by using a standard along with the test specimens.
- Theoretically, the total protein content of serum should be less than that of plasma by about 0.3 g/dL. If oxalate-fluoride is used as an anticoagulant, water diffuses out of the erythrocytes to compensate for the increased salt concentration. This shift occurs within 15 min and is proportional to the concentration of anticoagulant used. With the concentrations of the anticoagulant employed the dilution that occurs yields a plasma protein concentration usually no higher and sometimes less than that of serum.
- Haemolysis causes a false high value of protein. The use of a tourniquet may also yield a false high value of protein.
- The Biuret reagent (stock and working) must be filtered at least weekly.
- The precision (repeatability) expected for this procedure is about ± 0.3 g/dL (±3.5%). The main source of error is pipetting the initial sample aliquot. This increases with the aliquot of 100 µL, if the automatic pipetter is not calibrated.
- A new calibration curve should be made for each individual colorimeter and when there is any change in the working of the instrument (e.g. change of bulb).
- Prepare a serum blank if the serum is highly pigmented (haemoglobin or bilirubin), milky (lipaemic), or turbid in appearance. Read the absorbance of the specimen, using water in place of reagent (4 mL) and subtract the value from the absorbance reading of the test solution. Another way to handle the problem is to take two readings at two wavelengths (530 and 540 nm or 540 and 560 nm) for both the test specimen (T) as well as the standard (S), and to take the difference for comparison. This is called the bichromatic method.
- Either bovine serum albumin or human serum albumin can be used as the standard.

Determination of serum albumin

Albumin is synthesized in the **liver**. Decreased levels of albumin in serum may be found in certain conditions such as cirrhosis of the liver and other liver disorders. **Loss of albumin** due to kidney disorder such as nephritic syndrome will also lead to a decline of serum albumin level as also with malnutrition, malignancy, and chronic protracted conditions like ulcerative colitis. Pathological conditions associated with increased levels of serum albumin are not known.

Normal Value   3.5–5.0 g/dL

Principle   Albumin binds bromocresol green dye in a suitable buffer making a shift in the dye's peak absorption wavelength. The increase in absorbance is read at 630 nm (range 620–640 nm) which is proportional to the albumin concentration. Commercial kits are available (see Appendix H for suppliers at the end of this Volume). Brij 35, a non-ionic detergent helps in stabilizing the reaction.

Specimen   Serum or plasma can be used for the testing procedure.

Interfering substances: Icteric and haemolysed specimens may interfere with the test. Serum bilirubin concentrations up to 15 mg/dL do not interfere with the test. The albumin concentration shows an increase of 0.1 g/dL for each 100 mg/dL of haemoglobin in the specimen.

Reagent
- *Succinic acid solution (5%, w/v)*
  Dissolve 5 g of succinic acid in about 80 mL of distilled water. Transfer this solution to a 100-mL volumetric flask and make up to the volume with distilled water.
- *Sodium hydroxide (0.25 N)*
  Weigh out quickly 10 g of sodium hydroxide and dissolve in 500 mL of fresh distilled water. Transfer to 1-L volumetric flask, and make the volume up to 1000 mL with fresh distilled water.
- *'Brij-35' (30%, w/v)*
  Dissolve 30 g of 'Brij-35' in about 30 mL of hot distilled water, transfer into a 100-mL volumetric flask and make up to 100 mL volume with distilled water.
- *Dye solution*
  100 mg sodium azide into a 1-L beaker. Add 900 mL of distilled water and 4 mL of 'Brij-35'; stir until dissolved. Adjust the pH to 4.20 ± 0.05 using sodium hydroxide solution for raising the pH or succinic acid solution for lowering the pH.
- *Sodium chloride–sodium azide solution*
  Weigh 9.0 g sodium chloride and 0.5 g of sodium azide. Transfer the salts into a 1-L volumetric flask. Dissolve and make the volume up to 1000 mL with distilled water.
- *Albumin standard (100 g/L)*
  Weigh out accurately 10 g of dry albumin powder and transfer into a 100-mL volumetric flask. Add slowly 80 mL of sodium chloride–sodium azide solution and mix by shaking the flask until the albumin is completely dissolved. Finally make the volume up to 100 mL with sodium chloride–sodium azide solution. Determine its exact concentration by comparing with good quality commercially available albumin standard (Ortho-Ethanor Ltd., Bombay).

Procedure
1. *Dilution of specimen and standard (1:20)*:
   (a) Place two test tubes (15-mL capacity) in a test tube rack and label them as 'T' and 'S' for holding the test specimen and standard respectively. Take more tubes if there are more specimens and mark them as T_1, T_2, etc.

(b) Add 9.5 mL of distilled water in both tubes (T and S).
(c) Transfer 0.5 mL of the test specimen and albumin standard (about 4 g/dL) into the respective tubes marked as T and S. Mix well.

2. *Colour reaction:*
   (a) Place three fresh test tubes (15-mL capacity) in the test tube rack and label them as 'T', 'S', and 'B' for the test specimen, standard and blank, respectively.
   (b) With the help of a dispenser, dispense 5.0 mL of the colour reagent in each of the tubes ('T', 'S' and 'B').
   (c) Transfer 0.25 mL of diluted test specimen and diluted standard [see (step 1)], respectively to the tubes marked as 'T' and 'S'. Add 0.25 mL of distilled water in the tube marked 'B'.
   (d) *Alternatively:* Directly use 25 µL of undiluted serum and standard, and 25 mL of water for the blank and mix with 5 mL of colour reagent as was done with the diluted specimen/standard. This method is not recommended for turbid specimens, and for specimens showing haemolysis or high bilirubin concentration. It yields erroneous results.
   (e) Mix the contents of tubes 'T', 'S' and 'B' [step (c)] thoroughly.
   (f) Allow to stand at room temperature for 10 min.

3. *Photometric reading:*
   Measure the absorbance of the test and the standard against the blank at 630 nm (for filter use the range close to 620–630 nm).

4. Calculation:
   Albumin concentration (g/dL) = $(A_t/A_s) \times 4$ A^m Absorbance (O.D.) of test solution A is Absorbance (O.D.) of standard solution 4 is concentration of standard (g/dL)
   Note: For conversion to SI units, use the formula g/dL × 10 = g/L

Preparation of calibration curve

1. Prepare four concentrations of albumin according to the following chart:

Tube No.	1 : 20 dilution of standard (mL)	Distilled water (mL)	Corresponding concentration of protein (g/dL)
1	1.0	3.0	1.0
2	2.0	2.0	2.0
3	3.0	1.0	3.0
4	4.0	0.0	4.0

2. Carry out albumin estimation of solutions in tubes labelled 1–4 following the testing procedure outlined earlier.
3. Prepare the calibration curve. It should be a straight line.
   Note: The calibration curve must be drawn with every new batch of reagent and must be made for each individual colorimeter used.

Additional information

- Bilirubin does not seriously interfere with the test.
- If a slight precipitate is formed in the colour reagent during storage, filter it before use. The reagent does not lose its sensitivity.
- Saline is not used in diluting the specimen. The addition of electrolytes decreases the absorbance. Neither billrubin nor succinate buffer seems to interfere.
- In case of low serum albumin levels, the results tend to be high owing to the attachment of dye to other proteins. The technician should be aware of this problem and the physician should be informed.

Calculation of Globulin Concentration of Serum Globulin concentration in serum is indirectly determined by subtracting the albumin concentration from the total protein concentration. The normal globulin concentration in serum is in the range of 2.3–3.5 g/dL.

DETERMINATION OF BLOOD UREA

Urea is a waste product formed in the liver following the breakdown of protein. It passes into the blood, is filtered out of the kidneys and excreted in the urine. If the kidneys do not remove urea, the concentration in the blood is increased. This can happen if the kidney tubules become damaged or if the volume of blood flowing through the kidneys is reduced. Thus determination of serum urea (or **blood urea nitrogen**, BUN) is the most widely used screening test for the evaluation of kidney function.

The test is frequently requested along with the serum creatinine test since simultaneous determination of these two compounds appears to aid in the **differential diagnosis** of pre-renal, renal, and post-renal uraemia (increased serum concentration of urea). Pre-renal causes could be cardiac-related or due to increased protein catabolism; renal causes include glomerulonephritis, chronic nephritis, nephrotic syndrome and other conditions. Acute upper gastrointestinal bleeding can cause increase in protein into the gut which after absorption may cause high level of BUN. Post-renal causes include obstruction of the urinary tract. Higher increase in urea than creatinine is often an indication of a pre-renal problem; a mild increase in urea as compared to increase in creatinine level is suggestive of renal disease. Post-renal problems lead to increase of both urea and creatinine proportionately. In other words, the ratio does not change significantly.

Normal value

8–18 mg/dL (values vary with diet).

Specimen

Serum specimen is commonly submitted for reporting blood urea concentration. Since urea may be lost through bacterial action, the specimen should be analysed within 2 h after blood collection or should be preserved by refrigeration.
Interfering substances: Avoid using haemolysed and icteric serum. Haemoglobin levels up to 100 mg/dL and bilirubin levels up to 15 mg/dL do not interfere with the test. If the serum specimen is haemolysed or icteric, deproteinize with TCA.

Diacetyl Monoxime Method

Principle

Diacetyl monoxime in a hot acid medium reacts with urea producing a specific pink coloured complex. The presence of ferric ions and other activators intensifies the colour. The intensity of the colour is measured colorimetrically at 520 nm (range 510–540 nm) and is proportional to the concentration of urea nitrogen in the specimen under test.

Specimen

Patient's whole blood (EDTA-anticoagulated), plasma and serum are submitted for analysis.

Equipment and supplies

- Colorimeter
- Conical tubes and test tubes to 20 mL
- Pipettes: 50 µL, 0.1 mL, 0.5 mL, 5 mL
- Measuring cylinder, 50 mL
- Water-bath at 100°C (boiling)

Reagents

- *TCA (5%) solution:*

TCA (CCl$_3$COOH)	10 g
Distilled water (q.s.)	200 mL

  Weigh the acid out quickly, it is highly deliquescent. Transfer to a beaker. Add 100 mL of distilled water and mix to dissolve the chemical. Transfer the solution to a 200-mL volumetric flask and make up to volume to 200 mL with distilled water. Label the volumetric flask as "TCA, 5%" and put the date. Warning: This solution is highly corrosive.

- *Acid reagent:*

Concentrated sulphuric acid (H$_2$SO$_4$)	44 mL
Orthophosphoric acid (H$_3$PO$_4$), 85%	66 mL
Cadium sulphate	1.6 g
Thiosemicarbazide	50 mg
Distilled water (q.s.)	500 mL

  Half fill a 500-mL flask with distilled water, add the sulphuric acid very slowly, stirring constantly, and follow with the orthophosphoric acid. Continue mixing the solution and add the thisemicarbazide and then the cadmium sulphate. Make up the volume to 500 mL with distilled water. Transfer the reagent to a brown bottle. Label the bottle "ACID REAGENT" and write the date. Store in the refrigerator (2–8°C). The reagent will keep for at least 6 months in the refrigerator. *Warning*: Sulphuric acid is highly corrosive.

- *Diacetyl monoxime stock solution*

Diacetyl monoxime*	2 g
Distilled water (q.s.)	500 mL

  Label the volumetric flask (or bottle) as "Diacetyl Monoxime Stock Solution" and write the date. The solution will keep for at least 6 months in the refrigerator (2–8°C).

- *Colour reagent:* **Make this immediately before use**

  Mix the stock solution of diacetyl monoxime and acid reagent in equal proportions (1:1).

Acid reagent	50 mL
Dacetyl monoxime reagent	50 mL

  Mix the acid reagent and stock solution in 100 mL stoppered flask. Label the flask as "UREA COLOUR REAGENT" with date. The quantities described earlier are sufficient for 33 assays. The reagent must be prepared daily. *Note:* Prepare at least 15 mL of colour reagent for each test. Which means 7.5 mL of each mixed in a small flask or in a big test tube?

- *Benzoic acid solution:* This is needed to prepare the urea reference solution.

Benzoic acid	1 g
Distilled water (q.s.)	1000 mL

  Measure 1000 mL of distilled water and heat to just below boiling. Add the benzoic acid and mix well until it is dissolved. Allow to cool. Transfer the solution to a 1000-mL gas-stoppered bottle. Label the bottle "BENZOIC ACID 0.1% SOLUTION" and write the date.

- *Urea reference (or standard) solution, 125 mmol/L*

Urea	750 mg
Benzoic acid, 1g/L (0.1%) (q.s.)	100 mL

  Dissolve the urea in about 20 mL of the benzoic acid solution in a 100-mL volumetric flask. Make up the volume to 100 mL with benzoic acid solution. Label the flask "**UREA STOCK REFERENCE**

---

*Also called 2,3-butanedione monoxime

SOLUTION, 125 mmol/L" and write the date. Store the solution in a refrigerator. The solution will keep for several months at 2–8°C.

Urea working reference (or standard) solution, 10 mmol/L

Urea stock reference solution	8 mL
Benzoic acid ($C_7H_6O_2$), 0.1% (q.s.)	100 mL

Mix the solution well in a 100-mL volumetric flask. Label the volumetric flask "UREA "WORKING REFERENCE SOLUTION, 10 mmol/L" and write the date. Keep in a refrigerator.

- *Blank reagent*

TCA (CCl_3COOH), 5%) solution	50 mL
Distilled water (q.s.)	100 mL

Mix and transfer the solution in a glass-stoppered bottle. Label the bottle "**BLANK REAGENT**" and write the date. Store the solution at room temperature. The reagent will keep for several months at room temperature.

Warning: TCA is highly corrosive.

- *Control serum*

A control serum (of known concentration) should be used with each batch of tests. If the result of the test with the control serum is correct, it can be assumed that the patient's results will also be correct.

Procedure

1. Prepare the colour reagent immediately before use, using a 1 : 1 mixture of the diacetyl monoxime stock solution and acid reagent. Prepare at least 15 mL of colour reagent for each test. Mix the colour regent in a large test tube or in a small flask.
2. Pipette into a conical centrifuge tube 50 μL of whole blood (EDTA anticoagulated), plasma or serum.
3. Add 1 mL of TCA solution and mix. Centrifuge at high speed (3000g) for 5 min to sediment the precipitated proteins and obtain a clear supernatant fluid.
4. Take three (or more if needed) large test tubes and label them as 'B' for blank, 'R' for reference, 'T' for test (patient's specimen). If there is more than one specimen, continue as T_1, T_2, etc. Make sure that each 'T' marked tube has patient's ID recorded.
5. Pipette into each tube as follows:
   Blank(B): 0.1 mL of bland reagent and 3.0 mL of freshly prepared colour reagent
   Reference(R): 0.1 mL of working reference solution and 3.0 mL of freshly prepared colour reagent.
   Test(T): 0.1 mL of supernatant fluid and 3.0 mL of freshly prepared colour reagent. Continue the same if there is more than one specimen.
6. Mix the contents of each tube. Place all the tubes in the water bath at 100°C for 15 min to allow the red colour to develop.
7. Remove the tubes and place them in a beaker of cold water until they have cooled to room temperature.
8. Measure the colour intensity at a wavelength of 520 nm against the blank.
   - Place the green filter (520 nm) in the colorimeter or choose the appropriate wavelength in a spectrophotometer.
   - Fill the cuvette with the blank solution ('B') and place it in the colorimeter.
   - Adjust the absorbance reading to '0' (zero) with the blank solution in place.
   - Pour out solution B and replace with a small amount of working reference solution in the tube 'R'. Pour this out (rinsing) and fill the cuvette with solution 'R'. Place the cuvette in the colorimeter and read the absorbance, A_R.
   - Pour out the reference solution, rinse the cuvette with the test solution ('T') and then fill it with the test solution-carrying patient ID. Read the absorbance, A_T.

9. *Calculation*: Calculate the urea in the blood as follows:
   Urea concentration (mmol/L) = $A_T/A_R \times C$,
   where A_T is absorbance reading of test solution (patient's specimen), A_R is absorbance reading of urea working reference standard and C is concentration of working reference standard (10 mmol/L).

For the **conversion of urea concentration** in mg/dL unit to the International unit of mmol/L, apply the following formula:
$$\text{mmol/L} \times 6 = \text{mg/dL}$$

Additional Note:
The reference range of urea concentration in blood is approximately 3–7 mmol/L (18–42 mg/dL). If a value is greater than 25 mmol/L (150 mg/dL), repeat the entire test with that specimen, using two-fold diluted specimen. Perform the test and calculate the results exactly as before, but multiply the result by two to obtain the true urea concentration.

DETERMINATION OF CREATININE

Creatinine is a waste product of creatine phosphate, a substance store in muscle and used for energy. Creatinine is removed from plasma through glomerular filtration and is then excreted in the urine without being reabsorbed by the tubules to any significant extent. When **renal function** is impaired, blood creatinine levels rise, but more than 50% of kidney unction must be lost before this happens. So **elevation** usually indicates significant **insufficiency**. Other reasons for the increase of serum creatinine level are shock, water imbalance, dehydration and ureter blockage. Simultaneous determination of urea and creatinine is desirable in order to trace the aetiology as both increases with decreased kidney function. Creatinine determinations have one advantage over urea determinations; they are not affected by a high protein diet as is the case for urea levels. Determination of creatinine clearance is a highly sensitive test for measuring the glomerular filtration rate.

Normal values

(non-specific alkaline picrate method)

Serum: 0.9–1.5 mg/dL
Urine: 90–150 mg/dL (100 times higher than serum).
Urinary discharge per day: 1.0–2.0 g/day

For the conversion of creatinine concentration in mg/dL unit to the International unit of μmol/L, apply the following formula:
$$\text{mg/dL} \times 88.4 = \text{μmol/L}$$

Alkaline Picrate Method

Creatinine gives a red colour with alkaline solutions of picric acid (**Jaffe reaction**). The reaction is not specific and other chromogenic substances present in urine or serum may give false high values. This error does not normally interfere in clinical diagnosis.

Specimen

The procedure described here can be followed for serum, plasma, or urine. For serum and plasma, a protein-free filtrate must be used. If urine is analysed, make a 1:400 dilution of urine with water.

Reagents

Picric acid (1.05% in water, 0.04 mol/L)

> Dissolve 10.5 g of picric acid (hydrated) or 9.3 g anhydrous picric acid in about 500 mL of hot water (80°C). Cool to room temperature and then dilute to 1000 mL in a volumetric flask. Exact standardization

of the acid is not required. For screening, a saturated solution of picric acid can be used. Make 1000-mL in a graduated 1-L beaker. The reagent is stable at room temperature but should be protected from sunlight.
- *Sodium hydroxide (0.75 N, 0.75 mol/L)*
  Dissolve 30 g of sodium hydroxide in 800 mL of water and make this up to 1000 mL with water. Store the solution in a tightly closed polyethylene bottle.
- *Sulphuric acid (0.66 N, 0.33 mol/L)*
  Add 18.8 mL concentrated sulphuric acid (pure grade, AR) to about 500 mL of water in a 1-L volumetric flask. When cool, dilute to 1000 mL.
- *Sodium tungstate (5% in water, 0.3 mol/L)*
  Dissolve 50 g of sodium tungstate in about 500 mL of water and dilute it to 1000 mL.
- *Hydrochloric acid (0.1 N, 0.1 mol/L)*
  Dissolve 8.55 mL of concentrated hydrochloric acid (11.7 N) in water and dilute to 1000 mL in a volumetric flask. This reagent is used in preparing the standard.
- *Creatinine standards*
  o *Creatinine stock standard* (1 mg/mL or 100 mg/dL):
    Dissolve 100 mg of pure grade creatinine in 100 mL of 0.1 N hydrochloric acid (see above). Keep refrigerated.
  o *Creatinine working standard* (20 µg/mL or 2 mg/dL):
    Dilute 2 mL of the stock standard solution to dL with water in a volumetric flask. Add a few drops of chloroform as a preservative. This solution is unstable. Keep it in the refrigerator and take it out for daily use; discard after one week.

Procedure

1. Preparation of protein-free filtrate:
   (a) Take in a clean test tube 1.0 mL of plasma or serum.
   (b) Add to the 1.0 mL of sodium tungstate, 1.0 mL of 0.66N sulphuric acid, and 1.0 mL of water.
   (c) Mix thoroughly.
   (d) Centrifuge at 2000 rpm for 5 min.
   (e) 2 mL of the supernatant is required for the test run.
   Note: If a urine specimen is to be analysed, dilute it by mixing 0.1 mL of the urine specimen with 40 mL of water in a graduated cylinder. Removal of protein will not be necessary for normal urine. Remove protein in case of proteinuria. The protein free filtrate of urine will be diluted 1:100 (instead of 1:400).
2. *Colour reaction*:
   (a) Take three test tubes and label them as 'T', 'S' and 'B' for test, standard and blank.
   (b) Make the additions to the labelled tubes as indicated in the following table

	Test (T) mL	Standard (S) mL	Blank (B) mL
Distilled water	2.0	3.5	4.0
Creatinine standard	0.0	0.5	0.0
Specimen	2.0*	0.0	0.0
Picric acid solution	1.0	1.0	1.0
Sodium hydroxide	1.0	1.0	1.0

* Contains 0.5 mL of the specimen (diluted 1 : 4) which is the same as the volume of the standard. Hence there is no dilution factor taken into consideration for the calculation.

(c) Allow the reaction mixture to stand for 20 min.

3. *Reading the absorbance*:
   Read the absorbance readings of samples and standard against blank at 520 nm (range 500–540 nm), exactly after 20 min. *Contains 0.5 mL of the specimen (diluted 1 : 4), which is the same as the volume of the standard. Hence there is no dilution factor taken into consideration for the calculation.
   Calculation:
   (a) For serum:
      Concentration of creatinine (mg/dL) = $(A_T/A_S) \times 2$
   (b) For urine:
      Concentration of creatinine in urine (mg/dL) = $(A_T/A_S) \times 2 \times 100$,
      where A_T is absorbance of the test specimen, A_S is absorbance of the standard, 2 is concentration' of standard (2 mg/dL) and 100 is 400/4; urine is diluted 400 times but the amount taken (2 mL) was four times the quantity of standard (0.5 mL) which was run simultaneously.

Determination of Creatinine Clearance

The group of tests generally referred to as renal clearance tests are useful in assessing the capacity of the kidney to eliminate (or clear) certain substances present in plasma. Two of these substances are routinely considered—creatinine and urea. Clearance study of creatinine has proved to be more reliable and reproducible because the serum level of urea varies considerably depending on the type of food taken by the patient. The request for the clearance study is made by the physician when the patient shows an increase of non-protein nitrogenous constituents of blood—mainly urea, creatinine and uric acid. The correct assessment of the functional capacity of the kidney comes from the clearance study (Chapter 34 in this Volume).

DETERMINATION OF BILIRUBIN

Bilirubin is a waste product of haemoglobin breakdown. The body eliminates this unwanted compound through the liver and bile into the intestine. It ultimately goes out of the body with the stool. Bilirubin is **insoluble in water** and hence cannot be eliminated through the urine. Albumin carries the insoluble circulating bilirubin to the liver where it conjugates into a soluble compound, **bilirubin-diglucuronide**. The conjugated bilirubin, also known as **direct bilirubin**, then goes into the intestine through the bile. Inside the intestine, with the help of intestinal microbes, conjugated bilirubin further degrades into other products, most important of which is urobilinogen. Most of the urobilinogen goes out of the body through the faecal material. Only a small fraction of the bilirubin metabolite—**urobilinogen** (formed in the intestine)—recycles through the body and excretes through the urine.

The term 'direct' comes from the way serum bilirubin is determined in the laboratory by its direct colour reaction. Total bilirubin in serum is determined after processing the specimen. The value of total serum bilirubin includes both conjugated and unconjugated bilirubin present in circulation. Unconjugated bilirubin (**indirect bilirubin**), also called '**free bilirubin**', is calculated as the difference between total and conjugated.

The reference range for total serum bilirubin is 0.1–1.2 mg/dL (2.0–21.0 µmol/L), and of direct bilirubin, 0–0.3 mg/dL (0–6 µmol/L). Bilirubin analysis is requested as a part of the **hepatic (liver) function test**. An increased bilirubin (total) concentration in the blood stream results in the clinical condition of jaundice. This increase may result from a number of causes. The estimation of direct (**conjugated**) and indirect or unconjugated bilirubin may help in the differential diagnosis of various types of jaundice—pre-hepatic (haemolytic), hepatic and post-hepatic (obstructive). In pre-hepatic or haemolytic jaundice, the unconjugated bilirubin increases due to the increased destruction of red cells, and the normally functioning liver is unable to cope with the increased demand for conjugation. Hence, the rise of unconjugated bilirubin (indirect) exceeds the rise of conjugated (direct) bilirubin. As a result, the normal ratio of unconjugated to conjugated (6 : 4) rises along with a rise of the absolute concentrations of each component. There is a normal variation (**Gilbert's Syndrome**) in certain people who lack an enzyme in the liver which allows conjugation of bilirubin causing rise of unconjugated bilirubin. In this condition the liver has no disease otherwise and life expectancy is normal. In case of hepatic jaundice, the conjugation of bilirubin is disturbed due to liver disorder, and as a result, the excretion of bilirubin in to bile greatly decreases. Non-passage of bilirubin through the liver increases the concentration of total bilirubin in blood. There is no appreciable change in the ratio of the two fractions, the unconjugated and conjugated bilirubin. The situation is quite different in case of post-hepatic or obstructive jaundice. Here the excretion of decreases due to stone formation or cancers blocking biliary drainage, and the concentration of bilirubin in the blood rises. Since bile mostly has conjugated bilirubin in obstruction its concentration in the blood is higher than that of unconjugated bilirubin. In premature newborn, deficient enzyme system in liver, leads to high bilirubin level.

Normal values

Adult:

Conjugated (direct)	0.0–0.2 mg/dL
Unconjugated (indirect)	0.2–0.8 mg/dL
Total	0.2–1.0 mg/dL

Infant:

Premature:	>10 mg/dL
Full term:	>4 mg/dL

Conversion to International unit: mg/dL × 17.1 = µmol/L

Specimen

Serum is the specimen of choice for the quantitative assay of bilirubin in blood. Blood is collected without any anticoagulant, allowed to clot for an hour at room temperature, and then centrifuged. Separate the supernatant fluid (serum) promptly. Analyse promptly, but in case of anticipated delay, refrigerate the specimen and analyse within 24 h. Always bring the specimen to room temperature before taking the aliquot for analysis.

A **haemolysed specimen** is unfit for bilirubin analysis. Serum submitted for bilirubin estimation is kept **away from strong light** since the ultraviolet light destroys bilirubin.

Jendrassik and Grof Method

This is the most widely accepted method for bilirubin analysis.

Principle

Bilirubin reacts with diazotized sulphanilic acid and yields a pink or purple colour due to the formation of azobilirubin. The intensity of the colour is proportional to the amount of bilirubin present. In a subsequent step, a strongly alkaline tartrate solution is added to convert the purple azobilirubin to a blue azobilirubin colour. In order to differentiate between the conjugated bilirubin (direct) and the unconjugated bilirubin (indirect) present in the serum, the specimen is first reacted with the diazo reagent without the presence of an accelerator (caffeine-benzoate reagent) and then in its presence. Conjugated bilirubin reacts with the diazo reagent while unconjugated bilirubin does not react with the diazo reagent in the absence of the accelerator (caffeine-benzoate). The colour reaction in the presence of the accelerator (or coupler) represents total bilirubin. The difference of the total and conjugated bilirubin represents free or unconjugated bilirubin.

For conjugated bilirubin, allow the **diazo reaction** to continue for 1 min and then terminated by **ascorbic acid**. Ascorbic acid destroys the excess diazo reagent. In case of total bilirubin, first treat the specimen with the **accelerator** (or coupler) and then allow the diazo reaction to continue for 10 min. Termination of the diazo reaction by ascorbic acid is not necessary. In both the cases, purple azobilirubin (acid medium) is converted to blue azobilirubin, by treating with sodium tartrate (alkaline medium), before measuring the absorbance at 600 nm. The colour is stable for 30 min.

Reagents

- *Saline (0.85% NaCl)*
- *Hydrochloric acid solution 0.05 mol/L (or 0.05 N):*
  Dilute 4.5 mL of concentrated hydrochloric acid to 1000 mL. It is stable at room temperature for indefinite period.
- *Caffeine-benzoate reagent*:
  Add 50 g of caffeine, 75 g of sodium benzoate and 125 g of sodium acetate (trihydrate) to 800 mL of warm water placed in a 1-L volumetric flask. Dissolve the ingredients, cool and dilute to 1000 mL. This solution is stable for months at room temperature.
- *Diazo reagent*
  (a) *Diazo I or sulphanilic acid solution (0.5% in HCl):*
  Add 5.0 g of sulphanilic acid to 15 mL of concentrated hydrochloric acid in a 1-L volumetric flask and dilute to the mark with distilled water. The solution is stable indefinitely.
  (b) *Diazo II or sodium nitrite solution:*
  Dissolve 500 mg of sodium nirite ($NaNO_2$) in 50 mL of distilled water placed in a 100-mL volumetric flask and dilute the solution to 100 mL. The solution is stable for two weeks when stored in a refrigerator.
  (c) Mix 10 mL of reagent (*a*) with 0.25 mL of reagent (*b*) immediately before use. Do not use this reagent after 30 min of its preparation.
- *Ascorbic acid solution (4% in water):*
  Dissolve 200 mg of ascorbic acid in 5 mL of water. This should be freshly prepared on the day of use. A convenient method is to pre-weigh (200 mg) ascorbic acid in small vials for ready use.
- *Alkaline tartrate*
  Dissolve 100 g of sodium hydroxide and 350 g of sodium tartrate in about 500 mL of distilled placed in a 1-L volumetric flask. When cool, dilute the solution to 1000 mL. Store it in a polyethylene bottle. The solution is stable for 6 months at room temperature.

Procedure

Direct bilirubin:
1. Dilute the specimen by mixing 1 mL of serum with 4 mL of saline (five-folds dilution).
2. Take two test tubes marked as 'T_D' and 'B_S' which corresponds to direct bilirubin test and serum blank (for direct bilirubin).
3. Add 1 mL of diluted serum and 2 mL of 0.05 hydrochloric acid in both the tubes.
4. The tube "T_D", add 0.5 mL of reagent (*c*) and immediately note the time.
5. After **exactly** 1 min, add 0.1 mL ascorbic acid. Mix and then add at once, 1.5 mL of alkaline tartrate, mix and read the absorbance after 5–10 min.
6. To tube 'B_S', the diluted serum blank, during the waiting period of step (4), add 0.5 mL of diazo I or reagent (*a*), 0.5 mL of ascorbic acid and 1.5 mL of alkaline tartrate; mix. No waiting period for the chemical reaction is necessary. Use the solution as the serum blank for the direct bilirubin.

Total bilirubin:
1. Take two test tubes (15-mL capacity) and mark them as 'T_T' and 'B_S' corresponding to total bilirubin test and serum blank.
2. Place 1 mL of diluted serum and 2.1 mL of caffeine-benzoate reagent in both the test tubes.

3. Add 0.5 mL of diazo mixture or reagent (c) in the test tube marked 'T_T', mix and note the time. The solution in T_T will be pink in colour due to the formation of azobilirubin.
4. Wait exactly for 10 min and then add 1.5 mL of alkaline tartrate (*Note:* Ascorbic acid is not added). The solution will turn blue. Mix and wait for 5–10 min.
5. During the waiting period of step (4), take the test tube marked 'B_S', holding diluted serum and caffeine reagent, and add 0.5 mL of diazo I (reagent *a*). Mix and then add 1.5 mL of alkaline tartrate. No waiting period for the chemical reaction is necessary. Use this as the serum blank.
6. Transfer the solutions in tubes 'T_T' [from step (4)] and 'B_S' [step (5)] into two matched cuvettes and read the absorbance of the 'T_T' (total bilirubin) against the serum blank ('B_S') which is used to set the zero absorbance.
7. Prepare a calibration curve as described in Chapter 4 in Vol. I, using the control serum. Do not use methyl orange artificial standard for the Jendrassik and Grof method.
8. Read the bilirubin values from the calibration curve.
9. *Calculation*:
   Total bilirubin – Direct bilirubin (conjugated) = Indirect (free or unconjugated) bilirubin

DIAGNOSTIC ENZYMOLOGY

Diagnostic enzymology deals with the quantitative measurement of those enzymes, which have clinical significance. In most modern clinical laboratories, enzyme analysis comprises nearly 30% of the workload. This is because the diagnostic enzyme assay is becoming more dependable and the information that it provides regarding functional disorders of various organs of the body is not available by other laboratory procedures. The reason behind enzyme analysis is that various organs of the body contain specific enzymes as their cellular components to carry on their specific biochemical functions. When these organs are in distress, a leakage of the organ-specific enzymes into the blood stream occurs especially with inflammation and cell death. Quantitative biochemical analyses of the blood and other body fluids can thus assist the physician to evaluate the severity of the diseased organ. Because of its growing significance, some of the basic facts of enzyme assay need to be discussed here.

Enzymes are organic catalysts that accelerate various biochemical reactions. They are needed in small quantities and apparently, they are not used up in the reaction. The whole thing can be explained with a comparable story, meant for beginners.

Once upon a time there was an Arab Sheikh who had 17 camels. He left a will for his three sons to share the camels after him in such a way that the distribution would be in the ratio of 1/2, 1/3 and 1/9. After the Sheikh's death the sons began to fight as they found that it is not possible to split the 17 camels without killing them. So they went to the Kaji, the wise man. The Kaji added his own camel to the 17 camels of the Arab; that resulted in 18 camels, and then he could distribute the camels to the three sons as follows (Fig. 33.2):

$$17 \quad + \quad (1) \quad \rightarrow \quad 18 \quad \rightarrow \quad (9+6+2) \quad + \quad (1)$$
$$\text{Substrate} \quad + \quad \text{(Enzyme)} \quad \rightarrow \quad \text{Substrate-Enzyme-Complex} \quad \rightarrow \quad \text{(Products)} \quad + \quad \text{(Enzyme)}$$

After distributing the camels he took away, his own camel as it was left over. This illustrates the way an enzyme works as an organic catalyst. It temporarily combines with the substrate until the product is formed, and at the final stage the enzyme is free to work again without any apparent loss of activity.

In any enzymatic reaction, the substrate or the starting material is converted to the product. Enzymes are protein molecules and often substrate specific, degenerated by heat, metals, strong acid, or alkali. Enzyme reactions are reversible; the direction of the reaction, however, depends on the type and concentration of substrate, the pH and other conditions. Quantitative assay of enzymes requires the measurement of the rate of activity of the enzyme, rather than its weight or volume. The rate of enzyme activity, however, depends on many variable factors. Therefore, test conditions are chosen in a way that the reaction rate will depend only on the amount of enzyme present in the sample to be measured. The substrate is in excess, and all other factors that influence the reaction rate should be optimized and controlled.

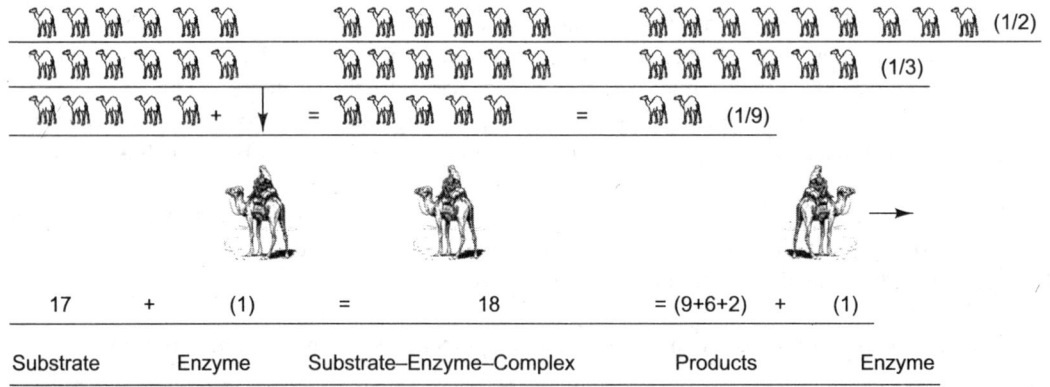

Fig. 33.2 *The story of the camel illustrates that the enzyme is temporarily bound to the substrate to yield the products and comes out unchanged.*

Many of these reactions involve the coenzyme **nicotinamide adenine dinucleotide** or **NAD**. Coenzymes are small organic non-protein molecules that carry chemical groups associated to the specific enzymes. They do not form a permanent part of the enzyme but are required by the enzyme for its activity. Therefore, they are sometimes referred as cofactors or co-substrates. During the course of enzymatic reaction, NAD (oxidized state, with no absorptivity at 340 nm) will be reduced to NADH (reduced state, high absorptivity at 340 nm). As a result, optical density of the reaction medium increases: which can be measured at 340 nm wavelength (in the ultraviolet range). From the change of optical density (ÄA), one can measure the rate of enzyme activity per unit time. It is expressed in the International Unit (IU) of enzyme activity, which is defined as the amount of substrate consumed in micromoles (μmole) or amount of product formed in micromoles (μmole) in 1 min. The results are expressed in IU/L (International Unit per litre of specimen) at 37°C or any other specified temperature, which may be 25°C or 30°C.

This is exemplified in the following reaction in which lactic dehydrogenase (LDH) converts lactic acid into pyruvic acid whereby NAD forms NADH:

$$\text{Lactic acid} + \text{NAD} \xleftrightarrow{\text{LDH}} \text{Pyruvic acid} + \text{NADH}.$$

Two methods are currently followed in the measurement of enzyme activity—two point method and continuous method. In the two-point method, the reaction is terminated after a specified time, and the amount of substrate used or product formed is measured by a suitable analytical procedure. The enzyme activity is computed from the change in the concentration of the substrate (used) or the product (formed) in micromoles during a 1 min period; taking into consideration the unit volume of serum specimen. On the other hand, in continuous assay, the enzymatic reaction is not terminated, and the change in substrate or product concentration is constantly monitored while the reaction is in progress. The former can be compared with the measurement of distance (d) travelled between the starting and finishing time (t) and expressed as d/t; while the latter can be compared with the radar system for tracking the speed of a moving object. In order to accomplish the continuous assay of the enzyme, the reaction mixture must be tested without disturbing the enzyme activity. Two co-enzyme pairs in their oxidized and reduced states—NAD/NADH and NADP/NADPH—are commonly used in the continuous assay. This has been mentioned earlier for lactic dehydrogenase.

Occasionally these co-enzymes are not directly used in the principal enzyme reaction; and they are '**coupled**' with a secondary reaction to accomplish the continuous analysis of the principle enzyme under study (e.g. ALT or GPT).

Routine Analysis of Diagnostic Enzymes

Following routinely requested enzymological assays would be discussed in the following pages.
- *Alkaline phosphatase* (ALP): Liver
- *Transaminases* (AST and ALT): Liver
- *Creatine kinase* (CK): Heart
- *Lactic dehydrogenase* (LD): Heart and liver
- *Amylase*: Pancreatic function

Alkaline phosphatase

Phosphatases belong to the class of enzymes called hydrolase and they are characterized by their ability to hydrolyse a large variety of organic phosphate esters with the formation of an alcohol and a phosphate ion. From clinical point of view, they are of two kinds—ALP and acid phosphatase. Assay of ALP activity of serum is requested in case of suspected liver or bone disorder. ALP is also found in placenta and mild elevation is common in pregnancy. The enzyme works best in the reaction medium of pH 10 (alkaline). On the other hand, increased serum acid phosphatase (ACP) activity (pH of the medium, 5.0) may be related to prostrate cancer and in the investigation of rape case as the male semen contains abundance of acid phosphatase.

Increased ALP activity is diagnostic to liver and bone diseases. Very high ALP activity in serum is also found in patients with bone cancer and marked increase occurs in obstructive jaundice and biliary cirrhosis. Moderate elevations have been noted in case of Hodgkin's disease, congestive heart failure, infective hepatitis and abdominal problems. ALP analysis is routinely done and hence it is included here. Mild elevation of bone ALP is common in growing children till there is fusion of all epiphysis. Elevation is also noted in osteoporosis and pregnant woman as it is produced by the placenta.

Specimen Serum is the preferred specimen but plasma (heparinized) can also be used. A blood specimen after overnight fasting is recommended, but a specimen collected at any other time can also be used. Separate the serum promptly and store in a refrigerator if immediate analysis is not possible. ALP activity increases with storage, hence, as a general rule, it is best to analyse ALP specimens the same day they are drawn.

Normal range 20–130 U/L (p-nitrophenyl phosphate method)

Laboratory Assay by Colorimetric Method The method of **p-nitrophenylphosphate** is described here. The p-nitrophenylphosphate is not a natural substrate for the phosphatases. It is used because the enzyme uses this synthetic compound and gives a reasonably rapid rate of reaction. In addition, it is analytically convenient to measure the product formed (p-nitrophenol). The liberated phenol is yellow in colour in alkaline medium and is colourless in acid medium. Continuous assay can be done for ALP by measuring the rate of formation of p-nitrophenol at pH 10. The two point method described here is suitable for the routine laboratories of developing countries and the reagents are easily available. In this method the enzyme reaction is terminated by alkali treatment.

Principle The substrate, p-nitrophenyl phosphate (PNPP) is hydrolysed by ALP to p-nitrophenol and phosphoric acid. Some divalent ions like Mg^{++} are added to the system, which act as activators. PNPP is colourless in acid or alkaline medium while PNP is yellow in colour in the alkaline medium and colourless in the acid medium.

$$\text{p-Nitrophenyl phosphate} + H_2O \xrightleftharpoons{ALP/ACP} 2 \text{ p-Nitrophenol} + H_3PO_4$$
$$\text{(colourless)} \qquad\qquad\qquad\qquad \text{(yellow)}$$

Two types of **buffers** can be used for maintaining the pH of the reaction medium—glycine buffer and MAP (2-methyl-2-aminopropanol-1) buffer. The latter is recommended but difficult to get in the laboratories of developing countries and in addition, it is cumbersome to prepare and has a short shelf life. Glycine buffer, however, inhibits the ALP reaction and hence the values are lower than the activity measured in the MAP buffer. In the following pages, only the use of glycine buffer will be discussed.

Reagent

- *Stock substrate of PNPP (4 mg/mL or 15.2 µmol/mL)*
  Dissolve 0.4 g of p-nitrophenyl disodium phosphate in 100 mL water. The PNPP should be of highly pure quality and correct for hydration if it is a hydrated salt. The solution is unstable; prepare only as much as needed. Preweighed dry substrate can be kept in small vials for ready use. If the solution is refrigerated it stays for a few days without any appreciable change.
- *Sodium hydroxide solutions*
  (a) *1 N NaOH*:
      Dissolve 40 g sodium hydroxide in about 800 mL of water placed in a 1-L volumetric flask; dilute the solution to 1000 mL volume with water.
  (b) *Other strengths (0.1 N, 0.05 N, 0.02 N)*:
      Dilute 1N sodium hydroxide 1 : 10, 1 : 20 and 1 : 50 for getting 0.1, 0.05 and 0.02 N sodium hydroxide solutions. Take three 100-mL volumetric flasks. Add to these 10 mL, 5 mL and 2 mL of 1 N NaOH and dilute each to 100 mL. This will yield sodium hydroxide solutions of earlier strengths in the same sequence.
- *Glycine buffered substrate*
  (a) *Glycine buffer (alkaline)*: Mix 7.5 g of glycine, 0.095 g of magnesium chloride, 750 raL water, and 85 mL 1N sodium hydroxide in a 1-L volumetric flask. Dilute the solution to the 1000 mL mark. Keep in a refrigerator.
  (b) *Working substrate*: Mix equal volumes of glycine buffer and stock substrate of PNPP. Adjust the pH to 10.3–10.4 if necessary. The use of a pH meter is recommended. Adjustment of pH is done by slowly adding dilute HCl or NaOH as needed. If the reagents are of good quality, this may not be necessary.
- *Standard solution of p-nitrophenol (PNP)*
  (a) *Stock standard (1 mmole/L)*: Dissolve 139.1 mg of high purity PNP in water to make 1000 mL of solution in a 1-L volumetric flask. This solution is stable if kept in the dark. If high purity PNP is not available commercially, make a batch of purified PNP by re-crystallization from hot water; dry it overnight in a vacuum desiccator over silica gel or any other desiccant.
  (b) *PNP working standard (0.04 mmol/L)*: Pipette 1.0 mL of the stock standard into a 25-mL volumetric flask and dilute the volume with 0.05 N NaOH solution. Mix thoroughly. This should be prepared daily for the test.

Procedure

1. Pipette 1.0 mL of buffered substrate into each of two test tubes, labelled as 'T' and 'B' corresponding to test and blank. Use one pair of tubes for each specimen.
   Note: The blank ('B') is the serum blank.
2. Place the tubes in a water bath set at 37°C for 5–7 min to equilibrate the temperature.
3. With the timer set, add 0.05 mL serum to the 'T' tube and mix. Do not add serum to "B" tube.
   Note: Use a 1-mL graduated pipette with 0.01-mL graduation for taking the aliquot (0.05 mL). If an automatic pipetter is available, set it to 50 µL.

4. Incubate at 37°C for exactly 30 min.
5. At the end of 30 min, add 10 mL of 0.05 M NaOH to both tubes to stop the reaction and dilute the PNP formed. Mix well.
6. Add 0.05 mL of serum to the B tube (serum blank), and mix the contents thoroughly.
7. Pour the contents of the B and T tubes into appropriate cuvettes and read absorbances of the solutions at 405 nm. Use the B tube to zero the instrument.
8. Consult the calibration curve to determine the enzyme activity in International unit (U/L) or calculate as follows.
9. *Calculation*:
   (a) Determine the absorptivity factor (F) in terms of International unit for ALP enzyme. The procedure is as follows:
   - Dilute 1.0 mL of working standard of PNP (0.04 μmole) to 4.88 mL with 0.05N NaOH and read the absorbance (A_s) against 0.05N NaOH that is used for setting the zero absorbance.
   - The absorbance (A_s) is equivalent to 60 U/L (see additional information).
   - The absorptivity factor (F) = $60/A_s$ U/L.
   (b) Calculate the enzyme activity by the following formula:
   $$\Delta A = A_T - A_B$$
   $$\text{ALP activity (U/L)} = \Delta A \times F$$
   where A_T is absorbance of solution in tube 'T' under experimental conditions, after 30 min of enzymatic reaction, A_B is absorbance of solution in tube 'B' at 0 min (serum blank), ΔA is change in absorbance following enzymatic reaction = $A_T - A_B$ and F is absorptivity factor that corresponds to the absorption scale in terms of International units (U/L).

Additional information
- For daily tests, use the formula but check the calibration curve once a month.
- Molar absorptivity of PNP is 18,750, and then a solution containing 1.0 mmol/L or 1 μmole/mL will have an absorbance of 18.75. Therefore, the earlier solution (4.88 mL) with 0.04 μmole of PNP should have an absorbance close to 0.15 (18.75 × 0.04 × 1/4.88) that corresponds to 60 U/L (60 μmole/min/L of serum).

Preparation of calibration curve
As a part of the quality control program, check the calibration curve once a month. In case of discrepancy, check the reagents and the standards.

Reagents
- PNP working standard solution (0.04 mmol/L)
- Sodium hydroxide solution (0.05 N)
Details of preparing the reagents have been presented earlier

Procedure
1. Dilute 1.0, 2.0, 3.0 and 4.0 mL of working standard (0.04 mmol/L or 0.04 μmol/mL) to 4.88 mL with 0.05 N NaOH. In other words, mix 3.88, 2.88, 1.88 and 0.88 mL of 0.05 N NaOH with 1.0, 2.0, 3.0 and 4.0 mL of the working standard of PNP.
2. Transfer each solution to matched cuvettes and read the absorbances at 405 nm against 0.05 N NaOH solution as the instrument blank. If sufficient cuvettes are not available, use two matched cuvettes and use one for the blank (0.05 N NaOH) and the other use for PNP standards, beginning from the lowest concentration. Rinse with new solution (higher strength) each time after taking the reading of the previous solution.

3. Tabulate the results and plot the absorbance readings against the enzyme activity values of the standards—60, 120, 180 and 240 (see calculation).
4. *Calculation*: The solution with 1.0 mL of working standard contains 0.04 mmol of PNP in 4.88 mL of solution. If this quantity of PNP is formed in 30 min by the enzyme that was present in 0.05 mL of specimen and diluted to 11.0 mL, then the rate of PNP formation is: $11.0/4.88 \times 0.04 \times 1/30 \times 1000/0.05 = 60$ µmol/min/L of serum = 60 U/L,
where $11/4.88$ = volume ratio of the reaction mixture
  0.04 = µmole of product in the reaction mixture
  $1/30$ = rate per minute (reaction was allowed for 30 min)
  $1000/0.05$ = conversion to per litre for the amount of specimen taken.

Transaminases

Transamination is a process in which an amino group is transferred from an **amino acid to an alpha-ketoacid**. It is an important step in the metabolism of amino acids. The enzymes responsible for transamination are called transaminases (now called, **aminotransferases**). Two most useful enzyme markers of acute hepatocullular injury are ALT (alanine amino transferase) and AST (aspartate amino transferase). These were called GOT (glutamate oxalacetate transaminase) and GPT (glutamate pyruvate transaminase), respectively.

Increased serum transaminase activity is seen in **liver dysfunction**. Greater activity of AST (GOT) over ALT (GPT) is typical of myocardial infarction and muscle injury as in case of intramuscular injection and rhabdomyolysis.

Alanine Amino Transferase (ALT) and Aspartate Amino Transferase (AST) The enzymatic chemical reactions of ALT and AST are shown here:

$$\text{L-alanine} + \alpha\text{-oxoglutarate} \xrightarrow{\text{ALT}} \text{Pyruvate} + \text{L-glutamate}$$

$$\text{L-aspartate} + \alpha\text{-oxoglutarate} \xrightarrow{\text{AST}} \text{Oxaloacetate} + \text{L-glutamate}$$

For the quantitative assay of these enzymes, two methods are available:
- Spectrophotometric method
- Colorimetric method

Spectrophotometric method is now widely used and is ideal for the automated continuous assay. It is also more accurate. Unfortunately, it requires a spectrophotometer that will read absorbance at 340 nm. Some of the newer colorimeters are able to read at this range, which is not available to many peripheral laboratories. Hence, a colorimetric method is also presented here. The colorimetric method has proved to be cheaper.

Principle The basic principle of the spectrophotometric method is to measure the changing optical density of the reaction medium as the enzyme reacts on the substrate. The indicator system used are the coenzymes NAD-NADH (or, NADP-NADPH). In the colorimetric method, which is a two-point method, where the reaction is stopped and the amount of substrate formed (ketoacid) is chemically reacted to yield colour. The intensity of the colour developed per unit time is a measure of the enzyme activity.

Spectrophotometric method This method is more sensitive and accurate than the colorimetric method but is expensive to perform and also requires spectrophotometer that will work in the ultraviolet range (340 nm).

Specimen The serum specimen submitted for the enzyme assay of ALT and AST should be free from haemolysis. Collect the blood by venipuncture without anticoagulant and separate the serum promptly. If analysis cannot be done within an hour, refrigerate the specimen.

Normal ranges The adult reference range for both AST and ALT is roughly 10–40 U/L when measured at 37°C. Although men have slightly higher values than women do, most laboratories use a single range for both genders.

Principle When the enzymatic reaction of ALT is coupled with LD activity, it utilizes one of the products (pyruvate) as substrate. This is in collaboration with its coenzyme NADH. As a result the optical density or absorbance of the reaction medium changes due to the oxidation of NADH. (*Note:* NAD has minimal absorbance at 340 nm wavelength). By following the change (ΔA), the rate of ALT is determined.

$$\text{L-alanine} + \alpha\text{-oxoglutarate} \xrightarrow{\text{ALT}} \text{Pyruvate} + \text{L-glutamate}$$

$$\text{Pyruvate} + \text{NADH} \xrightarrow{\text{LD}} \text{Lactate} + \text{NAD}$$

Similarly, the enzyme assay for AST involves the coupled reactions of AST and MDH (malate dehydrogenase), using the substrates L-aspartate and á-oxoglutarate. Here again, the coenzyme NADH converts to NAD.

$$\text{L-alanine} + \alpha\text{-oxoglutarate} \xrightarrow{\text{ALT}} \text{Oxaloacetate} + \text{L-glutamate}$$

$$\text{Oxaloacetate} + \text{NADH} \xrightarrow{\text{MDH}} \text{L-malate} + \text{NAD}$$

Note:
- Because none of the reactants or products of these reactions absorbs in the ultraviolet or visible region of the spectrum, they must be coupled to indicator reactions for analysis. ALT requires LD, whereas AST requires MDH.
- The reactions are monitored by following the decrease in the absorbance at 340 nm as NADH is consumed in the reaction. (NAD has no absorbance).
- Pyridoxal phosphate, an additional coenzyme, is needed to run the above reaction, which is abundantly present in serum. It may have to be added in patients with vitamin B deficiency.

Reagent and supplies
- The commercial kit supplies all the required reagents
- Spectrophotometer
- Laboratory supplies required for chemical analyses

Procedure Strictly follow the instructions provided by the manufacturer.

Colorimetric Method The colorimetric method is commonly followed in the peripheral laboratories of developing countries. The reference laboratory, however, uses the spectrophotometric method.

Principle The activity of transaminases (aminotransferases) is determined by measuring the colour of the hydrazone (brown) which is formed by the reaction between 2,4-dinitrophenyl hydrazine (DNPH) and the ketoacid which is one of the products of transaminase reaction. The DNPH reacts with all oxoacids. These include oxoglutarate and oxalacetate, as well as pyruvate, which are on the two sides of the above equations. DNPH gives more colours with oxalacetate and pyruvate than with oxoglutarate, thus making the method feasible with an acceptable limit of error. In both estimations—ALT and AST, the substrates are suboptimal, to reduce the background colour given by the alpha-ketoglutarate (or oxoglutarate) in the reaction with DNPH. Though not as accurate as the spectrophotometric method (UV), the colorimetric method is easily adaptable to the local conditions of developing countries and is much faster to perform than the spectrophotometric method.

Reagents, equipment and supplies

- *Phosphate buffer, pH 7.4, 0.1 M:*
  - (a) *Disodium hydrogen phosphate dihydrate (0.1M):* Dissolve 8.9 g of disodium hydrogen phosphate dihydrate, $Na_2HPO_4 \cdot 2H_2O$ in 200 mL of water in a 500-mL volumetric flask and dilute to the mark (500 mL).
  - (b) *Monopotassium phosphate anhydrous (0.1 M):* Dissolve 1.36 g anhydrous potassium dihydrogen phosphate KH_2PO_4 in 50 mL distilled water and dilute the solution to 100 mL.
  - (c) *Buffer solution:* Mix 420 mL of disodium phosphate solution with 80 mL of monopotassium dihydrogen solution. Normally this will yield the desired pH of 7.4. Check the pH and adjust to pH 7.4, if necessary, using small amounts of the correct phosphate.

    Note: Disodium hydrogen phosphate increases pH and monopotassium dihydrogen phosphate decreases pH. Use only the analytical grade chemicals for preparing the buffer.

- *Substrate for ALT — DL-alanine (200 mM/L) and alpha-ketoglutarate (2mM/L):*
  Dissolve 1.78 g DL-alanine and 30 mg oxoglutaric acid or alpha-ketoglutaric acid in 20 mL of phosphate buffer containing 1.25 mL of 0.4 N NaOH placed in a small beaker (100-mL). Make up to 100 mL with buffer and adjust to pH 7.4 if necessary. Add 1 mL of chloroform as a preservative and store in the refrigerator. Discard the substrate if it becomes turbid.

- *Substrate for AST — DL-aspartate (200 mM/L) and alpha-ketoglutarate (2 mM/L)*
  Dissolve 2.66 g DL-aspartic acid and 30 mg oxoglutaric acid (or alpha-ketoglutaric acid) in 20.5 mL of 1 N NaOH placed in a 250-mL beaker. Adjust the pH to 7.4 (± 0.1) by adding NaOH drop wise and stirring. Transfer quantitatively with buffer to a 100-mL volumetric flask and make up to 100 mL with phosphate buffer (pH 7.4) solution. Add 1 mL of chloroform as a preservative and store in the refrigerator. Discard the substrate if it becomes turbid.

- *Pyruvate standard:*
  - (a) *Stock standard (20 mM/L):* Dissolve 220 mg sodium pyruvate in phosphate buffer and make up to 100 mL. This is discarded after preparing the working standard.
  - (b) *Working standard (2 mM/L or 2 µmole/mL):* Dilute 10 mL of the stock standard to 100 mL with phosphate buffer. Dispense small amounts (approximately 2 mL) of the working standard in test tubes (5-mL), stopper them, and keep them in the freezer. Use one tube at a time for preparing the calibration curve. Any remaining solution in the tube should be discarded. Sodium pyruvate is not stable in solution and care should be taken to ensure that the standard solution has not deteriorated.

- *2,4-dinitrophenylhydrazine or DNPH (1 mM/L):*
  Dissolve 200 mg DNPH in 1 N HCl (warm up, if necessary) and make up to 1 L with 1 N HCl. Store in the refrigerator.

  1 N HCl: Prepare by diluting 90 mL concentrated HCl (12 N) to 1 L with distilled water.

- *Sodium hydroxide solutions (1 N and 0.4 N):*
  1 N: Dissolve 40 g of sodium hydroxide in 500 mL of water and make up to 1000 mL in a volumetric flask.
  0.4 N: Dilute 40 mL of 1 N NaOH to 100 mL with water in a 100-mL volumetric flask.

- Colorimeter or spectrophotometer
- Laboratory supplies for chemical analysis

Procedure This procedure describes the simultaneous determinations of ALT and AST

1. Label 2 test tubes as 'T' and 'B', corresponding to test and blank. If both enzymes are to be determined simultaneously, use 4 test tubes and label them as 'AL_T', 'AL_B' and 'AS_T', 'AS_B' corresponding to the ALT and AST—test and blank respectively.

2. Pipette 1.0 mL of the desired substrate into the respective tubes—ALT substrate for 'AL$_T$' and 'AL$_B$' tubes and AST substrate for 'AS$_T$' and 'AS$_B$' tubes. Place all the test tubes in a 37°C water bath for about 5 min for temperature equilibration.
3. To the tubes marked 'AL$_T$', and 'AS$_T$' add 0.2 mL serum, set the timer concurrently.
4. Mix rapidly by swirling and place the tubes back in the water bath. If there are more specimens, space the timing accordingly.
5. After exactly 30 min remove the tubes marked AL$_T$ and AL$_B$ and immediately add 1.0 mL of 2,4-dinitrophenylhydrazine and mix, thereby stopping the reaction and developing the colour. Leave the tubes at room temperature until the 'AS$_T$' and 'AS$_B$' tubes are ready in the following step.
6. Continue incubation (37 °C) for the tubes marked 'AS$_T$' and 'AS$_B$' until exactly 60 min after adding the serum. Add 1.0 mL of hydrazine and mix, as done in the previous step for AL$_T$.
7. Remove the tubes from the water bath and add 0.2 mL of serum to the tubes for the serum blank, marked 'AL$_B$' and 'AS$_B$'.
8. After 20 min at room temperature, following the addition of hydrazine, add 10 mL of 0.4 N NaOH to all the tubes, stopper them and mix by inversion.
9. Leave the reaction to continue for at least 5 min but no longer than 30 min.
10. Read the absorbance of the test solutions ('AL$_T$' and 'AS$_T$') and the serum blanks ('AL$_B$' and 'AS$_B$') against water at 505 nm or use a green filter (490–520 nm).
11. Determine the changes in absorbance ($\ddot{A}A$) by subtracting the blank readings from the corresponding test readings.
    (a) For AL$_T$ = AL$_T$ – AL$_B$
    (b) For AS$_T$ = AS$_T$ – AS$_B$
12. Refer to the calibration curve for reporting the enzyme activity in International Units (U/L).

Preparation of calibration curve

1. Take five test tubes and mark them #1 to #5.
2. Add the substrates and water according to the following table.
   Note: The total quantity of the serum, substrate and pyruvate solution is 1.2 mL, the same quantity as the reaction mixture in the test.
3. Add 1 mL of hydrazine reagent to each tube, mix, leave for 20 min at room temperature, and add 10 mL of 0.4 N sodium hydroxide. Mix thoroughly. Leave for at least 5 min.
4. Read the absorbance within 5–30 min after the addition of NaOH, at 505 nm or use a green filter. Use tube 1 (without the standard) as a blank to set the zero absorbance.
5. Tabulate the results with varying enzyme units against the corresponding absorbances.
6. Plot a calibration curve of absorbance against transaminase units as given in the table for ALT and

Tube No.	Pyruvate standard (mL)	Water (mL)	Substrate* (mL)	ALT U/L	AST U/L
1	0	0.2	1.0	0.0	0.0
2	0.1	0.2	0.9	13.4	11.5
3	0.2	0.2	0.8	27.4	29.3
4	0.3	0.2	0.7	46.6	54.7
5	0.4	0.2	0.6	72.0	91.2

*Use specific substrate—ALT or AST (2 µmole/mL).

Note: The units are not proportional to the amount of the standard added because the colour developed is not strictly linear.

Creatinine kinase

The request for reporting the **Creatinine kinase** (CK) activity of serum is made in case of suspected **myocardial infarction** and **muscle disease**. After a myocardial infarction CK activity rises rapidly to relatively high levels, but it also falls rapidly. The increase in CK activity occurs before the rise of AST and is unchanged in case of liver disorders. It can be elevated in case of muscle injury and even an intramuscular injection and cause confusion.

Creatine kinase is also called **creatine phosphokinase**. The enzymatic action of creatine kinase is represented by the following equation:

$$\text{Creatine} + \text{ATP} \xleftrightarrow{\text{CK}} \text{Creatine phosphate} + \text{ADP}.$$

The reaction mixture used for the enzyme activity should contain, along with the substrates, magnesium salt and a sulphydryl compound (cysteine, glutathione and mercaptoethanol). The magnesium ion acts as the activator, and the sulphydryl compound reactivates the CK activity lost in serum because of sulphydryl oxidation.

Two commonly employed methods of CK assay in serum—Spectrophotometric method and colorimetric method. Only the colorimetric method will be discussed here. Kits are available for the spectrophotometric method along with manufacturer's instruction to perform the test. The kits are expensive and the method also requires an expensive spectrophotometer that reads absorbance in the ultraviolet range.

CPK MB (or CK MB) is mostly produced in cardiac muscle and thus a more reliable marker of cardiac muscle injury. This is frequently analysed in western laboratories.

Troponins T and I: These are contractile proteins of the myofibril. The cardiac isoforms are very specific for cardiac injury and are not present in serum from healthy people. These are the preferred markers for detecting myocardial cell injury in western labs.
- Rises 2–6 h after injury
- Peaks in 12–16 h
- It stays elevated for 5–10 days, T for 5–14 days

Myoglobin is released from muscles and can be measured to estimate myocardial injury but this less specific. Other investigational tests will not be discussed here. CK and LDH measurements are elaborated as follows:

Normal CK values   30–174 U/L

Colorimetric Method for CK   This simple and easy procedure can be followed in any routine laboratory. Chemicals are available through the dealers of Sigma chemicals (St. Louis, Mo.) or other suppliers.

Principle

$$\text{Creatine phosphate} + \text{ADP} \xleftrightarrow[\text{Mg}^{++}]{\text{CK}} \text{Creatine} + \text{ATP}$$

The creatine produced, as a result of CK activity, is measured colorimetrically with alpha-naphthol and diacetyl. In spectrophotometric method, ATP is taken through two coupled reactions involving hexokinase and glucose-6-phosphate dehydrogenase. In the second enzymatic reaction, NAD is reduced to NADH that allows the measurement of the absorbance of the reaction medium at 340 nm.

Reagents, equipment and supplies
- *Tris buffer (0.1 M, pH 7.4):*
  (a) Dissolve 12.1 g tris (hydroxymethyl) aminomethane, and 3.7 g magnesium sulphate heptahydrate in approximately 500 mL of water in a beaker. Warm to 30 °C, if necessary, in order to facilitate the preparation of the solution.

(b) Adjust the pH to 7.4 with 5 N HCl.

  Note: Tris buffer is affected by temperature; hence, follow the manufacturer's instructions for the pH meter in order to obtain the correct pH.

(c) Transfer the buffer [step (b)] into a 1-L volumetric flask and dilute to 1000 mL with water. The reagent is stable.

- *Buffered cysteine solution*: Prepare tris-cysteine solution fresh on the same day: Pour suitable amount of buffer and add cysteine so that there is the equivalent of 0.7 g of cystein in 100 mL of buffer.
- *Phosphocreatine (0.012 M)*: Dissolve 0.25 g of phosphocreatine in about 75 mL water, adjust the pH to 7.4 with 0.1 N HCl or 0.1 N NaOH, transfer quantitatively into a 100-mL volumetric flask and dilute to 100 mL with water. This solution should be stored in the freezer. Prepare a fresh solution every two weeks.
- *Adenosine diphosphate solution*: Dissolve 0.17 g ADP in about 75 mL water, adjust pH to 7.4 with 0.1 N NaOH, transfer quantitatively to a 100-mL volumetric flask and dilute to 100 mL with water. Keep the solution frozen.
- *Substrate*: Mix equal volumes of buffered cysteine (reagent 2), phosphocreatine (reagent 3), ADP (reagent 4) and distilled water. Divide the substrate in small aliquots (volume to be decided by the amount used daily) in separate test tubes. Take out one test tube each day for daily use. Discard the remaining substrate after the day's work. Do not use the substrate if there is evidence of free creatine (high absorbance of serum blank against water blank).
- *p-Chloromercuribenzoic acid solution:* Dissolve 1.1 g of chloromercuri-benzoic acid in 25 mL of 1 N NaOH placed in a 100-mL volumetric flask. Add 1 N HCl until precipitate just forms. On dilution to 100 mL with water the solution will clear.
- *Barium hydroxide solution (4.5%)*: Dissolve 45 g of barium hydroxide octahydrate [$Ba(OH)_2 \cdot 8H_2O$] in 1000 mL of distilled water. Balance the barium hydroxide solution against zinc sulphate solution (see next paragraph).
- *Zinc sulphate solution (5%)*: Dissolve 50 g of zinc sulphate heptahydrate ($ZnSO_4 \cdot 7H_2O$) in 1000 mL of distilled water. Balance the zinc sulphate solution against barium hydroxide solution.

  Balancing of barium hydroxide solution with zinc sulphate solution:

  The actual concentrations of these solutions are not critical but they must be balanced. In other words, equal volumes of these solutions should exactly neutralize each other.

  (a) Take 5 mL of zinc sulphate solution into a 50-mL Erlenmeyer flask. Add two drops of phenolphthalein.

  (b) Take the barium hydroxide solution in a burette and titrate the zinc sulphate solution against barium hydroxide slowly and with constant swirling to the first permanent pink.

  (c) If the solution does not match, dilute the more concentrated solution (zinc sulphate or barium hydroxide) proportionately with water.

  Example: If 4.3 mL of barium hydroxide are needed to neutralize 5.0 mL of zinc sulphate, dilute the barium hydroxide in the ratio of 5 : 4.3 or 1.16 times. Hence, add 16 mL water to 100 mL of barium hydroxide solution. On the other hand, if 6.1 mL of barium hydroxide is needed, dilute zinc sulphate solution 6.1/5 or 1.22 times. Hence, add 22 mL water to 100 mL of zinc sulphate solution.

- *Stock alkali solution*: Dissolve 60 g NaOH and 128 g NaCO in water and dilute to 1 L with water.
- *Alpha-naphthol*: Prepare a fresh solution of alpha-naphthol by dissolving 0.8 g in 10 mL of stock alkali solution and filter.
- *Creatine standard (1.7 µmol/mL)*: Dissolve 22.3 mg creatine in 50 mL water contained in a 100-mL volumetric flask. Dilute to 100 mL with water. Store frozen in small aliquots (1 mL). The solution is stable for one month or longer.

- Colorimeter or spectrophotometer
- Laboratory supplies for chemical analysis

Procedure
1. Take three centrifuge tubes and label them as 'T', 'S' and 'B' corresponding to test, standard and blank, respectively.
2. Take out the frozen substrate, allow it to equilibrate with room temperature and transfer 1 mL of the substrate into each of the above centrifuge tubes. Place the tubes in a water-bath kept at 37 °C.
3. Add 0.1 mL of serum in the tube marked 'T', mix and simultaneously set the timer for 30 min.
4. While the enzymatic reaction is in progress, add 0.1 mL of creatine standard in the tube marked 'S', and 0.1 mL water to the tube marked 'B'. Mix both the tubes 'S' and 'B', and leave them in the water bath at 37 °C, along with the 'T' tube.
5. After 30 min of incubation at 37 °C, take out all the tubes from the water bath and treat them in the same way as described in further steps.
6. Add 0.5 mL of p-chloromercuribenzoic acid and mix.
7. Add 0.5 mL each of barium hydroxide and zinc sulphate solutions with mixing after each addition.
8. Centrifuge the tubes or filter. Filtration leads to higher error due to evaporation. While centrifuging, cover the tubes with aluminium foil, or plastic caps. Centrifuge at high speed (2500g) for 15 min.
9. Transfer 0.5 mL of supernatant into another centrifuge tube.
10. Add 1.0 mL of alpha-naphthol and mix.
11. Place the tubes in the water bath (37 °C) for 15–20 min.
12. Add 2.5 mL water, mix, and centrifuge for a few minutes.
13. Decant the supernatant into a cuvette and read the absorbance against the reagent blank ('B') at- 540 nm.
14. *Calculation*:

$$\text{CK activity (U/L)} = (A_T/A_S) \times 1/30 \times 0.17 \times 1000/0.1$$

where A_T is absorbance of the test ('T'), A_S is absorbance of the standard ('S'), 1/30 is conversion to 1 min, 0.17 is µmol of creatine present in the reaction mixture and 1000/0.1 is conversion to 1 L of serum.

Lactic dehydrogenase

The enzyme lactic dehydrogenase (LD) is present in all cells. Its increased activity in serum is not specific for disease of any tissue, although it may support a diagnosis that is based on other findings, e.g. myocardial infarction, renal infarction, hepatitis, megaloblastic anaemia, muscular dystrophy, or metastatic cancer. Hence many physicians use the LD data as supportive evidence rather than primary diagnostic tool. This is used rarely now and not included in most automated panels in west.

The chemical forward reaction of lactic dehydrogenase can be presented by the following equation:

$$\text{Lactic acid} + \text{NAD} \xrightarrow{\text{LD}} \text{Pyruvic acid} + \text{NADH}.$$

The reaction is reversible but the conditions for the reverse reaction are different than those for the forward (e.g. the pH for the forward reaction is 8.8–9.8 and for the reverse reaction is 7.4–7.8). Using the above reaction at pH 8.3–8.9 the amount of enzyme is measured by the rate of increase in absorbance at 340 nm as NADH is produced. The absorbance is measured in a spectrophotometer. Note that the alkali pH pulls the reaction forward. Commercial kits provide all the reagents to run the test when the laboratory is equipped with a spectrophotometer that can read in the ultraviolet range. Follow manufacturer's instruction in performing test by the spectrophotometric method. We will, however, describe the affordable colorimetric method although the method is not as accurate as the spectrophotometric method.

Colorimetric Method of LD Assay LD activity can be determined colorimetrically using 2,4-dinitrophenylhydrazine (2,4-DNPH) as the chromogen in alkaline medium. It is a discrete or two-point method and requires an ordinary colorimeter to make the measurement. The method is not as sensitive as the spectrophotometric method.

Normal ranges

Adults: 70–240 U/L

Children: 150–590 U/L

Specimen Haemolysed serum should never be used for LD determination, since red cells contain 150 times more LD activity than the serum. For the same reason, separate the serum promptly (within 1–2 h) after the blood specimen has been drawn. If immediate analysis is not possible, store at room temperature for 2–3 days. If the serum has to be stored for a longer period, store it in the refrigerator with NAD (10 mg/mL).

Principle The enzyme lactate dehydrogenase catalyses the conversion of lactate in the buffered substrate into pyruvate in the presence of NAD. The increased concentration of the product (pyruvate) is measured colorimetrically using 2,4-dinitrophenylhydrazine. The latter reacts with the pyruvate and gives a brown colour in alkaline medium, which is proportional to the amount of pyruvate present in the reaction mixture.

Reagents

- Preparation of substrate
    (a) Glycine buffer (0.1 M): Dissolve 3.753 g glycine (amino-acetic acid) and 2.922 g NaCl (AR) in 200 mL of water and make up to 500 mL in a volumetric flask. Keep the solution in the refrigerator.
    (b) Sodium lactate solution (357 w/v): Mix 52 mL of lactic acid (AR) with 21.5 g of NaOH dissolved in 120 mL distilled water. Add a few broken glass pieces and boil carefully for about 30 min. Cool and make up to 200 mL with distilled water. Keep in a refrigerator.
    (c) Sodium hydroxide solution (0.1 N or 0.1 M): Dilute 0.4 N NaOH (see later) four-fold: Take 25 mL of 0.4 N NaOH in a 100-mL volumetric flask and make it up to 100 mL with water. Mix thoroughly by inversion.
    (d) Buffered substrate: In a 250-mL beaker mix 120 mL of glycine buffer, 20 mL NaOH solution and 10 mL of sodium lactate solution. Adjust the pH to 10.0, using 0.1 N NaOH. Keep the final solution in the refrigerator.
- Nicotinamide adenine dinucleotide (NAD): Dissolve 10 mg of NAD in 2.0 mL of distilled water. Keep in the refrigerator. After using replace immediately in the refrigerator. The solid NAD should be kept in the freezer.
- Standard solution of sodium pyruvate (1 µmole pyruvate/mL): Dissolve 220 mg sodium pyruvate (analytical grade) in glycine buffer and make up to 100 mL. Dilute 5 mL of this solution to 100 mL with glycine buffer to give the working standard of 1 µmol/mL. The remaining solution of the stock can be discarded.
- 2,4-dinitrophenylhydrazine reagent (2,4-DNPH): Dissolve 200 mg of 2,4-DNPH in 1 N HCl (warm). Prepare 1 N HCl by diluting 85 mL of concentrated HCl (approximately 12 N) to 1000 mL with distilled water.
- Sodium hydroxide (0.4 N): Dissolve 16 g of NaOH in 500 mL of water and dilute to 1000 mL with distilled water in a 1-L volumetric flask.

Procedure

1. Dilute the serum five-fold with saline by mixing 0.2 mL of serum with 0.8 mL of 0.97, NaCl (saline).
2. Label two test tubes as 'T' and 'B', corresponding to test and blank.

3. Pipette 1.0 mL of buffered substrate and 0.2 mL of NAD solution in both tubes and place them in a water bath (37°C) for 5 min in order to equilibrate the temperature.
4. Set the timer, add 0.1 mL of serum in the tube marked 'T', mix and simultaneously start the timer.
5. Exactly after 15 min of incubation at 37°C add 1.0 mL of hydrazine solution to both the tubes. Do not take out the test tubes from the water-bath.
6. Add 1.0 mL of serum in the tube marked B (serum blank).
7. Mix the contents of each tube and continue incubation for another 15 min (exact timing is not necessary).
8. Add 10.0 mL of sodium hydroxide solution (0.4 M) to both the tubes, and mix.
9. Wait for an additional 10 min and then read the absorbance of the test and serum blank solutions against water at 505–510 nm (green filter). Use the water blank for setting the instrument.
10. Determine the change in absorbance (AA) by subtracting the absorbance reading of the serum blank ('B') from that of the test solution ('T'):

$$\Delta A = A_T - A_B$$

11. Determine the absorbance of the standard (A) in the following way:
    (a) Mix 1.0 mL of substrate and 0.3 mL of water in a test tube. Label the tube as 'B' (blank).
    (b) Mix in another test tube 1.0 mL of substrate, 0.1 mL of pyruvate standard and 0.2 mL of water. Label this as 'S' (standard). The standard is equivalent to 333 U/L (see calculation)
    (c) Add 1.0 mL of hydrazine solution in both tubes, leave for 15 min at 37 °C and then add 10 mL of NaOH (0.4 N).
    (d) Determine the absorbance of the standard (A_g) against the blank (B).
12. *Calculation*:

LD activity in serum (U/L) = $(A_T - A_B)/A_S \times 333$

where A_T is absorbance of test solution, A_B is absorbance of blank B and 333 is value of the standard (U/L).*

*Calculation of the value of standard

$$0.1 \times 1/15 \times 1000/0.02$$

0.1 = µmole of pyruvate in the reaction mixture
1/15 = Per minute (when the observation is taken for 15 min)
1000/0.02 = Conversion of aliquot of specimen taken to 1 L
Note: 0.1 mL of diluted (1:5) serum has 0.02 mL of undiluted serum.

Preparation of calibration curve It is not necessary to prepare the calibration curve every day but the working of the system must be checked once a month by running the calibration curve. For daily use the above formula may be applied as the values are linear over a wide range.

1. Take seven test tubes and mark them 1–7.
2. Add pyruvate standard, buffer and water as shown in the following table:

Tube No.	Pyruvate standard (mL)	Buffered substrate (mL)	Water (mL)	LD activity (U/L)
1	0.0	1.0	0.3	0
2	0.1	0.9	0.3	333
3	0.2	0.8	0.3	666
4	0.3	0.7	0.3	999

Note: The quantity of the reaction mixture is 1.3 mL prior to the addition of chromogen and sodium hydroxide solution.

3. Add 1.0 mL of hydrazine solution to all the tubes, leave for 15 min at 37°C and then add 10.0 mL of 0.4 N NaOH (as for the test run).

Additional information
- Lactate dehydrogenase can be inactivated by improper handling of the specimen. This will result in false low values.
- Repeated freezing and thawing is harmful for the enzyme.
- If the enzyme activity of the serum is more than 1000 U/L, dilute the serum or reduce the time of reaction. Include the dilution factor in calculation.

Amylase

Amylase, Lipase and Trypsin are enzymes present in normal pancreatic glands which are secreted in pancreatic juice for digestion of starch, fat and protein respectively. Amylase is the most frequently assayed test to evaluate pancreatitis and pancreatic injury. Amylase is a hydrolytic enzyme that splits complex carbohydrates such as starch and glycogen into simpler molecules of sugars (e.g. glucose). Amylase is present in saliva and pancreatic juices. This enzyme is elevated in a variety of situations. Elevations ranging from 4 to 50 times can occur in acute pancreatitis. Mild elevation can occur in abdominal emergencies such as perforated ulcer, intestinal infarction and rupture of tubal pregnancy. The enzymatic chemical reaction (hydrolysis) of amylase can be shown as follows:

$$\text{Starch + water} \xrightarrow{\text{Amylase}} \text{Sugar(s)}.$$

The clinical significance of the estimation of amylase lies almost entirely in the diagnosis of acute pancreatitis, in which the enzyme level frequently exceeds more than 10-times the Normal range (60–180 Somogyi Units/dL, iodometric). Levels in excess of 550 units/dL (SU) strongly support a diagnosis of acute pancreatitis. The rise is rapid and transient, reaching a peak within the first 12–24 h after onset and returning to normal usually in 2–3 days. Some of the other causes of high amylase activity in serum include salivary gland disorders, abdominal disturbances affecting the pancreas, and intake of some drugs (morphine). In these cases, the rise of the amylase activity is not as high. Chronic pancreatitis and carcinoma of the pancreas are rarely associated with a raised serum amylase.

Normal Ranges

Iodometric: 60–180 Somogyi Units (SU)/dL

International unit: 95–290 IU/L

Iodometric Method   There are two principles applied in determining amylase activity—the **amylolytic** method that determines the depletion of starch (substrate) and the **saccharogenic** method that determines the rise of sugar level (product). The saccharogenic method is now obsolete. Most modern methods are based on the forward reaction of amylase, i.e. breakdown of starch. Starch reacts with iodine and gives a stable colour. Depletion of starch is assessed by a decreased reaction with iodine (iodometric method), which is described here. Use of special **dye-linked starch** as substrate and measuring the amount of dye released because of amylase activity is limited to advanced laboratories. The iodometric method described here is simple and inexpensive but not as accurate as the dye-linked method.

Principle   The iodometric method is based on the ability of iodine to form a vivid blue colour in combination with starch. The by-product of amylase action may also form coloured substances with iodine but at different wavelengths from the characteristic starch–iodine complex. In this method, iodine colour reagent is added to the substrate-sample mixture after an incubation period. The greater the amount of amylase activity, the lighter will be colour of the final solution.

Reagents
- **Buffered starch substrate (pH 7.0):**
  (a) Dissolve 13.3 g of anhydrous disodium phosphate (Na_2HPO_4) and 4.3 g of benzole acid (C_6H_5COOH) in approximately 250 mL of distilled; water.
  (b) Heat to boiling.
  (c) In a separate beaker, dissolve 0.200 g of soluble starch in 5 mL of cold water. Add this starch solution to the boiling buffer (b). Stir and rinse the beaker repeatedly to ensure complete transfer of starch (**quantitative**).
  (d) Allow the mixture to cool to room temperature and dilute to 500 mL with water. Store the mixture in the refrigerator.
  (e) The solution should remain clear. One should assess its stability by measuring the absorbance of mixed reagents (observing for a significant decline in the reagent blank value from run to run).
- *Iodine solution:*
  (a) *Stock iodine solution (0.1 M):* Dissolve 3.567 g of potassium iodated (KIO_3) and 45 g of potassium iodide (KI) in 800 mL of water. Add slowly 9 mL of concentrated HCl (12 N) slowly to the mixture with constant stirring. Dilute to 1000 mL and store in an amber bottle in the refrigerator. The solution is stable for 12 months.
  (b) *Working iodine solution (0.01 M):* Dilute 50 mL of stock iodine solution (a) to 500 mL. Store in an amber-colour bottle at 4°C. The solution is stable for 2 months.
- Saline (0.9% NaCl).

Procedure
1. Dilute the serum 1:10 with 0.9% saline.
2. Take two large-size test tubes (25 mL) or volumetric flasks and label them as 'T' and 'S', corresponding to test and standard.
3. Add 1 mL of the buffered substrate in both the tubes ('T' and 'S') and place them in a water bath at 37°C.
4. After 3 min add 0.1 mL of diluted serum in tube 'T', mix immediately and start the stopwatch.
   Note: Do not add anything in tube 'S' at this point; an equivalent amount of water will be added in step (7).
5. Gently incubate for exactly 15 min.
6. Remove the test tube from the bath, and add 0.4 mL of working iodine solution; mix well.
7. Then add 8.5 mL of water in tube 'T' and 8.6 mL of water in tube 'S'. Some technicians add 8.5 mL of water and 0.1 mL of serum, instead of 8.6 mL of water at this step. This compensates for any colour or turbidity of the serum. Mix the contents of the tubes and proceed to the measurement of the intensity of the colour developed.
8. Transfer the contents of the test tubes in two matched cuvettes marked as 'T' and 'S'.
9. Read the absorbances of 'T' and 'S' solutions at 660 nm using water as a blank.
10. Calculation:
    Note: International Unit is not used here because of the variability in the molecular weight of starch.
    Amylase activity (SU/dL) = $(A_S - A_T)/A_S \times (C_S \times 100/V_{SR})^*$
    = Absorbance ratio × 8000^* × Dilution factor,**
    where A_S is absorbance of standard solution, A_T is absorbance of test solution, V_{SR} is volume of serum in the reaction mixture (0.01 mL) and C_S is concentration of standard in Somogyi Unit (SU, as calculated later).

    Calculation of C_S (amylase unit factor):
    (a) 1 Somogyi unit (SU) of amylase activity = 5 mg starch hydrolysed under aforesaid conditions (enzymatic reaction for 15 min at 37°C at pH 7.0).

(b) Amount of starch present in the reaction mixture = 0.4 mg
(c) C_S = 0.4/5 amylase units (Somogyi)
Enzyme activity factor (amylase activity/dL serum)
= $C_S \times 100/V_{SR}$ = 0.4/5 × 100/0.01 = 8000

**Dilution factor*: If the test solution ('T') reads less than half the standard (or control, 'S'), it indicates that the amylase activity is too high for the test. The test should then be repeated, starting with a more dilute mixture of serum and physiological saline.

Additional Information
- The amylase of serum is activated by chloride ions, so that dilutions of serum must be made in physiological saline.
- Use cotton wool plugs in the mouth pieces of all pipettes to avoid traces of saliva causing falsely high amylase values.

LIPID PROFILE

Routine tests of lipid profile include cholesterol, high-density lipoprotein (HDL) and low-density lipoprotein (LDL) and triglycerides. The physician for the patients with coronary artery disease and other atherosclerotic conditions requests these tests. Some of the screening tests are now available in the physician's office but the reference laboratories of the developing countries are better equipped for complete analysis. The smaller peripheral laboratories are now able to participate with the greater availability of the biochemical kits. The older colorimetric methods, involving long chemical procedures of extraction and hydrolysis have now been abandoned.

Specimen
Although serum is preferred, plasma can also be used. Serum specimen for cholesterol determination should be used as far as possible on the same day. The specimen is stable for a week if refrigerated (2–8°C) and for one month if frozen (–10°C). The samples should be brought to room temperature before use.

Serum or plasma appearance
The appearance of a serum or plasma sample after it has remained undisturbed for 4–6 h at 4–8°C may prove to be helpful in classifying and ultimately treating hyperlipidaemic patients. However, the appearance reveals little about the HDL and LDL cholesterol levels. This test is inexpensive and simple to perform but requires that specimens be stored in clear tubes with very little of the label obstructing the cross-sectional view through the tube, especially at the meniscus of the specimen. A creamy layer forming at the surface of the serum contains chylomicrons, which is an indication of either a non-fasting specimen or a serious defect in lipoprotein lipase production or function. Varying degrees of cloudiness, called lipaemia, are usually associated with elevated triglyceride levels,. In such cases, a dilution of he specimen may be required to bring the triglyceride levels within the linear range of the analytical method. Consequently, the appearance provides observable data that aid in the correlations and validation of laboratory results.

Total Cholesterol
Cholesterol is a lipid, classified as a sterol. It is widely distributed in various animal tissues and vegetable oils and consumed with food. It can also be synthesized in the liver, is a normal constituent of bile, and is the principal constituent of most gallstones. It is important in metabolism serving as a precursor of various steroid hormones, e.g. sex hormones and adrenal corticoids.

Serum cholesterol (total) is found in two forms—esterified cholesterol and non-esterified (free) cholesterol. As esterification of cholesterol is closely related to liver function, a fall of esterified cholesterol reflects liver disorder. The level of cholesterol is affected by stress, age, sex, hormonal balance and pregnancy.

Normal Value Normal values vary with age, diet, sex, and geographic or cultural region.

Test	Category	Adults (fasting)	Children and adolescent (12–18 years)
Total cholesterol (mg/dL)	Desirable level	140–199	<170
	Borderline high	200–239	170–199
	High	>240	>200
HDL (mg/dL)*	Men	35–65	
	Women	35–80	
LDL (mg/dL)	Desirable level	<130	<110
	Borderline high	140–159	110–129
	High	>160	>130

Note: HDL (good cholesterol) above 75 mg/dL is most desirable. The risk of coronary heart disease increases as the level drops below 45 mg/dL.

Conversion factor to International Unit: Cholesterol concentration (mg/dL) = 38.7 × (mmol/L)

Desirable Limits Total cholesterol level of 199 mg/dL or less is desirable for reducing the risk of coronary heart disease or stroke. Less than 180 mg/dL is probably real good and sought by most cardiologists. Levels higher than 240 mg/dL, almost doubles the risk of heart disease. Sub groups of cholesterol are also important and HDL (High Density Lipoprotein) cholesterol has a protective effect and higher than 40 mg/dL is desirable. Very low density lipoprotein (VLDL) cholesterol and LDL cholesterol affects coronary risk adversely. Elevated triglyceride levels also add to the risk.

Principle Early methods for cholesterol analysis were subject to a high degree of analytical variance, primarily due to the poor reactivity of many of the cholesterol esters. Newer method now utilize cholesterol esterase a s pre-treatment, which breaks all the ester linkage to generate from cholesterol and eliminate much of the previous problem in testing.

The first step is an enzymatic hydrolysis of cholesterol ester by cholesterol esterase (CE):

$$\text{Cholesterol ester} + H_2O \xrightarrow{CE} \text{Cholesterol} + \text{Fatty acid.}$$

The free cholesterol (nonesterified) is then oxidized by cholesterol oxidase to a ketone, with the production of hydrogen peroxide (H_2O_2) that can be measured in a peroxidase-catalysed reaction that oxidizes a reduced dye (4-aminophenazone) with phenol to a coloured product (quinoneimine) that absorbs at 500 nm. The commercial reagent kits generally combine all enzyme and other required components, and the formulations vary. The method has been optimized in various automated systems.

Cholesterol determination without extraction

Most of the classical methods (Liebermann–Burchard, Salkowski reaction and others) were time-consuming and hazardous requiring manual organic phase extractions and manipulations using strong acids, considerable skill, and technologist's time. The strong acid reagents necessitated working in fume hood, careful manipulation to prevent spills, and logistic problems of storage and transport of reagents. The enzymatic methods have largely replaced them and the laboratories are able to get the commercial kits from local vendors. Considering the difficulties of peripheral laboratories in remote places, an easier colorimetric method is suggested here.

Reagents
- *Glacial acetic acid (analytical grade)*
- *Ferric chloride reagent (2.5% in phosphoric acid):* Dissolve 2.5 g of ferric chloride $FeCl_3 \cdot 6H_2O$, in 100 mL of phosphoric acid (85%). Store the reagent in a glass-stoppered bottle. Label with date. This solution is stable indefinitely.
- *Cholesterol standard*
   (a) *Stock standard*: Dissolve 250 mg of pure grade cholesterol in 50 mL of glacial acetic acid in a 100-mL volumetric flask and dilute it to 100 mL volume with the same.….
   (b) *Working standard*: Dilute the stock standard 1 : 20 with glacial acetic acid (0.1 mL of standard mixed with 1.9 mL of glacial acetic acid). *Note:* For preparing calibration curve, greater amount will be needed and hence, mix 0.5 mL of standard with 9.5 mL of glacial acetic acid.

Procedure
1. Dilute serum 1:20 by mixing 0.1 mL of serum with 1.9 mL of distilled water.
2. Arrange three large-size test tubes (15-mL capacity) in a test tube rack and label them as 'T', 'S' and 'B' corresponding to test, standard and blank respectively.
3. Add 5.0 mL of ferric chloride reagent in all the tubes ('T', 'S' and "B').
4. Add 0.5-mL of diluted serum in the 'T' marked test tube, 0.5 mL of standard in 'S', and 0.5 mL of distilled water in 'B'.
5. Mix the contents of each tube simultaneously for 10 sec by shaking the test tube rack.
6. Immediately place the rack in a boiling water bath for exactly 90 sec.
7. Cool immediately in running tap water (or cold water) for 5 min; mix well the contents of each tube and measure the absorbance of the test (A_T) and standard (A_S) against the blank at 560 nm (560–600 nm).
8. Complete the readings within 15 min.
9. *Calculation*:
   Cholesterol concentration (mg/dL) = $A_T/A_S \times 250$
   Conversion to International Unit: mg/dL $\times$ 0.0259 = mmol/L.

Additional information
- The reagent with the specimen should not be left at room temperature for longer than 10 sec after mixing, since reaction also takes place at room temperature.
- There may be a slight difference in the colour of the ferric chloride reagent with the serum sample (orange purple) and with the standard (purple). This is because of the presence of serum proteins in the sample. This difference in colour does not cause any variation in the values of cholesterol.

Preparation of calibration curve
1. Prepare various concentrations of the standard by further dilution of the working standard (as mentioned in the reagent preparation).

Tube No.	Working cholesterol (Standard) (mL)*	Glacial acetic acid (mL)	Concentration of cholesterol (mg/dL)
1	0.5	2.0	50
2	1.0	1.5	100
3	1.5	1.0	150
4	2.0	0.5	200
5	2.5	0.0	250

*1 : 20 diluted stock standard.

2. Carry out cholesterol estimation of solutions in tubes labelled 1–5 by following the testing procedure outlined earlier.
3. Tabulate the absorbances (optical density) with the corresponding cholesterol concentrations.
4. Prepare a calibration curve. It should be linear and the curve must go through the origin.
5. Prepare a new calibration curve with every new batch of reagent. An independent calibration curve should be made for each colorimeter in use.
6. Dilute the sample with distilled water if the concentration is above 400 mg/dL; repeat the test and multiply the result by the dilution factor.

Lipoproteins—HDL and LDL

HDL and LDL are now analysed by enzymatic and immunochemical methods. These analyses are available only through the reference laboratories.

Serum Triglycerides

Triglycerides are true fats, esters of glycerol and fatty acids that belong to the organic group of compounds called **lipids**. Most animal and vegetable fats are triglycerides. Upon hydrolysis, by the lipase enzyme (LPS) they yield glycerol and fatty acids and the quantitative analysis of glycerol forms the basis of triglyceride assay. Elevated level of triglycerides in serum is a risk factor related to atherosclerotic disease that causes thickening of the walls of larger arteries. This may lead to a heart attack. Some of the clinical conditions that cause hyperlipaemia are glycogen storage disease, nephrotic syndrome, diabetes mellitus, chronic hepatitis and alcoholism. Excessive elevation of triglycerides when more than 1000 can cause acute pancreatitis by causing activation of pancreatic amylase in side pancreatic cells hence causing cell death and inflammation.

Specimen Although serum is preferred, plasma can also be used for determining triglycerides. Anticoagulants such as EDTA should be used in case of the enzymatic method. For the colorimetric method, fluoride-oxalate can be used.

Fasting (12–14 h) samples are recommended for this analysis. Hence, blood is collected before breakfast. The analysis should be done on the same day or the sample should be stored in the refrigerator for not more than 2–3 days.

Interfering substances: Haemoglobin and bilirubin in high concentrations may interfere with the triglyceride analysis. Avoid a haemolysed serum specimen. Gross contamination of the samples at any stage makes them unsuitable for use. The samples should be brought to room temperature prior to use.

Laboratory Assay Serum triglyceride determination is essential in evaluating **hyperlipidaemic** patients and their risk of cardiovascular disease. Early methods were long and tedious that involved extractions with organic solvents that were not easily adaptable to automation. As with cholesterol testing, the advent of enzymatic method has proved to be a relief. Reagents are now available that contain all enzymes, buffers, and cofactors needed for the assay.

In all the different reagent kits, the first step is nearly always a lipase-mediated hydrolysis of triglycerides to glycerol and fatty acids.

$$1 \text{ triglyceride} + 3 \text{ H}_2\text{O} \xrightarrow{\text{LPS}} 1 \text{ glycerol} + 3 \text{ fatty acids}.$$

In the following steps glycerol is taken through a series of chemical reactions with the mediation of three enzymes glycerol kinase (GK), glycerol phosphate oxidase (GPO) and horseradish peroxidase (P). In this method, the peroxidase frees oxygen radical that oxidizes a reduced dye to a coloured end product. This can be read in the visible wavelength of light. The three enzymatic reactions, after the hydrolysis of triglycerides, are shown here.

$$\text{Glycerol} + \text{ATP} \xleftrightarrow{\text{GK}} \text{Glycerol-3-phosphate} + \text{ADP}$$

$$\text{Glycerol-3-phosphate} + O_2 \xleftrightarrow{\text{GPO}} \text{DHAP} + H_2O_2$$

$$H_2O_2 + \text{Reduced dye} \xleftrightarrow{\text{P}} \text{Oxidized dye}^* + H_2O$$

*Absorbance is measured at visible wavelength of light depending on the chromogen uses.

An alternative method is to use glycerol phosphate dehydrogenase (GPD) in place of glycerol phosphate oxidase. In this method NAD is used which is reduced to NADH, allowing the measurement of absorbance at 340 nm. Various automated systems adapt the same procedure for triglyceride assay. The major problem with this type of assay is the ability of the spectrophotometers to distinguish absorbance differences at that wavelength. Sample blanks are necessary to reduce interferences from other UV-absorbing pigments in the sample.

Reagent, Equipment and Supplies
- Use commercial kit which supplies all the required reagents.
- Spectrophotometer
- Laboratory supplies for chemical analysis

Procedure
Follow manufacturer's direction in performing the test.

Normal Range 10–190 mg/dL serum (0.11–2.15 mmol/L)

Conversion to International Unit
$$\text{mg/dL} \times 0.0113 = \text{mmol/L}$$

Note: Conversion factor based on triolein, molecular weight 885.

ELECTROLYTES

Electrolytes are substances that ionize in solution and conduct electricity. Acids, bases and salts are electrolytes. Electrolyte imbalance in the body or disturbance in homeostasis can bring about serious consequences. Electrolytes enter the body through the diet and leave the body primarily through the kidney, although other routes are also important such as sweat and the gastrointestinal tract. Hormones, secreted by the endocrine glands, control the absorption of electrolytes by the renal tubules and thus play a vital role in maintaining homeostasis.

One of the most important functions of electrolytes is to maintain the acid–base balance of the body. Such electrolytes as sodium, potassium, chloride, phosphorus, bicarbonate and carbonic acid are in some way related to this process. Osmotic balance is maintained by sodium, potassium and chloride; in addition, potassium plays a crucial role in the active transport of materials against the concentration gradient. Some of the electrolytes also form important constituents of the body structure (calcium and phosphorus) while others act as catalysts or form a part of some enzymes (magnesium, zinc and copper).

The clinical condition that may very likely bring about electrolyte imbalance in the body is fluid loss through diarrhoea, vomiting and sweating. Disturbance in endocrine function is one of the most important causes of electrolyte imbalance. This is particularly true for sodium and potassium. Analysis of electrolytes is a stat (emergency) procedure. Severe drift from the homeostatic level of electrolytes may result in disordered cardiac rhythm and cardiac arrest or other serious complications. Serum is the most common specimen submitted for electrolyte analysis.

Several methods are applied in the analysis of electrolyte—titrimetry, photometry and electroraetry.

Sodium and Potassium

Sodium is the major extracellular cation (Na) of the body. Compare with the very beginning of unicellular life floating in the ocean with salt rich fluid in the exterior and potassium kept inside. Sodium salts are necessary to preserve a balance between calcium and potassium to maintain normal heart action and the equilibrium of the body. Sodium salts regulate the osmotic pressure in the cells and fluids and guard against an excessive loss of water from the tissues. Almost all the blood sodium is found in the plasma; there is very little in the red cells. In normal persons, plasma sodium values lie between 137 and 148 mEq (or mmol/L). Very low values are found in acute Addison's disease. Conditions in which extracellular fluid is lost (e.g. vomiting, diarrhoea), lead to a salt deficiency and hence to low plasma sodium values which may be exaggerated if water losses are replaced without adequate salt therapy. A non-specific fall in plasma sodium values also occurs in many chronic diseases.

Unlike sodium, potassium is the major intracellular cation of the body. It is high in red blood cells and hence, haemolysed blood should be discarded for potassium analysis. In addition, the serum should be promptly separated, or it may yield a false, elevated value. Potassium in conjunction with sodium and chloride, aids in the regulation of osmotic pressure and acid–base balance. A proper balance of potassium, calcium and magnesium is accessory for the normal function of the heart and muscle tissues. Potassium is also known to play a significant role in the conduction of nerve impulses.

The plasma of a normal person contains 3.9–5.0 mEq K/L, (or mmol K/L). This is a very constant value. Raised values are found in Addison's disease and when excretion is limited by advanced chronic renal disease or acute oliguria. Low values are found in excessive use of diuretics and profuse loss in diarrhoea. Insulin causes inward shift of glucose and potassium and used in very high level of Potassium in conjunction with intravenous glucose water. Reduced plasma potassium concentration often causes electrolyte shifts with persistent alkalosis, which is restored, to normal by potassium replacement.

Specimen Serum, plasma, and urine are all acceptable for sodium measurements. In case of plasma, heparin or oxalate is used as anticoagulant. Haemolysis does not affect the results of sodium but will yield false high value of potassium. Heparinized plasma is preferred for potassium assay (clotting effects *K*-value). Specimen for potassium determination should be kept at room temperature and assayed promptly.

Laboratory assay: Ion selective electrode

Use of **ion selective electrode** (ISE) is the most common way to determine sodium and potassium. The older methods of flame photometry and atomic absorption spectrophotometry are limited to reference and research laboratories. Chemical methods have been abandoned. Peripheral laboratories are not usually involved in the determinations of sodium and potassium.

Normal Range Serum, plasma: Sodium 136–145 mmol/L; Potassium 3.4–5.0 mmol/L
Urine: Sodium 40–220 mmol/day, varies with diet. Potassium 25–125 mmol/day
CSF: Sodium 136–150.

Calcium

Calcium and inorganic phosphate are the major constituents of bone and have a reciprocal relationship in serum. A higher proportion of non-skeletal calcium is present within cells than in extracellular fluids, and most of this intracellular calcium is bound to proteins in the cell membrane. Calcium in serum is present in ionized form or as a complex with protein or other inorganic substances such as citrate, phosphate and others. Intracellular ionized calcium is physiologically active and functions as an intracellular messenger by binding to or being released from specific intracellular proteins, a process that changes protein conformations and hence its activity or function.

Calcium plays many important roles in the physiology of the body; it activates many enzymes and its role in blood coagulation has been discussed earlier. Of the many factors that affect serum calcium level, parathyroid hormone, and vitamin D are most important. Decreased activity of parathyroid hormone decreases the calcium level of blood and vitamin D increases the internal absorption of calcium and phosphate.

Calcium measurements are used in the diagnosis and treatment of parathyroid diseases, a variety of bone diseases, chronic renal failure and tetany. Increased serum calcium levels are associated with primary hyperparathyroidism, multiple myeloma, metastatic bone lesions and hypervitaminosis D. Hypocalcaemia is associated with hypoparathyroidism, nephrotic syndrome, and rickets and renal failure.

Specimen Serum is the preferred specimen. Haemolysed and heparinized samples are unsuitable for this method. Similarly, plasma prepared using EDTA, oxalate or citrate must not be used as these preservatives cause removal of calcium by chelation. Calcium in serum is stable for 12 h at room temperature (25–35°C), one week at 2–8°C and for a longer period up to 3 months at –20°C.

Laboratory assay

Calcium can be determined by different methods—titrimetric, colorimetric, fluorometric or by atomic absorption. The titrimetric method is tedious and time-consuming and is not widely used. Reference laboratories use ion selective electrode but it only reports ionized calcium. The methods best suitable for the laboratories of developing countries are the colorimetric methods, using dye *o*-cresolphthalein complexone (CPC) or arsenazo III.

Cresolphthalein Complexone Method The cresolphthalein complexone method is highly sensitive which sometimes makes the method inadaptable to the conditions existing in developing countries. The use of calcium-free glassware and water are important and the use of disposable plastic ware is recommended.

Principle The metal-complexing dye *o*-**cresolphthalein complexone** (CPC) forms a red complex with calcium in alkaline solution;:

$$Ca^{++} + o\text{-CPC} \rightarrow Ca^{++} - o\text{-CPC (red)}.$$

The inclusion of HCl helps to release calcium bound to proteins and **8 hydroxy-quinoline** eliminates the interference by magnesium. 2-amino, 2-methyl, 1-propanol (AMP) provides the proper alkaline medium for the colour reaction. The intensity of the colour is measured at 540 nm/yellow green filter.

Equipment and supplies
- Spectrophotometer or filter photometer (540 nm/yellow green filter)
- Laboratory supplies of volumetric glassware
  All glassware used in this method must be scrupulously cleaned, soaked overnight in 3% (V/V) HCl to remove traces of calcium, thoroughly rinsed with distilled water and dried before use.
- Test tubes (18 × 150 mm) and test tube racks.
- Timer

Reagents All chemicals must be pure grade
- *Concentrated hydrochloric acid (HCl)*: Concentrated hydrochloric acid is usually 12 N. See the bottle for actual strength. Dilute with distilled water to make 6N strength.
- *AMP Buffer pH 10.7*
  Measure 37.8 mL of AMP reagent and add 150 mL of distilled water and mix. Adjust the pH to 10.7 with 6N HCl and make up to 250 mL with distilled water. Store the buffer solution in the refrigerator in a brown coloured glass bottle. Label with date. This is stable for 3 weeks.

- *o-Cresolphthalein complexone solution (colour reagent)*
  (a) Add 15 mL concentrated HCl to a 250 mL volumetric flask containing about 25 mL of distilled water. Mix by swirling.
  (b) Quantitatively transfer 25 mg o-cresolphthalein complexone powder (wash down with distilled water) into the hydrochloric acid solution (a). Mix to dissolve.
  (c) Add 250 mg of 8 hydroxyquinoline and dissolve and then make up to 250 mL with distilled water.
  (d) Store the colour solution in a brown coloured glass bottle at room temperature (25–35°C). Label the bottle with date. This is stable for about one month.
- *Stock calcium standard 50 mg/dL*: Before weighing, dry calcium carbonate at 100°C for 2 h. Allow to cool in a desiccator.
  Dissolve 625 mg of dried calcium carbonate in 50 mL of distilled water taken in a 500 mL volumetric flask and add 3.5mL concentrated. HCl. Mix to dissolve and make up to 500 mL with distilled water. Store the stock standard in a brown bottle at room temperature (25–35°C). Label with date. It is stable for about 6 months.
- *Working standards*
  Into four 100 mL volumetric flasks transfer 10, 15, 20 and 25 mL of stock calcium standard and dilute each to 100 mL with benzoic acid to get working standards containing 5, 7.5, 10, and 12.5 mg/dL calcium, respectively. Store the working standards in brown bottles at room temperature (25–35°C). Label the bottle with date. These are stable for 2 months.
  Note: Use 10 mg/dL as single working standard for daily run (see step #2 of procedure).

Procedure
1. Mark three test tubes as 'B', 'S' and 'T', representing test, standard and blank respectively.
2. Add 01. mL of distilled water in tube marked 'B', 0.1 mL of working standard (10 mg/dL) in tube marked 'S' and 0.1 mL of serum in tube marked 'T'.
3. Add 2 mL colour reagent in each tube and mix well.
4. Then add 2.0 mL of buffer in each tube and mix well.
5. Incubate at room temperature (25–35°C) for 15 min.
6. Set the spectrophotometer /filter photometer to zero using blank at 540 nm/yellow green filter.
7. Measure the absorbance of standards (A_S) and test (A_T).
8. *Calculation:* The following calculation is valid only when the standard curve is linear. Check the linearity once a month. If a new reagent is made, recheck the standard curve. Once linearity is proved, it is just enough if a single standard such as S_{10} (10 mg/dL) is used and the concentration in the patient's sample is calculated using the formula :

$$A_T/A_S \times 10 \text{ (mg/dL)} = \text{Serum calcium concentration (mg/dL)}.$$

Preparation of standard curve
1. Label 5 test tubes (18 × 150 mm) labelled B for blank, and S_5, $S_{7.5}$, S_{10}, $S_{12.5}$, for four standards and QC (control serum).
2. Add reagents, working standards (S_5 = 5 mg/dL, $S_{7.5}$ = 7.5 mg/dL, S_{10} = 10 mg/dL, $S_{12.5}$ = 12.5 mg/dL) and QC serum in the order indicated into appropriately labelled tubes.

Tube No.	Blank	S_5	$S_{7.5}$	S_{10}	$S_{12.5}$	Control serum (QC)
Distilled water (mL)	0.1					–
Standard (mL)	–		0.1	0.1	0.1	–
Control serum (mL)	–					0.1
Colour reagent	2.0	2.0	2.0	2.0	2.0	2.0
			Mix Well			
Buffer (mL)	2.0	2.0	2.0	2.0	2.0	2.0
			Mix Well			

3. Construct a calibration graph by plotting the absorbance of the standards against their respective concentrations.
4. Plot the absorbance values of control serum QC on the calibration graph and read off the concentration. The measurable range with this graph is from 1.0 to 12.0 mg/dL.
5. It is advisable to plot a calibration graph whenever the reagents are freshly prepared.

Quality control Include one internal QC in every batch of samples analysed each day irrespective of the number of samples in a batch. Since calcium is analysed single batch in a day in an intermediate laboratory, it will not be possible to analyse several QC samples and calculate within-day precision. However, even if only a single QC sample is analysed in a day, this value can be pooled with the preceding 10 or 20 values obtained in the previous days and **between-day precision** can be calculated. Ensure that this is well within the acceptable limit, i.e. 8%. Quality control serum with its corresponding calcium concentration is commercially available.

Normal range Serum Calcium 8.5–10.4 mg/dL 2.2–2.78 mmol Ca/L

Additional Note:
- Haemolysed and lipaemic sera interfere with the measurement of calcium. Set up an appropriate blank for such samples by adding 0.1 mL of serum to 4 mL of distilled water. The absorbance obtained against distilled water is then subtracted from the test absorbance before the test result is calculated.
- Control sera, with known calcium concentration, must be run every day in order to obtain reliable results. Control sera is commercially available (Boehringer Mannheim and others)

Chloride

Chloride is the major extracellular anion of the body. Blood serum contains 99–108 mEq/dL or 351–383 mg/dL, principally as sodium chloride. Its primary role in the body is to maintain proper water distribution, osmotic pressure, and normal anion–cation balance in the external fluid (plasma). A decrease in plasma chloride occurs in conditions where there is a low plasma sodium or when the bicarbonate is raised as in metabolic alkalosis. Chloride concentration of red cells is lower than that of whole blood. The chloride ion is ingested through the food and filtered or re-absorbed by the kidney according to the body's need. Chloride, to some extent, may be lost through sweating. Prolonged vomiting, from any cause, may result in a significant loss of chloride and ultimately a decrease in serum and body chloride.

Loss of serum chloride is associated with nephritis, diabetic acidosis or excessive fluid loss. Increased chloride concentration of serum is seen in case of congestive heart failure and decreased renal blood flow. Estimation of chloride are of value as a check on the accuracy of the other plasma electrolytes, in case of electrolyte imbalance (disturbance in homeostasis), since the sum of sodium and potassium (in mEq per L) is usually 20 more than the sum of chloride and bicarbonate.

Specimen Use serum that has been separated from the blood clot soon after drawing. Grossly haemolysed serum should not be used as it may create false decreased values. Avoid contamination of blood with tissue fluid. Store the serum in tightly capped tubes. Chloride is stable in serum for one day at room temperature, up to one week in refrigerator and for three months if frozen.

Laboratory assay

There are several methodologies available for measuring chloride, including ion selective electrode (ISE) which is most commonly used by reference laboratories. The older amperometric (coulometric) titration and mercurometric titration are no longer in use for various reasons. Colorimetric assay of chloride is most suitable to peripheral laboratories of developing countries. The kits are now available and it is easy to follow.

Colorimetric Method The method described here does not require protein free filtrate.

Principle

$$Hg(SCN)_2 + 2Cl^- \rightarrow HgCl_2 + 2SCN^- 3SCN^- + Fe^{3+} \rightarrow 4\ Fe(SCN)_3 \text{ (red complex)}$$

Chloride ions form a soluble non-ionized compound with mercuric ions and displace thiocyanate ions from non-ionized mercuric thiocyanate. The released thiocyanate ions react with ferric ions to form a colour complex that absorbs light at 480 nm. The intensity of the colour produced is directly proportional to the chloride concentration.

Equipment and supplies

- Spectrophotometer or colorimeter (480–520 nm)
- Standard laboratory glassware
- Laboratory supplies for chemical assays

Reagent Commercial kit from a reliable company is recommended. The reagents are in ready to use form and stable at room temperature until the expiration date stated on the label. Clearly mark the reagent bottle as **POISON**. It contains hazardous chemicals (mercury and methanol). If swallowed, it can be fatal. Do not pipette by mouth. Do not dispose the reagent in the sink. Take appropriate disposal procedures. The reagents are stable until the expiration date stated on the label. Store the reagent at room temperature. Protect from light. Do not use the reagent if the colour changes to red-brown and/or cloudy. The reagent should be clear, pale-yellow solution. Standard solution is also included.

- *Chloride reagent* (*active ingredient*)

Mercuric nitrate	0.058 mM
Mercuric thiocyanate	1.75 mM
Mercuric chloride	0.74 mM
Ferric nitrate	22.3 mM

    Non-reactive ingredients and stabilizers in dilute acid and methanol.
- *Standard solution (100 mEq/L)*: Weigh dry 5.850 g of NaCl (analytical grade) and quantitatively transfer into a 1-L volumetric flask (wash down with distilled water), dissolve by mixing and make it to the volume (1 L).

Procedure

1. Label test tubes as 'B' (blank), 'S' (standard) and 'T' (test). If there are more tests, number them as T_1, T_2, etc.
2. Put them in a test tube stand.
3. Pipette 1.5 mL chloride reagent to each tube.
4. Add 0.01 mL (10 µL) of standard and sample to respective tubes. Mix.
5. Incubate at room temperature for at least 5 min.
6. Set the spectrophotometer to 480 nm (filter 480–520 nm) and zero with reagent blank.

7. Read and record the absorbance readings of all tubes—A_S, A_T (A_{T1}, A_{T2}, etc).
8. *Calculation:*

$$A_T/A_S \times \text{Concentration of standard} = \text{Concentration of chloride (mEq/L)}$$

Note: Follow manufacturer's instruction, if different from what is described here.

Calibration It is not necessary to determine a standard curve with this procedure since the reaction is essentially linear in a range of 70–140 mEq/L

Quality control Normal and abnormal control sera of known concentrations of chloride should be analysed routinely with each group of unknown samples.

Additional Notes:
- Samples with chloride values above 140 mEq/L should be diluted 1:1 with distilled water. Rerun, and resulting values are multiplied by 2.
- Hydrochloric acid fumes and fumes from chloride bleach may cause high results.
- Bromide and fluoride can cause falsely elevated chloride values.
- Lipaemic and/or icteric sera do not interfere in the reaction.

Normal range

Serum: 98–106 mmole/L (or mEq/L)
Sweat: 5–35 mmole/L (or mEq/L)
Urine: 110–250 mmole/day (varies with chloride intake)

Note: These values should only be taken as guidelines. It is recommended that each laboratory establish its own range of expected values since differences exist between instruments, laboratories and local population.

ACID–BASE BALANCE AND BLOOD GASES

Acid–base and electrolyte balance govern the **homeostatic** mechanism of the body. Two organs are closely associated with this balance—lungs and kidney. They communicate through the mediation of hormones. The acid–base balance is finally reflected by the pH, which is delicately maintained at pH 7.4 in blood. These biochemical information, obtained through blood analysis, are used to assess patients in life-threatening situations (Table 33.2). Although the technicians working in peripheral laboratories are rarely involved with the analyses of blood gases and the parameters of acid–base balance, but a physiological knowledge of body's complicated balancing act help them to understand the crucial role played by the laboratories. This section is devoted towards the understanding of acid–base physiology and the way the laboratories interact with the attending physicians. Before we pitch into this complicated discussion, we need to require a review of several basic concepts: acid–base, buffer, pH, pK, the principles of equilibrium and the law of mass action.

Definitions

Such as electrolytes, acids and bases, when in solution, are ionized. The ions carry an electrical charge, + or – and migrate towards the opposite poles when held in an electrical field. For example, the electrolyte sodium chloride (NaCl) ionizes into Na^+ and Cl^-, the hydrochloric acid (HCl) ionizes into H^+ and Cl^- and the alkali sodium hydroxide (NaOH) or a base, ionizes into Na^+ and OH^-. An **acid** is a substance that can yield a hydrogen ion (H+) or hydronium ion when dissolved in water. Hydrochloric acid H^+Cl^- is a familiar example. A **base** is a substance that can yield hydroxyl ions (OH^-). Sodium hydroxide (Na^+OH^-) is a base. The base with OH^- ion is capable of accepting the H+ ion of the acid. The union of these two ions—H and OH—produces water, with no charged ions.

$$\text{HCl} + \text{NaOH} \rightarrow \text{NaCl} + \text{H(OH)}$$
$$\text{Acid} + \text{Base} \rightarrow \text{Salt} + \text{water (H}_2\text{O)}$$

Total strength of an acid or base is determined by its **normality (N)**. Thus equal volumes of hydrochloric acid and sodium hydroxide, both of 1 N strength, will neutralize each other, yielding water and sodium chloride. They have lost their powers as acid or base. However, the total strength (normality) does not truly express their reactivity. To give an example, if you put your finger into a 6 N hydrochloric acid it will burn your finger but if you do the same with same strength (6 N) boric acid, you will not get hurt.

To make things clear, let us take an example from our daily life. Imagine two friends and both own $100. One of them (A) has $98 in the wallet and $2 in bank while the other (B) has $6 in the wallet and $94 in the bank. Now they arrive in a shop, which only accepts cash for any purchase. Who is richer in this situation? Obviously, it is the friend A. The same situation is with hydrochloric acid and boric acid. 98% of H+ ions of hydrochloric acid are in ionized state while with boric acid it is only 6% although both of them may be of same strength of normality ($100). Therefore, boric acid is **weak acid** and hydrochloric acid is a **strong acid**. In other words, the concentration or activity of hydrogen ions in a solution determines the acidity or reactivity of the acid. The same holds good for alkali. Sodium hydroxide is a strong alkali whereas bicarbonate is a weak alkali. The degree of ionization is defined by a constant, **K**, which characterizes the strength of the acid. The larger the value of K, the stronger the acid and the greater is the tendency of it to dissociate.

Hydrogen ion activity of a solution also determines the pH of the solution. In other words, pH is a symbol relating to the hydrogen ion (H^+) concentration. Numerically the pH is approximately equal to the negative logarithm of the hydrogen ion (H^+) activity in aqueous solution.

$$pH = \log_{10} \frac{1}{H^+}.$$

By virtue of its logarithmic nature, pH is a dimensionless quantity. Thus, pH decreases as [H^+] increases and, conversely, pH increases as [H^+] decreases. The pH ranges from 1 to 14, where 1 is the strong acid and 14 is the strong base. The water (neutral) has a pH of 7.0 where H and OH ions are in equal proportion. As the pH goes above 7.0, it gets increasingly alkaline which can be scaled as decreasing H^+ ion (increasing OH). On the other hand, when the pH goes below 7.0, there is increasing amount of H^+ ion (decreasing OH). Since this relationship is also logarithmic in nature, the correlation between pH an [H^+] is not linear. As illustration of this point, a decrease of 1 pH unit represents a 10-fold increase in the hydrogen ion activity.

A **buffer**, composed of a weak acid or weak base and its corresponding salt, is a system that resists change in pH. The **law of mass action** applies to the dissociation reaction equilibrium is established between the weak acid and its dissociated ions. Like pH, pK is defined as the negative log of the **ionization constant** (K). Strong acids have pK values less than 3.0, whereas strong bases have pK values greater than 9.0. For acids, raising the pH above the pK will cause the acid to dissociate and yield a [H^+]. For bases, lowering the pH below the pK will cause the base to release [OH^-]. The lower the value of pK, the stronger is the acid; likewise, the higher the pK, the weaker is the acid.

Handerson–Hasselbalch equation explains how the buffer system works to stabilize the pH of the body fluids in circulation:

$$pH = pK + \log\left(\frac{\text{Bicarbonate}}{\text{Carbonic acid}}\right)$$

Carbonic acid (H_2CO_3) is a weak acid with bicarbonate (HCO_3^-) serving as its conjugate base. When acid is added to this system, the hydrogen ions react with bicarbonate to form more carbonic acid and thus minimize changes in pH.

Note: Both bicarbonate and carbonic acid can be expressed in mEq/L. Carbonic acid, however, can also be expressed as PCO_2. The mathematical relationship is given in this equation:

$$H_2CO_3 = 0.03 \times PCO_2 \text{ mm Hg}.$$

At body temperature, the pK of the buffer pair bicarbonate-carbonic acid is 6.1 and the ratio of bicarbonate (HCO_3^-) and carbonic acid (H_2CO_3) is maintained by the body precisely at 20 : 1. Thus, under normal conditions, the above equation can be written as:

$$pH = 6.1 + \log 20 \quad Or, \quad pH = 6.1 + 1.3^* = 7.4$$

*The value of log 20 = 1.3.

The variation of this ratio is the cause of pH imbalance. The bicarbonate level of the blood is maintained by the kidney (metabolic), whereas the carbonic acid, or PCO_2 level is regulated by the lungs (respiratory).

There are four **clinically important buffers systems** that maintain the normal pH balance in the body between the narrow range of 7.35 and 7.45. These buffers, in order of decreasing physiologic importance, are the bicarbonate–carbonic acid buffer system, haemoglobin, plasma proteins, and phosphates. Although not considered to be the most important physiologically, haemoglobin accounts for the majority (80%) of the chemical buffering capacity of the blood. Plasma proteins are the next most abundant buffer, representing approximately 14% of the chemical buffering capacity of the blood. The remainder of the buffering capacity is represented by the bicarbonate–carbonic acid system (~5%) and inorganic phosphates (~1%). In the body, most buffering takes place inside the cell, where all of the four major buffer systems are found. Outside of the cell, plasma buffer include bicarbonate, proteins and inorganic phosphates.

Lungs participate in the intake of oxygen and removal of carbon dioxide, the product of oxidative respiration. Oxygen is transported primarily through the haemoglobin of the red cells and it also releases the carbon dioxide. Both these gases are bound to haemoglobin to meet the demand of numerous cells of the body. Partial pressure of the oxygen in blood determines to a great extend how much oxygen the haemoglobin will carry. The other two factors are the normal effective haemoglobin and affinity of the available haemoglobin. The affinity of haemoglobin for oxygen shifts, increased–decreased, with change in pH, PCO_2, 2,3-DPG (2,3-diphosphoglycerate) and temperature. The analysis of PCO_2 helps to understand the H_2CO_3 status which is controlled by lungs. Blood gas analysers determine PCO_2. The value of pH gives the end result of the acid–base imbalance and is determined by potentiometry. Bicarbonate level (HCO_3^-) is regulated by the kidney. Thus ventilation by lungs and discharge of bicarbonate by kidney regulate the bicarbonate–carbonic acid ratio of the body's buffer system. For the normal function of the body, this ratio must stay close to 20 : 1.

The **acid–base (pH) imbalance** in blood leads to four major clinical conditions—metabolic acidosis, metabolic alkalosis, respiratory acidosis and respiratory alkalosis. The trend of laboratory reports and the causes of these pathologic conditions are shown in Table 33.2. The fall of plasma bicarbonate is often associated with metabolic acidosis. Metabolic acidosis can also be caused under untreated diabetic conditions due to building up of ketone bodies (Chapter 29 in this Volume). This leads to increased anion gap.

Table 33.2 Laboratory findings in acidosis and alkalosis

Clinical condition	Bicarbonate	PCO_2	pH	PO_2	Cause
Metabolic acidosis	Fall	Fall*	Fall	Normal	Excessive discharge of urinary bicarb. High anion gap.
Metabolic alkalosis	Rise	Rise	Rise	Rise	Poor discharge of urinary bicarb.
Respiratory acidosis	Rise* or Normal	Rise	Fall	Fall	Hypoventilation and CO accumulation
Respiratory alkalosis	Fall*	Fall	Rise	Normal	Hyperventilation and fall of CO_2 level

*May be late in compensation.

Anion gap is a concept used to estimate electrolyte (anion and cation) levels in the serum and conditions that influence them. The anion gap ranges from 8 to 15 mEq/L in normal patients. This is estimated by subtracting the sum of the anions chloride and bicarbonate ($Cl^- + HCO_3^-$) which is (103 + 27) mEq/L from the sum of the cations sodium and potassium ($Na^+ + K^+$) which is (140 + 4) mEq/L. Because the potassium cation is low in serum (4.5 Eq/L), the anion gap is calculated by the formula $Na^+ - (Cl^- + HCO_3^-)$ or 140 − (103 + 27) = 10 mEq/L of anion gap. With the building up of ketone bodies (which contains organic acids), the acid level of blood increases (pH falls below 7.4) and the anion gap increases. This is called diabetic acidosis.

The laboratory determinations of pH, PCO_2 (partial pressure of carbon dioxide in mmHg), PO_2 (partial pressure or tension of oxygen in mmHg), oxygen saturation of haemoglobin (%) and bicarbonate concentration (mEq/L) help in the understanding of the acid–base imbalance. The concentration of 2,3-DPG (diphosphoglycerate), an intermediate metabolite in red cells, is not determined because of technical difficulties. With the easy availability of blood gas analysers, bicarbonate determination by titrimetry has practically become obsolete. Because of cost involvement, most peripheral laboratories in developing countries cannot afford blood gas analysers. Hence, titrimetric assay of bicarbonate is described here.

Specimen

Heparinized venous blood is commonly submitted to the laboratory on ice for the analysis of blood gases. Arterial blood is recommended but is difficult to obtain.

Determination of Blood Gases

Blood gases and pH are determined electrochemically (Chapter 31 in this Volume). Determinations of pH and PCO_2 are done by the potentiometric method. The blood analyser is convenient to use; it is accurate but expensive under conditions of developing countries. On the other hand, the use of a microgasometer is not only cumbersome but often proves to be erroneous due to a number of factors inherent in the technique. An alternative procedure is to determine the pH and bicarbonate and consult the nomogram (Fig. 33.3) to find out the PCO_2. Titrimetric analysis of bicarbonate is presented here.

Only the blood gas analysers do determination of the partial pressure of oxygen (PO_2). The clinical significance of PO_2 determination is to assess the oxygen carrying capacity of haemoglobin. An elevated PO_2 may be related to decreased oxygen affinity of the haemoglobin, low plasma pH, and high PCO_2. Because of the non-availability of the blood gas analyser in routine laboratories of developing countries, we will confine our further discussion to the determination of pH and bicarbonate. Determination

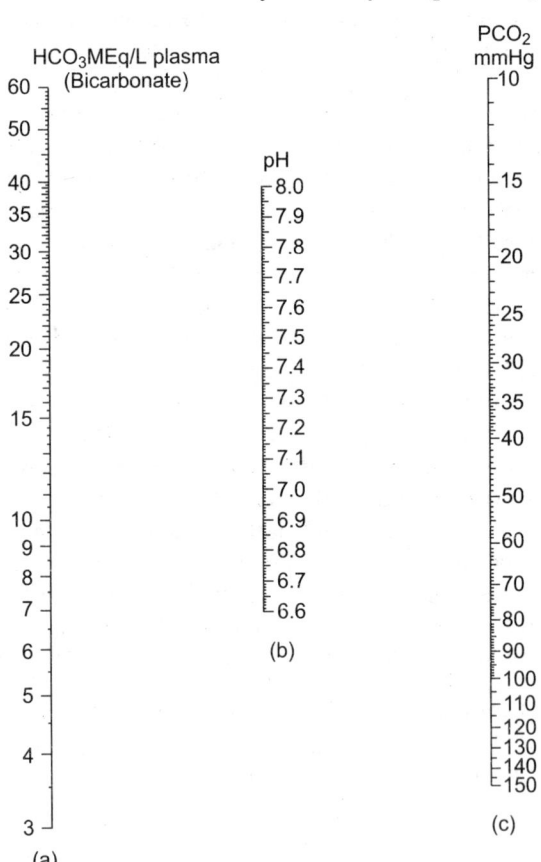

Fig. 33.3 *Siggaard Andersen alignment nomogram for the determination of acid-base values. Determine the bicarbonate and pH. Locate the values on the left and middle scales, join the points with a ruler, and extend the line to the PCO_2 scale to determine the corresponding value.*

of SO_2 by pulse oximetry (SpO_2) has become very popular. It is a non-invasive procedure and the instrument is not expensive. The devise pass light of two or more wavelengths through the tissue of the toe, finger, or ear. The pulse oximeter differentiates between the absorption of light as a result of oxyhaemoglobin and deoxyhaemoglobin in the capillary bed and calculates oxyhaemoglobin saturation. The results are not totally reliable and dependent on the pulse rate. A low oxygen saturation, below 95%, may be associated with breathing difficulties.

Normal Values

pH (serum or plasma):	7.35–7.45
Bicarbonate:	19–28 mmole/L
PCO_2:	35–45 mm Hg
PO_2:	83–108 mm Hg (varies with age)
SO_2:	95–99%

Determination of serum/plasma bicarbonate by titrimetry

If the blood gas analyser is available, determination of PCO_2 and PO_2 become easy and is recommended because of the high degree of accuracy in the results. The alternative titrimetric method, which is described here, is suitable for the laboratories of developing countries. The values of the bicarbonate concentration of serum or plasma (heparinized) and pH, as determined by titration and potentiometry, respectively, help to determine the PCO_2 level from the nomogram (Fig. 33.3).

Specimen

1. Obtain 3 mL or more of blood by venipuncture in the usual manner.
2. Place in a clean dry tube of about 3–5 mL volume.
3. Stopper the tube and allow a clot to form.
4. After the clot retracts, the serum may be obtained directly or by centrifuging. Exposure to air should be minimal until the serum has been separated from the cells. Heparinized plasma may also be used.
5. Keep the serum in sealed containers or under liquid paraffin. If the specimen is processed promptly, this may not be necessary.

Principle Serum is added to pre-standardized hydrochloric acid and the loss of strength is considered to be due to bicarbonate. Although the serum buffer system may affect neutralization, it is considered here as minor. The difference in the strengths of HC1 is determined by titrating against NaOH (0.01 N), using a mixed indicator. The titration is then standardized by the use of standard bicarbonate solution in place of serum. *Note:* Heparin is expensive and unstable in hot climate. Some laboratories use oxalated blood (5 mg/5 mL) for plasma bicarbonate determination. Oxalated blood cannot be used for pH determination.

Reagents

- *Hydrochloric acid standard (0.1 N):* Purchase concentrated volumetric solution (e.g. 1 N HC1) from a local dealer and dilute it to the desired strength of 0.1 N.
- *Sodium hydroxide standard:*
  - *Stock standard (0.1 N):* Dissolve 5.0 g (approximately) of sodium hydroxide pellets in freshly boiled and cooled water (CCL free) and make up to about 1000 mL. Sodium carbonate will settle to the bottom in a few days; use the supernatant for titration. Determine the strength by titrating against 0.1 N HCl or 0.1 N H_2SO_4 using methyl orange or phenol red as the indicator. Dilute the alkali to obtain 0.1 N NaOH. Store in a polythene bottle. The strength is likely to decrease with time due to absorption of atmospheric carbon dioxide. Alternatively, purchase 1 N NaOH from a local dealer and dilute it to 10-fold volume.

o   *Working standard of sodium hydroxide (0.01 N):* Make a 10-fold dilution of the stock standard with freshly boiled and cooled distilled water. Determine the correct strength of the stock standard before dilution.
- *Mixed indicator:*
  o   Neutral red solution (0.065% in methyl alcohol): Dissolve 65 mg of neutral red in 50% methyl alcohol and make up to 100 mL.
  o   Methylene blue (0.065% in methyl alcohol): Dissolve 65 mg of methylene blue in 50% methyl alcohol and make up to 100 mL. *Note:* If it is difficult to weigh a small quantity of indicator, prepare a stronger solution and dilute it to the above concentration.
  o   Mixed indicator: Mix 50 mL of (a) with 15 mL of (b).
  Note: Some laboratories use phenol red indicator (0.1%, aqueous). Use one drop for titration.
- *Phenol red indicator (0.1%):* Dissolve 100 mg of water soluble sodium salt of phenol red in water and make it up to 100 mL; use one drop for titration.
- *Standard bicarbonate solution (25 mEq/L):* Weigh 2.100 g dry sodium bicarbonate, dissolve in water, and make it up to 1000 mL. The sodium bicarbonate should be AR grade and dried for several hours in an oven at about 80°C. Before weighing, allow to cool to room temperature in a closed vessel. Discard most of the solution; 100 mL is sufficient to keep for use. Keep the standard solution tightly stoppered in a glass bottle.

Procedure

1. Prepare a fresh working standard of sodium hydroxide (0.01 N) and determine the exact normality by titrating against 1.00 mL of 0.1 N HCl, using one drop of phenol red indicator. Normality of NaOH = (0.1 × 1)/Titre-volume of NaOH
2. Check the bicarbonate concentration of standard:
Pipette 1.0 mL of 0.1N HCl into a titration flask (Erlenmeyer, 25-mL) and add 1.0 mL standard bicarbonate solution (0.025 mEq/L), swirl for about 30 sec and then leave to stand for 5 min. Titrate with sodium hydroxide (0.01 N).
Bicarbonate conc. (mEq/L) = 100 − (Difference in NaOH titration volumes × 10)
   Note: 100 = Strength of acid (0.1 N in mEq/L)
              10 = Conversion of 0.01 N NaOH to mEq/L
The difference of NaOH titration volume should be 7.5 mL if the bicarbonate standard is 25 mEq/L.
3. Take three titration flasks (25-mL); label them as 'B' (blank), 'S' (standard) and 'T' (test).
4. Add 5 mL of working HCl acid solution (0.01N) in all the three flasks.
5. Add 1 mL of bicarbonate standard (25 mEq/L) in the flask marked 'S' and 1 mL of serum in the flask marked 'T'.
6. Add 0.5 mL of mixed indicator in each flask and mix thoroughly.
7. With the help of a micro burette, titrate the blank acid solution against 0.01 N (10 mEq/L) NaOH until the solution is of a permanent green colour.
8. *Note the burette readings:* T_B for blank (acid only); T_S for bicarbonate standard and T_T for test serum specimen.
9. *Calculation:*
   (a) Using bicarbonate standard:
       Bicarbonate (mEq/L) = $(T_B − T_T)/T_S × 25$
   (b) Without bicarbonate standard: In this case it is important that the strength of hydrochloric acid is correctly determined.
       Bicarbonate concentration (mEq/L) = 100 − (D ×10)
       100 = Strength of acid (0.1N) in mEq/L

D = Difference in the NaOH titration value ($T_B - T_T$), using 0.01N NaOH
10 = Conversion of 0.01N strength of NaOH to mEq/L

Additional information Determination of serum or plasma bicarbonate is of little value for the differentiation of metabolic acidosis and respiratory alkalosis where the bicarbonate level falls. The bicarbonate concentration can, however, be used for the determination of PCO_2 level (Fig. 33.3).

Review Questions

1. List the routine biochemical analyses of serum and give the principle on which the analyses are based.
2. What is the clinical significance of each of the following biochemical analysis of serum: Glucose, protein, bilirubin, phosphorous and cholesterol?
3. What is the clinical significance of determining the transaminase level of serum? How are the results correlated with other biochemical findings?
4. How would you determine true glucose? What is the clinical significance of true glucose determination?
5. Under which clinical conditions would you expect a rise of serum protein level?
6. Why do you need fluoride as the anticoagulant for the determination of plasma glucose and BUN?
7. What are the laboratory findings in case of obstructive jaundice?
8. How are the following related: Diabetes mellitus, anion gap and metabolic acidosis?
9. What is the significance of serum bicarbonate determination?
10. A haemolysed sample will cause falsely increased levels of each of the following, EXCEPT: Potassium, sodium, phosphate and magnesium.
11. What is the significance of Henderson–Hasselbalch equation?
12. What is the role of lungs in maintaining pH balance in blood?
13. Name some of the important buffer system of the body.
14. How is SO_2 determined? What is its significance?
15. *Case study 1*: A 64 year old woman with chronic obstructive pulmonary disease (COPD) was admitted to the emergency department with extreme shortness of breath. She had a bluish colour that was particularly pronounced on her lips and nail beds and she displayed a weak and persistent cough with diminished, but rattling breath sounds. Home medication included bronchodilators, steroids, lasix (a loop diuretic that does not conserve plasma potassium), and digitalis.
    Vital signs: Heart rate, 148; blood pressure, 100/88; temperature, 37°C and respiratory rate, 38. *Blood gas results:* pH, 7.289; PCO_2, 91 mm/Hg; PO_2, 53 mm Hg; bicarbonate (HCO_3^-), 43 mmol/L.
    What is the patient's acid–base status?
    In addition to COPD, what condition likely contributed to her poor gas exchange (hypercarbia and hyoxemia)?
16. *Case study 2*: Her parents brought a 15-year-old girl in a coma to the emergency. She was diabetic and insulin dependent. The parents stated that she had several episodes of hypoglycaemia and ketoacidosis in the past, and their daughter has often been 'too busy' to take her insulin injections. Her blood and urine studies revealed the following abnormalities:
    Venous blood: Potassium ↑ Chloride ↓ Bicarbonate ↓ Glucose ↑ Urea ↑ Lactate ↑
    Arterial blood: pH ↓ PCO_2 ↓
    Urine: Glucose ↑ Ketone ↑
    What is the reason for the fall of chloride and bicarbonate? What is the significance of elevated potassium? What is the diagnosis?

34

Biochemical Test Profiles

◆

Subir Paul

Chapter Outline

Analytes commonly tested in chemistry
- ◆ *Protein (For General Checkup)*
  - *Total serum protein*
  - *Albumin*
  - *A/G ratio*
- ◆ *Electrolytes*
- ◆ *Mineral Metabolism*
  - *Calcium*
  - *Phosphorus*
  - *Iron*
- ◆ *Kidney (Renal) Function Tests*
  - *Creatinine*
  - *Blood urea nitrogen*
  - *Uric acid*
- ◆ *Liver Function Tests*
  - *Bilirubin*
  - *Liver enzymes*
- ◆ *Cardiac Function Tests*
- ◆ *Lipid Metabolism*
  - *Cholesterol*
  - *Triglycerides*
- ◆ *Carbohydrate Metabolism*
- ◆ *Thyroid Function Tests*
- ◆ *Other Tests of Organ Function*

- *Creatinine clearance for kidney function*
  - Calculation of clearance rate
    - Uncorrected
    - Corrected
- *Gastric Function tests*
- *Pancreatic Function Tests*
- *Tests for Malabsorption*
  - D-xylose absorption test
- *Review Questions*

The physician orders the biochemical tests as a single test or as a **chemistry profile**. A chemistry profile is a group of tests performed simultaneously on a patient specimen to provide an assessment of the patient's general condition. The physician can use the results of the chemistry profile, in conjunction with the physical examination, to assess the overall health of the patient.

Tests included in a **routine chemistry profile** reflect the state of carbohydrate and lipid metabolism, as well as kidney, thyroid, liver and cardiac function. Profiles or panels that assess one particular biological system, such as renal or liver function are also performed. Examples of chemistry panels are shown in Table 34.1. These tests are requested when a particular diagnosis is suspected or treatment must be monitored. Many automated instruments used in advanced laboratories are designed to provide '**panel test**' results. In developing countries, however, individual tests are handled independently.

ANALYTES COMMONLY TESTED IN CHEMISTRY PROFILES

Nearly 15 biochemical tests are routinely done in peripheral laboratories of developing countries. Others are sent to reference laboratories. Results of these tests can be used in more than one panel. Before we discuss the '**organ function tests**', an overview of the basic tests may be helpful.

PROTEIN (FOR GENERAL CHECKUP)

Two major groups of serum proteins are the **albumins** and the **globulins**. Albumins comprise approximately 60% of total serum protein and globulin about 40%. The albumins are made in liver, serve as transport proteins and help maintain the fluid balance in the body. Antibodies, blood coagulation proteins, enzymes and proteins that transport iron (transferrin) are all serum globulin.

Total Serum Protein

Total serum protein (6.0–8.0 g/dL) represents the sum of many different proteins. Total protein levels are increased in patients with dehydration, chronic inflammatory conditions or certain blood cancers. A decrease of serum protein can be related to malnutrition, loss through urine (proteinuria caused by kidney disorder) or lack of synthesis due to liver disorder. Most serum proteins are made in the **liver**.

Albumin

Albumin is produced by the **liver** and is the main protein in the blood. It gives the blood its **oncotic pressure** or colloid osmotic pressure, which prevents leakage of plasma fluid from the small blood vessels or capillaries into the tissues, thereby causing edema. Albumin also functions to bind drugs to **transport** them via the blood to body tissues. Decreased albumin levels may be due to its reduced synthesis in liver disease, or from loss through the gastrointestinal tract or urine in diseases of the bowel or kidneys. High levels can occur with dehydration.

Table 34.1 Biochemical test profiles

Panels	Tests
General (1) (Overall check up)	Glucose
	Total protein
	BUN
	Bilirubin (Total)
	Albumin Calcium
	Phosphorus
	Uric acid
	Alkaline phosphatase
	SGOT
	LDH
	Cholesterol
	A/G ratio
	Globulin
Thyroid (2) (Thyroid function)	T3
	T4
	T7
Renal (3) (Kidney function)	Creatinine
	BUN
	Uric acid
	Sodium
	Potassium
	CO_2
	Chloride
	Glucose
	Albumin,
	Total bilirubin,
Hepatic (4) (Liver function)	Direct bilirubin,
	Alkaline phosphatase,
	Total protein,
	ALT/SGPT,
	AST/SGOT
	LDH
	Globulin
Lipid (5)	Cholesterol,
	Triglyceride,
	HDL,
	LDL
Cardiac (6) (Heart function)	SGOT
	LDHCK
	(Isoenzymes done if CK is elevated)
Iron (7)	Total iron
	Total iron binding capacity
	Unsaturated iron binding capacity
Electrolytes (8)	Sodium,
	Potassium,
	Chloride,
	Carbon dioxide

A/G Ratio

The **albumin/globulin ratio** is often computed from the values of total protein and albumin. Globulin is the difference between total protein and albumin (Total protein – albumin = globulin). A fall of A/G ratio may be due to increase in globulin concentration in serum (viral infection) or decrease in albumin concentration due to loss (proteinuria) or poor synthesis (liver damage). So, a change in the A/G ratio indicates one of the many disorders whose further investigation must be initiated.

ELECTROLYTES

In clinical chemistry, the term electrolytes refers to the **major cations**—sodium (Na^+) and potassium (K^+) and the **major anions**—chloride (Cl^-) and bicarbonate (HCO_3^-). Electrolytes have a great effect on acid—base (pH) balance, as well as on heart, brain and muscle function. Fluid volume status in the body can affect electrolytes. Electrolytes measurement is included in most routine chemistry profiles and renal profiles.

MINERAL METABOLISM

Minerals are necessary for good health. Calcium, phosphorus (phosphate) and iron are examples of minerals often measured in chemistry profiles. **Calcium and phosphorus** are necessary for proper bone and tooth formation. Calcium is also required for blood coagulation. **Iron** is essential for haemoglobin production and is an integral component of some enzymes.

Calcium

Of all the minerals found in the body **calcium** is present in highest concentration. Approximately 99% of the body's calcium is bound in calcium complexes in the skeleton and is not metabolically active. Only unbound calcium ions are metabolically active and are measured in the calcium assay. Calcium is required for proper blood coagulation and for normal neuromuscular excitability. Vitamin D, parathyroid hormone, estrogens and calcitonin influence the calcium balance. These control dietary absorption of calcium, calcium excretion by the kidneys, and calcium movement in and out of bone.

Hypercalcemia (increased level of blood calcium) occurs in hyperparathyroidism, malignancies, certain hormonal disorders, excessive calcium and vitamin D intake, sarcoidosis and immobilization. It can cause calcium to be deposited in soft tissues, vascular wall, heart valve and other organs, leading to complications such as calcification and **kidney stones**. **Hypocalcemia** (decreased level of blood calcium) can be **life threatening** and should be reported to the physician immediately. This may be caused by hypoparathyroidism, hypothyroidism, vitamin D deficiency, poor calcium absorption due to intestinal disease and kidney disease.

Phosphorus

Most phosphorus in the body is in the form of inorganic phosphate. Approximately 80% is in the bone and the rest is mostly in **high-energy compounds** such as adenosine triphosphate (ATP). Calcium and certain hormones influence phosphorus levels. Elevated blood phosphors levels could be seen as an artefact of sample haemolysis but can also signify kidney diseases, hypoparathyroidism, severe muscle injury or certain bone conditions.

Iron

Iron is essential for **haemoglobin synthesis**. Iron is absorbed from dietary sources and is highly conserved by the body. Iron levels differ with age, gender and time of day, being higher in the morning than in the evening or night.

Iron deficiency can lead to **anaemia**. The deficiency can be due to insufficient iron in the diet, poor iron absorption, impaired release of stored iron or increased iron loss due to bleeding. Serum iron levels can be elevated with haemolytic anaemias, increased iron intake or blocked synthesis of iron-containing compounds, such as occurs in lead poisoning.

KIDNEY (RENAL) FUNCTION TESTS

The primary functions of the kidney are to remove the waste materials of metabolism and to preserve an optimum internal environment for cells (pH, water balance, electrolyte balance and fluid osmotic pressure). Thus substances are excreted into and reabsorbed from urine to help maintain **homeostasis**. These physiological processes are largely controlled by various hormones. Apart from this, kidneys are also the production sites for certain essential hormones of the body. The serum and plasma concentration of certain substances such as creatinine, BUN, sodium, potassium, bicarbonate, phosphorus and uric acid are altered in certain kidney diseases.

Currently used **kidney function tests** are as follows:

- **Serum creatinine**: Waste product formed in muscle. It has a relatively constant excretion rate and its concentration in serum is a fairly good measure of glomerular filtration rate. Creatinine is not reabsorbed by the tubule; therefore, any condition, which reduces glomerular filtration rate, will result in reduced excretion in urine with a consequent increase in plasma.
- **Blood urea nitrogen**: Urea is a waste product of protein break down which appears in the glomerular filtrate but approximately 40%, is reabsorbed in the tubule. In addition, its plasma concentration is strongly influenced by diet and other physiological conditions not connected with renal function. Hence, serum creatinine is considered as a better indicator of renal function. However, the serum concentration of urea (or BUN) rises in impaired renal function just as creatinine does.
- **Uric acid**
- **Glomerular filtration rate (GFR)**: This is also known as clearance test. It determines the filtration capacity of the nephrons. Marked decrease of GFR indicates kidney disorder. This will be discussed separately with 'Other Functional Tests'.
- **Urine analysis (physical and microscopic)**: This provides the general picture of the kidney function; excellent for screening. Presence of casts (microscopic examination), proteinuria, decreased volume and increased specific gravity indicate kidney failure. This has been discussed under Urinalysis (Chapter 25 in Vol. II).
- **Blood electrolytes**: Blood electrolytes (especially chloride) tend to accumulate if they are unable to get out of blood circulation through the renal route. Thus an increased concentration of blood electrolytes may indicate renal disorder. This will be discussed in the chemistry section.

Here we will focus on three commonly analysed serum components that directly indicate kidney disease—creatinine, BUN and uric acid. In addition, we will discuss the methodology for determining GFR separately.

Creatinine

Creatinine is a waste product of **creatine phosphate**, a substance stored in muscle and used for energy. Creatinine is excreted by kidney. When renal function is impaired, blood creatinine levels rise. Creatinine level is not affected by diet or hormone levels. Hence, the rise of blood creatinine level diagnoses the impairment of urine formation or excretion, which occurs in renal disease, shock and water imbalance or urinary blockage.

Blood Urea Nitrogen

In human body, surplus **amino acids** are converted to **urea,** which is excreted by the kidneys. This surplus is measured as **BUN**.

Diet, hormones and kidney function influence the level of BUN. Therefore, BUN level is not as good as indicator of kidney disease as is the **creatinine level**. BUN level can be low during starvation, pregnancy, and a low-protein diet. Increased BUN concentration can occur during a high-protein diet after administration of steroids, and in kidney disease.

Uric Acid

Uric acid is formed from the **breakdown nucleic acids** and is excreted by the kidneys. It has low solubility and tends to precipitate as uric acid crystals, or urates. Uric acid measurement is principally used to diagnose and treat **gout**, a disease in which uric acid precipitates in tissues and joints, causing pain. Uric acid levels can also increase after massive radiation or chemotherapy because of increased cell destruction.

LIVER FUNCTION TESTS

The liver is both a **secretory** and **excretory** organ of the body and has numerous metabolic functions. The liver is closely associated with **carbohydrate metabolism** (synthesis of glycogen from glucose), **protein metabolism** (most plasma proteins are made in liver) and **lipid metabolism** (source of cholesterol). The liver stores a number of essential substances and makes them available when needed—glycogen, vitamins, iron and others. It also destroys old cells by phagocytosis and causes detoxification of many substances.

Significant liver function must be lost or impaired before some laboratory tests show abnormality. Numerous tests are used to estimate liver function. Most are not specific for a particular disease but only reflect liver tissue damage or liver dysfunction. The tests which are routinely followed for assessing liver function are as follows:

- **Serum bilirubin (total and direct)**: Diagnoses conjugation disorders and bile duct obstruction.
- **Serum enzymes**: transaminases or amino transferases (SCOT or AST, SGPT or ALT) and ALP (alkaline phosphatase): Confirms the damage in the liver that has caused the release of the liver enzymes.
- **Serum total protein and albumin**: Examines the liver's function in the synthesis of albumin.
- **Urine bilirubin**: Confirms bile duct obstruction resulting in the rise of conjugated bilirubin in serum and its excretion through the kidney.
- **Urine urobilinogen**: Suggests increased haemolysis, bilirubin production and discharge of urobilinogen through the kidney.
- **Serum cholesterol (total)**: Assesses the liver's function in lipid metabolism.
- **Prothrombin time**: Assesses the liver's function in producing coagulation factors.

In the following sections, we will focus on **bilirubin** and **liver enzymes** which are routinely used for assessing the liver function.

Bilirubin

Bilirubin is a waste product from **breakdown of haemoglobin**. It is formed in the tissues, then transported to liver and excreted in the bile. In the liver, most bilirubin becomes bound to glucuronide and is then excreted into the bile—this is called **conjugated** or **direct bilirubin**. Bilirubin that is not conjugated is called **indirect bilirubin**. Total serum bilirubin equals direct bilirubin plus indirect bilirubin. Bilirubin assays usually measures both total and direct bilirubin. Indirect bilirubin is then calculated from those two numbers.

Bilirubin is measured to screen for or to monitor liver or gall bladder and **billiary tract** dysfunction. Since bilirubin levels are normally low, only increases in serum bilirubin are significant. Bilirubin can be increased when there is excessive destruction of haemoglobin such as in the haemolytic anaemias, impaired excretion by the liver such as in biliary obstructions including gall bladder stone, or impaired bilirubin processing as in hepatitis.

Liver Enzymes

A rise in liver enzymes generally reflects injury to tissue, since most enzymes are intracellular. Some enzymes are widely distributed in many body tissues, whereas others are found in only a few tissues. The measurement of enzyme levels is not always specific for damage to particular organ but is most helpful when used with other tests, clinical symptoms and patient history.

Enzymes used to assess **liver function** include the following:
- Alkaline phosphatase (ALP)
- **Alanine aminotransferase (ALT)**: formerly called serum glutamic pyruvic transaminase (GPT or SGPT)
- **Aspartate aminotransferase (AST)**: formerly called serum glutamic oxaloacetic transferase (GOT or SGOT)
- Gamma glutamyl transferase (GGT)
- Lactate dehydrogenase (LD or LDH)

Alkaline phosphatase (ALP or AP) is widely distributed in body, especially in bone and the liver ducts. Serum ALP level can greatly increase with liver tumours and lesions and can show a moderate increase with diseases such as hepatitis.

Aminotransferases (ALT and AST) are found in abundance in liver tissues. When liver tissues are injured, these enzymes are released in circulation. Serum concentrations of these enzymes change with time, rising during acute liver disease and falling as recovery occurs. Generally, only one enzyme need be measured—ALT or AST (aspartate aminotransferase). **ALT** levels are low in cardiac tissue and high in liver tissue. This enzyme usually rises higher than AST in liver disease, with moderate increases (up to 10 times normal) in cirrhosis, infections or tumours, and increases up to 100 times normal in viral or toxic hepatitis. **AST** is present in many tissues, particularly cardiac, muscle and liver. It is elevated after myocardial infarction, as well as in liver disease.

Gamma glutamyl transferase (GGT) is found in kidney, pancreas, liver and prostrates tissue. The GGT can be more helpful than AP in determining liver damage because GGT remains normal in bone disease. It is more useful than AST because it remains normal in muscle disorders. GGT measurement is often used to monitor recovery from hepatitis.

Lactic dehydrogenase (LD or LDH) is widely distributed in body tissue. The LD level increases in blood during liver disease and following myocardial infarction. Haemolysis of a blood sample will cause increased LD levels in the serum because of LD release from red blood cells.

A summary of the biochemical findings and their possible diagnosis for liver disorders is presented in Table 34.2.

CARDIAC FUNCTION TESTS

Most commonly used enzyme assay for the diagnosis of myocardial infarction is **creatine kinase** (CK), also called **creatinine phosphokinase** (CPK). It is present in large amounts in muscle and the brain, but in small amounts in organs such as the liver and kidneys. Following **heart attack**, CK is released from the damaged heart muscle. The serum CK level peaks in about 24 h, reaching 5–10 times the upper limit of normal (30–170 U/L). It falls rapidly back to normal levels within 3–4 days. Serum CK levels also increase following skeletal muscle damage and brain injury. It is determined routinely in emergency patients in patients with chest pain and when acute renal failure is suspected. For the differential diagnosis of heart and liver, CK is requested along with SGOT and LDH. Lowered CK can be an indication of alcoholic liver disease and rheumatoid arthritis. Determination of isoenzymes helps to determine the source of the injury. The physician requests for the **isoenzymes** when CK is elevated.

Table 34.2 Findings of biochemical profile in the diagnosis of liver disorders

Test	Acute hepatitis	Chronic hepatitis	Obstructive jaundice
Alkaline phos. (ALP)	1+	1+	3+
AST (SCOT)	3+	1+	1+
ALT (SGPT)	3+	1+	1+
Serum bilirubin			
Conjugated	2+	V	2+
Unconjugated	2+	V	2+
Urine bilirubin	2+	2+	2+
Cholesterol	0	0/1–	2+
Icterus index	2+	V	2+
Protein			
Total	0	0/2–	0
Albumin	2–	2–	0
Prothrombin time	2+	2+	2+
Urobilinogen			
In urine	2+*	2–	2–

Note: 1+, slight increase; 2+, increase; 3+, marked increase; 1–, slight decrease; 2–, decrease; 3–, marked decrease and 0, no change.
V, variable.
*In early stage.

LIPID METABOLISM

Lipids are synthesized in the body from dietary fats. The commonly measured lipids are cholesterol and triglycerides. These are of interest primarily because of their association with cardiovascular disease (CVD).

Cholesterol

Cholesterol is present in all tissues, and the serum concentrations tend to increase with age. Elevated cholesterol levels can increase the risk of coronary, cerebral and peripheral artery disease. It is recommended that total serum cholesterol levels be maintained below 200 mg/dL. Cholesterol fractions such as low-density lipoprotein (**LDL**) cholesterol, high-density lipoprotein (**HDL**) cholesterol and very low density lipoprotein (**VLDL**) cholesterol are also measured.

Triglycerides

Hyperlipidemia is an excess of fatty substances called **lipids**, largely cholesterol and triglycerides, in the blood. Triglycerides are the main form of lipid storage in humans, comprising approximately 95% of fat (adipose) tissue. Triglycerides are **transported** in the plasma bound to **lipoproteins**, molecules composed of lipid and protein. This is the only way that these fatty substances can remain dissolved while in circulation.

The best-known lipoproteins are **LDL** and **HDL**. Excess LDL cholesterol contributes to the blockage of arteries, which eventually leads to cardiovascular events including heart attack and stroke. Population studies have clearly shown that the higher the level of LDL cholesterol, the greater the risk of heart disease. This is true in men and women, in different racial and ethnic groups, and in all adult age groups. Hence, LDL cholesterol has been labelled the 'bad' cholesterol.

Increased blood levels of triglycerides cause the plasma to have a milky appearance. Blood to be tested for triglycerides should be collected when the patient has been fasting for 12–14 h, such as in the morning before breakfast.

CARBOHYDRATE METABOLISM

Glucose metabolism is largely regulated by **insulin** which is a hormone produced by the pancreas. Other hormones such as growth hormone, glucagons and cortisol also influence glucose metabolism. Glucose is a commonly tested blood constituent. **Diabetic patients** have high glucose level in blood (hyperglycaemia) which needs to be regulated in order to avoid other complications.

THYROID FUNCTION TESTS

Endocrine glands are ductless and internally secrete hormones into the blood stream that regulate many physiological processes of the body. They are the sites for the production of various hormones that regulate different physiological processes of the body. Thyroid gland is one of those sites. It produces various thyroid hormones that stimulate metabolism by increasing protein synthesis and oxygen consumption by the tissues. Thyroid hormones are synthesized from **iodide** and the amino acid **tyrosine**. In the blood, more than 99% of thyroid hormones are bound to serum proteins and are metabolically inactive. Grave's disease is an example of a disease caused by **hyperthyroidism**, or excessive secretion of **thyroid hormone**. On the other hand, decrease of thyroid function (**hypothyroidism**) causes a condition called myxedema.

The two major thyroid hormones are **thyroxine**, also called T_4, and **triiodothyronine**, also called T_3. Measurement of thyroid hormones is a special test done through specialized laboratories. They are mentioned here because of its importance in clinical biochemistry. Thyroid profiles or endocrine panels will include measurement of free or total T_4, free or total T_3 and thyroid stimulating hormone (TSH) levels. TSH is an anterior pituitary hormone that regulates thyroid gland activity. Measurement of the minute quantities of these hormones is usually done through immunological techniques.

OTHER TESTS OF ORGAN FUNCTION

Creatinine Clearance for Kidney Function

The best currently available method for measuring kidney function is the **creatinine clearance test**. It is also known as '**Measurement of glomerular filtration rate (GFR) for creatinine**'. It estimates the amount of blood, which passes through the glomerulus in 1 min with complete removal of the creatinine. That amount of creatinine is then measured in a timed collection of urine. The method is sensitive and can be easily followed in any laboratory with facilities to determine creatinine.

The expression of GFR in '**millilitres per minute**' indicates the amount of substance cleared by the kidney during a period of 1 min. Ideally the GFR is determined by measuring the clearance of a completely filterable substance that is neither absorbed nor excreted by the renal tubules. Urea clearance is of no value as a measure of GFR, because it is influenced by too many variables.

Calculation of clearance rate

Clearance calculated without considering the body weight will be considered as uncorrected. Except for children, the correction is not ordinarily done.

Uncorrected Clearance (uncorrected) can be mathematically expressed by the following formula:

$$\text{Uncorrected clearance (mL/min)} = (U_{cr} \times V)/P_{cr},$$

where U_{cr} is concentration of creatinine in urine, P_{cr} is concentration of creatinine in plasma (or serum) and V is the volume of urine passed per minute, expressed in mL.

Corrected The **GFR** is roughly proportional to the size of the kidney and the **body surface area** of the individual. Therefore, the calculation for the clearance of any given substance should provide for correction for deviations from the average adult body surface. This is done by multiplying the clearance by the factor 1.73/A, where 1.73 is the generally accepted average body surface in square metres and A is the body surface of the patient under investigation. The formula for calculating the **renal clearance**, therefore, expands as follows:

$$\text{Corrected clearance rate (mL/min)} = (U_{cr} \times V)/P_{cr}{}^* \times 1.73/A$$

*The uncorrected value of creatinine clearance.

The body surface area (A) may be determined conveniently from the nomogram (Fig. 34.1).

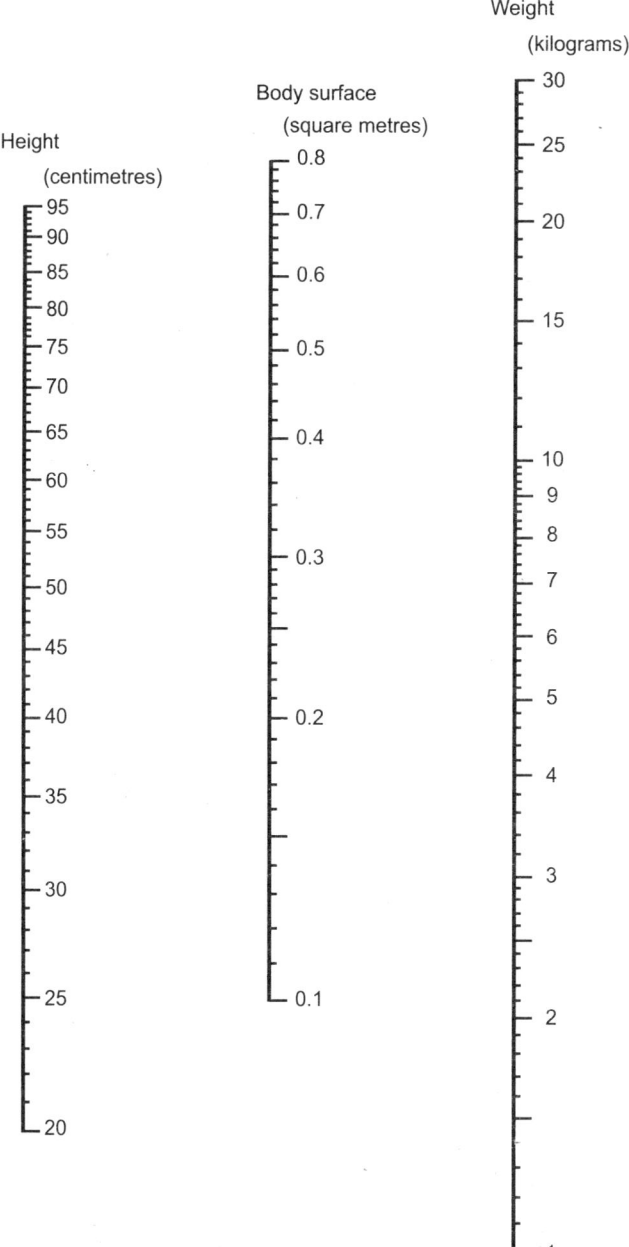

Fig. 34.1 *Nomogram to determine the body surface (A) of children: Take a scale and place it across the values of height (cm) and weight (kg). The point where the middle scale (body surface) intercepts is the body surface in square metres.*

Example

A patient discharged 228 mL of urine in 5 h period. The plasma concentration of creatinine was found to be 2.1 mg/dL and that of urine was 110 mg/dL. If the weight and height of the patient is respectively 70 kg and 150 cm ($A = 1.65$) calculate the creatinine clearance rate.

Calculation

$V = 228/5 \times 60 = 0.76$ mL/min; $U_{cr} = 110$; $P_{cr} = 2.1$

Uncorrected $GFR_{cr} = (110 \times 0.76)/2.1 = 39.8$ mL/min

Corrected $GFR_{cr} = 39.8 \times 1.73/1.65 = 41.7$ mL/min

Thus with average height and weight, the uncorrected value is not too different from the corrected value. Hence, it is not necessary. However, the same data for a child will be much higher as shown in the following example:

Example

If the body weight is 4 kg (infant) and height 37 cm, the body surface (A) will be 0.17.

Corrected clearance rate (mL/min) = $39.8 \times 1.73/0.17 = 405$

This shows that correction for body surface is absolutely mandatory if the body surface of the patient differs greatly from that of the average person. The error otherwise introduced is substantial in case of infants. GFR decreases with increasing renal failure.

Normal Value Men: 140 mL/min (± 27)
Women: 112 mL/min (± 20)

Procedure Perform the test in the morning. Give the patient three glasses of water to drink to guarantee adequate urine flow during the test period. Have the patient empty the bladder completely, discarding this urine. Note the exact time (including minutes). Thereafter, all urine should be collected for the next 5 h. Immediately afterwards obtain a blood sample for the creatinine determination. Send specimens, urine and blood, to the laboratory, where the urine volume is accurately measured and the creatinine levels of serum and urine are determined. Calculate the clearance rate by the above formula.

Sources of error
- Faulty timing or improper collection of the urine specimen is the most common source of error.
- Improper hydration of the patient.
- Exercise during the test.

GASTRIC FUNCTION TESTS

The use of **gastric analysis** as a diagnostic method has in recent years fallen under a cloud and, while descriptions of new modifications of test meals continue to appear, they receive at best a half-hearted reception. The reason for this is not far to seek. Variations in gastric secretion are so wide in healthy people that very little specific diagnostic information can be elicited in disease. Recent studies, however, indicate that patients with peptic ulcer show that basal acidity with duodenal ulcer often exceeds the highest control values; hence, this measurement has definite diagnostic value. Measurement of **basal secretion** is suggested as the simplest and most useful procedure in the study of clinical gastric physiology. If basal anacidity exists, the test should be supplemented by histamine stimulation.

Although many textbooks on medical technology have eliminated this chapter because of its questionable utility, we have chosen to describe the test here because of renewed interest. One should keep in mind that the physician or an experienced collects the specimen. The laboratory technician is only involved in the visual physical examination, microscopic examination and chemical examination, which includes—screening tests and titration for acidity. Microscopic examination of gastric juice is presented in Chapter 26 in Vol. II.

Clinical significance

Gastric secretion contains hydrochloric acid, intrinsic factor, digestive enzymes (pepsin and lipase) and electrolytes. The secretion is under hormonal control. Analysis of gastric juice is important in the diagnosis of gastric ulcers, carcinoma of the stomach, pernicious anaemia, **Zollinger–Ellison syndrome** and others.

Specimen

Patient preparation: The patient should fast (no food or liquid for 12 h), is not permitted to smoke in the morning of or during the test, and should avoid any form of exercise.

Collection of specimen: A gastric juice specimen is obtained by inserting a lubricated gastric **Levin tube**, orally or through the nose. The attending physician (or an experienced nurse) collects the specimen. The laboratory technicians are rarely involved in this. Two types of specimens arrive in the laboratory, gastric juice without stimulation (**basal secretion**), and following the subcutaneous administration of histamine dihydrochloride (**maximal secretion**).

Normal value

Gastric acidity:
 Basal acidity (H^+): < 2 mEq/L
 Maximal acidity: 1–20 mEq/L

Laboratory Investigation

Physical examination

Physical examination of the gastric juice is done without filtration. Report the physical conditions in the following line:

Amount   Measure the volume in a graduated cylinder. The normal volume is 50–80 mL. Over 100 mL volume is considered pathologic. Decreased volume is also considered to be abnormal.

Colour   Normal gastric juice is colourless. Bile will stain it yellow-green and **blood** will produce a **red to brown colour**. Presence of blood suggests a gastric ulcer. If the presence of blood is suspected, perform the occult blood test (see chemical screening). Microscopic examination of gastric juice may also reveal the presence of red blood cells, which suggests bleeding. Usually they are haemolysed.

Odour   Normal gastric juice has a sour odour. A faecal or rancid odour should be reported.

Fluid Character   Standing gastric juice separates into three layers—mucus (top), opalescent fluid in the centre and sediment at the bottom. The amount of mucus increases in gastric carcinoma, in gastritis and pyloric obstruction. Sediment is the amount of undigested food.

Chemical screening

Test for Starch
Supplies
- Pasteur pipette
- Watch glass

Reagent   *Potassium iodide solution (1% aqueous)*
- You can dilute the iodine solution, sold as 'antiseptic agent' (2%, see the label), two-folds with water in order to make it of 1% strength. This is good for the spot test. This, however, contains some amount of **alcohol**.

- If you want to make it yourself, take a few potassium iodide crystals in a beaker with 100 mL water. Add to this 1 g of iodine. *Caution*: Iodine is highly volatile.

Procedure
1. Place two drops of gastric juice in a watch glass.
2. Add iodine reagent on gastric juice held in the watch glass.
3. Watch instantly. A blue colour indicates presence of starch.

Test for Blood
Reagent *o-tolidine reagent* (4% aqueous)

Dissolve 4 g *o*-tolidine in 95% ethyl alcohol (just sufficient to dissolve) in a 100-mL volumetric flask; make the volume to 100 mL with water.

Procedure
1. Add 4 drops of *o*-tolidine reagent in the gastric juice held in a watch glass.
2. Add 4 drops of glacial acetic acid and 4 drops of water. If colour develops, it is due to contamination.
3. Add 1–2 drops of hydrogen peroxide. A green or blue colouration suggests the presence of blood. Presence of blood can be due to trauma or gastric ulcer.

Determination of Gastric Acidity
The physician occasionally requests quantitative determination of gastric acidity by **titration.** Many laboratories prefer centrifuged specimen while others feel that this procedure removes some of the hydrogen ions through the sediment. In order to remove the gross food particles, filter the specimen through two layers of gauze. Use the filtrate for the determination of free acid by titration.

Principle A known amount of gastric residue is titrated with 0.1 N NaOH to a pH of 3.5. If a **pH meter** is not available, add two drops of **Topfer's reagent**, which changes to a salmon colour when all the free hydrochloric acid is neutralized. The total acidity, however, is determined by titration using phenolphthalein as indicator.

Reagents
- *Sodium hydroxide solution (0.1 N):* Stock sodium hydroxide (1.0 N) is diluted 10-fold. Alternatively, dissolve 4 g of NaOH in fresh distilled water and make to 1000 mL.
- *Phenolphthalein solution (1%, alcoholic):* Dissolve 1 g of phenolphthalein in 100 mL of 95% alcohol.
- *Topfer reagent (dimethylaminoazobenzene)-0.5% alcoholic solution*: Dissolve 0.5 g of Topfer reagent in 100 mL of 95% alcohol.

Procedure
1. Take a porcelain-evaporating dish and transfer 10 mL (measure with a graduated cylinder) of gastric juice specimen. In case of high acidity, mix 1 mL of gastric juice with 5 mL of distilled water.
2. Add 1–2 drops of Topfer reagent.
3. Observe for colour change; a bright red colour will appear if free hydrochloric acid is present.
4. Add 1–2 drops of phenolphthalein to the gastric juice with Topfer reagent.
5. Titrate with 0.1 N NaOH from a burette, mixing after each addition until the last trace of red colour disappears and is replaced by a canary yellow colour.
6. Read from the burette the number of millilitres of NaOH used. This represents the amount of free hydrochloric acid.
7. Continue the titration until the red colour of phenolphthalein appears (deep pink), titrating to the point at which further addition of alkali does not deepen the colour.
8. Take the burette reading (mL NAOH) for the total acidity, counting from the original reading.

9. *Calculation*:
    (a) Free hydrochloric acid (mEq/L)
        $X \times 10$ (acid) $= 100 \times$ mL alkali (0.1 N NaOH $-$ 100 mEq/L)
        or, $X =$ mL 0.1 N NaOH $\times 10$,
        where $X =$ strength of free hydrochloric acid, 10 is volume of acid (gastric juice) taken for titration and 100 is conversion of 0.1 N NaOH to mEq/L.
    (b) Total acidity (mEq/L)
        $Y =$ mL of 0.1 N NaOH $\times 10$.
        Note: If the volume of gastric juice (V) taken for analysis is different from 10, or the normality of NaOH is not exactly 0.1 N, apply the following formula for calculating free acidity and total acidity:
        X (or Y) $\times V = N \times 100$
        X (mEq/L) $= (N \times 100)/V$,
        where X is free hydrochloric acid (mEq/L), Y is total acidity (mEq/L) and V is Volume of gastric juice (mL).
    (c) Combined acidity (mEq/L)
        Total acidity (Y) $-$ Free hydrochloric acid (X) $=$ Combined acidity
        Combined acidity is due to HC1, organic acids (e.g. lactic acid, amino acids and acid salts).
        Note: Free and total acidity are determined for both basal secretions as well as for maximal secretion (stimulated).

Interpretation Increased values of **basal acidity** (free and total) suggest **gastric ulcer** (2–5 mEq/L), duodenal ulcer (>5 mEq/L) or **Zollinger-Ellison syndrome** (>20 mEq/L). Chronic gastritis may be associated with an increase in free HC1 while achlorhydria is diagnosed by the lack of maximal total acidity (0 mEq/L). Higher values of **maximal total acidity** may be related to duodenal ulcer (20–60 mEq/L) and Zollinger-Ellison syndrome (>60 mEq/L). If there is no free HC1 after administering histamine (maximal), pernicious anaemia or cancer of the stomach may be considered. Presence of blood is a significant sign of ulcer.

PANCREATIC FUNCTION TESTS

This test may be performed to determine the activity of the pancreas in people with diseases that affect the pancreas (for example, pancreatitis, cystic fibrosis or pancreatic cancer). In developed countries use of computed tomography (CT) scans, abdominal ultrasound, endoscopy and magnetic resonance imaging (MRI) have replaced much of the old-fashioned laboratory tests. They are also less invasive and hence more comfortable to patients. It also provides better information for treatment. However, unfortunately, these are expensive procedures and hard to adapt to the existing conditions of underdeveloped countries. The following are some of the laboratory tests currently used and many of them are good for preliminary diagnosis.

Blood Tests

Blood tests can evaluate the function of the gallbladder, liver and pancreas. Levels of the pancreatic enzymes **amylase** and **lipase** can be measured. Blood tests can also check for signs of related conditions including infection, anaemia (low blood count) and dehydration. The physician makes special requests for the above enzymes to the biochemistry laboratory.

Faecal Test

Faecal trypsin

Trypsin is a digestive enzyme secreted by pancreas. It is present in the stool of a normal person. The trypsin has the ability to dissolve **gelatine** (a protein) which is used on the X-ray films. Small strips of exposed X-ray films are dipped into a test tube holding patient's stool suspension and left overnight. If the stool clears off the film after overnight exposure, the patient is considered normal. Lack of clearance of the film is considered as abnormal and is related to the deficiency of trypsin or malfunction of pancreas.

Faecal elastase test

The **faecal elastase test** is another test of pancreas function. The test measures the levels of elastase, an enzyme found in fluids produced by the pancreas. Elastase digests (breaks down) proteins. In this test, a patient's stool sample is analysed for the presence of elastase. Commercial kits are used which is based on EIA procedure.

Laboratory Investigation of Pancreatic Juice

Pancreatic juice (duodenal content) analysis can assess the **exocrine function** of the pancreas. The sample is obtained from a fasting patient in a similar way as described under the gastric function test after inserting the stomach tube further down into the duodenal area. The attending nurse, under the supervision of a physician, does this.

The basic method of pancreatic juice analysis has been further improved by **secretin stimulation test.** The secretin stimulation test measures the ability of the pancreas to respond to secretin. Secretin is a hormone made by the small intestine. Secretin stimulates the pancreas to release a fluid that neutralizes stomach acid and aids in digestion. Secretin is administered after the initial sampling. The contents of the duodenal secretions are aspirated (removed with suction) and analysed over a period of about 2 h. The laboratory examines and analyses the duodenal secretions and report the results to the physician for diagnosis. People with diseases involving the pancreas (for example, pancreatitis, cystic fibrosis or pancreatic cancer) might have abnormal pancreatic function.

Laboratory investigation comprises of physical examination, measurement of specific gravity, microscopic examination and chemical screening. Normal pancreatic juice is colourless or yellow with a specific gravity of 1.007–1.042 and pH of 8.0–8.3. Presence of **trypsin** and **amylase** is expected.

Physical examination

Report: colour, specific gravity (use hand refractometer) and pH as done for other body fluids (Chapter 26 in Vol. II).

Chemical screening for pancreatic enzymes

Deficiency of pancreatic digestive enzymes (trypsin, amylase and elastase) indicates a pathologic condition of the pancreas.

Trypsin Make the duodenal content slightly alkaline with 2% (aqueous) sodium carbonate. Check with **phenolphthalein**, which gives a faint pink colour. Place small amounts of the duodenal fluid in three test tubes labelled 'N' (negative control), 'P' (positive control) and 'T' (test). Boil the first tube ('N'), add trypsin to the second ('P'). Place small pieces of gelatine square in each. Incubate overnight at room temperature or in an incubator (35°C). Gelatine will dissolve in the tubes marked 'P' and 'T' (normal). Alternatively, cut-strips of exposed X-ray films can be used in place of gelatine strips. Clearing of the film indicates normal trypsin activity.

Amylase Dilute the duodenal content 10-fold with saline. Mix equal portions of the diluted duodenal content and 1% starch solution (2 mL each) in a test tube. Incubate for 30 min at 37 °C. Use 1 drop of **iodine solution** (1 g iodine and 2 g potassium iodide dissolved and diluted to 100 mL). A blue colour indicates amylase deficiency.

Elastase Several reports have indicated that faecal elastase determination is a new, sensitive, and specific non-invasive pancreatic function test. Commercially available kits are now available which are based on immunologic principles (ELISA, Roche Diagnostics).

TEST FOR MALABSORPTION

Malabsorption tests are done to determine if a patient has dietary malabsorption or maldigestion and to help differentiate between these two conditions. Malabsorption occurs when the gastrointestinal (GI) tract cannot take up a dietary compound. This may be caused by malfunction of the organ or lack of important digestive enzymes. Genetic disorder could lead to this situation or may be caused by injury to the tissue that provides the enzyme (i.e. the **pancreas**), alterations in pH that make the enzymes inactive, or due to surgery. In general, clinicians speak of both disorders as malabsorption disoders since they both result in a lack of absorption of nutrients.

D-xylose Absorption Test

The D-xylose absorption test measures the level of D-xylose, a type of sugar, in a blood or urine sample. This test is done to help diagnose problems that prevent the small intestine from absorbing nutrients in food. The intestines normally absorb D-xylose easily. When problems arise with absorption, the intestines do not absorb D-xylose. Hence, its level in blood and urine remains low due to the abnormality. The purpose of the test is to:

- Check to see if malabsorption syndrome is causing symptoms, such as chronic diarrhoea, weight loss and weakness. A person with malabsorption syndrome is unable to absorb nutrients, vitamins and minerals from the intestinal tract into the bloodstream.
- Find the cause of a child's failure to gain weight, especially when the child seems to be eating enough food.

The D-xylose absorption test is a convenient method of **diagnosing malabsorption**. The patient is orally administered a standard quantity (25 g) of d-xylose. The amount excreted in the urine over the following 5-h period is determined. The d-xylose absorption test is useful in a differential diagnosis between malabsorption which is intestinal in origin, and malabsorption which is pancreatic in origin. In malabsorption due to pancreatic insufficiency absorption of the pentose d-xylose will be essentially normal. In intestinal dysfunction, d-xylose absorption will be substantially decreased. The test results are abnormal in 80% of patients with malabsorption syndrome. The test may be invalidated by renal retention, myxedema or incomplete urine collection.

Patient preparation and after care

The health professional will provide information about the **routine medications** taken by the patient. Some of them may **interfere**. Do not eat or drink anything except water for 8–12 h before having this test. Children younger than 9 years old should not eat or drink anything except water for 4 h before the test. Asking patients to collect urine or faeces over a long time period can cause problems with compliance. It is important to make sure that the patient understands the test and the necessity of his/her compliance. Clinical laboratories will reject any samples that appear to have been collected or stored incorrectly.

Some amount of **aftercare** is needed when the test is done. Some patients may feel sick after the procedures since they are being exposed to compounds that they may have trouble absorbing. Nurses should be careful to discuss any side effects with the patient beforehand, and the patient should be given the smallest amount of substance possible to avoid problems. In addition, patients may be malnourished and need something to eat and drink once the procedure is over.

Specimen collection

1. In the morning, the patient should void to empty the bladder. This urine is discarded. The patient is then given 25 g of d-xylose dissolved in 250 mL of tap water. Immediately the patient is given another 250 mL of water. Note the time. *Note*: For children weighing less than 25 kg, give 0.5 g d-xylose per 225 g body weight.
2. Collect and pool all urine over the next 5 h. Keep the urine on ice or refrigerated prior to sending to the laboratory. *Note*: Many laboratories conduct blood analysis simultaneous with the urine analysis. This is not included here. Blood is collected by venipuncture.

Test procedure

The amount of **D-xylose** in urine samples is measured before and after the patient drinks a D-xylose solution. To begin the test, a sample of the first urine of the day is collected. This is followed by patient's intake of D-xylose solution by mouth. All urine specimens are then collected for 5 h after drinking the sugar solution. Sometimes urine is collected for 24 h. Some laboratories collect blood samples along with urine for comparison. This is not described here.

For adults, a blood sample is usually taken 2 h after drinking the solution. For children, a blood sample may be taken 1 h after drinking the solution. Another blood sample may be drawn 5 h after drinking the solution.

Normal values

Adult
   Dosage: 25 g
   Discharge:
   (a) Under 65 years: 4 g/ 5-h urine
   (b) Above 65 years: 3.5 g/5-h urine

Child
   Dosage: 0.5 g/225 g body weight
   Discharge: 16–33% of ingested xylose

Principle

Chemical determination depends on dehydration of the **pentose to furfural** in the presence of acid and heat followed by condensation of furfural with **p-bromoaniline** to form a pink coloured compound. At 70 °C, very little furfural is formed from precursors other than the available pentose. Thiourea acts as an antioxidant, which helps prevent the formation of interfering coloured compounds.

Equipment and supplies

- Spectrophotometer
- Water bath (70°C)

Reagents

- *p-Bromoaniline colour reagent*: Saturate glacial acetic acid with thiourea by adding approximately 4 g of thiourea to 100 mL of glacial acetic acid, decant. The clear supernatant is stable and may be prepared in advance. The colour reagent is prepared fresh before use by adding 2 g of p-bromoaniline to 100 mL of glacial acetic acid saturated thiourea.
- *Saturated benzole acid solution*: Dissolve 2.5 g benzole acid (CP) in 1000 mL distilled water by boiling in a 1500-mL beaker; cool and make up loss by evaporation.
- *d-Xylose stock standard (2 mg/mL):* Place 500 mg of d-xylose into a 250-mL volumetric flask. Add sufficient benzole acid solution to dissolve the d-xylose and dilute to the mark with saturated benzole acid. Keep in a refrigerator.

- *d-xylose working standards*: Dilute stock d-xylose standard with saturated benzole acid as shown below. Keep the solutions refrigerated.
- 5 mL of stock standard diluted to 100 mL. This is equivalent to 0.1 mg/mL.
- 10 mL of stock standard diluted to 100 mL. This is equivalent to 0.2 mg/mL.

  Standardization procedure: With each run, two standard levels are analysed in the same manner as are the unknowns. The standard used in the calculations should be that one whose net absorbance is closest to the net absorbance of the unknown test. To check the linearity and chemistry of the procedure, treat the remaining standard as an unknown and calculate its concentration to see how well it checks with its known concentration.

Procedure

1. Measure the volume of urine collected during 5-h period.
2. Prepare two dilutions of urine specimen : t[AV1] (i) 1 : 50: Mix 0.1 mL of urine with 4.9 mL of water, (ii) 1 : 200: Mix 0.1 mL of urine with 19.9 mL of water.
3. Pipette the following into four tubes labelled as 'SB', 'ST', 'UB', 'UT' that correspond to standard blank, standard test, unknown blank and unknown test, respectively.

	Standard		Unknown	
Reagent	Blank (SB)	Test (ST)	Blank (UB)	Test (UT)
Working standard	0.5	0.5	–	–
Dilute urine	–	–	0.5	0.5
p-Bromoaniline2.5	2.5	2.5	2.5	2.5

4. Mix, place all of the test reaction tubes in a 70 water bath for 10 min and all blank reaction tubes in the dark at room temperature.
5. Following incubation, cool the test reaction tubes in running water until they reach room temperature.
6. Place all tubes (tests and blanks) in the dark for 70 min.
7. Read the absorbance at 520 nm of all the tubes (standard blank and test plus unknown blank and test) against the water blank.
8. *Calculation and results*:

   Excretion of d-xylose (g) = $(A_t/A_s) \times C_s \times F \times V/1000$,

   where A_t is net absorbance of test solution.
   Difference of absorbance readings of tubes marked 'UT' and 'UB' against the water blank.
   A_s is net absorbance of standard.
   Difference of absorbance readings of tubes marked, 'ST' and 'SU' against the water blank.
   C_s is concentration of the standard.
   Note: Consider only that standard (0.1 or 0.2 mg) whose net absorbance reading is closest to the net absorbance reading of the unknown or test solution.
   F is Dilution factor (50 or 200), V is volume of urine during 5-h period, 1000 is used to convert milligrams to grams in the calculation.

Note: Urine whose net absorbance is greater than approximately 0.9 should be repeated on a greater dilution (more than 200) as the colorimetric chemical reaction is not linear at higher concentrations.

Interpretation:
D-xylose absorption should be greater than 1.2 g/5 h with a 5 g dose of D-xylose and 4.0 g/5 h in an adult given a 25 g dose of D-xylose. The D-xylose test will be normal if the patient has normal absorptive capacity in the intestine, or if the patient has malabsorption that is caused by a pancreatic problem. It will be low if the

patient has celiac disease, tropical sprue, Crohn's disease, advanced AIDs or pellagra (**niacin** deficiency). Falsely low results with the D-xylose test will be seen if the patient has been vomiting, has gastric stasis, fluid build up (ascites), fluid retention (edema) or bacterial overgrowth. There is a decrease in urinary excretion of D-xylose with aspirin, colchicines, digitalis, MAO inhibitors, food consumption, neomycin and opiates. In addition, excretion is lower in those with impaired renal function and in elderly patients

Review Questions

1. What are the functions of the following organs: Liver, kidney, pancreas and stomach?
2. A clinic patient had total protein and albumin assays performed on his blood. When the physician was given the test results, total protein 6.5 g/dL and albumin 3.0 g/dL, she asked the technician to calculate the A/G ratio.
3. Dr. Tiwari ordered the following chemistry tests for a patient: creatine kinase, AST and cholesterol fractions. Which of the following do you think Dr. Tiwari suspects—heart disease, renal disease, liver disease or thyroid disease?
4. What three enzymes are useful in diagnosing liver disease?
5. How would you assess the malfunction of the above organs in the clinical biochemistry laboratory?
6. What are the two major types of serum proteins and what are their functions?
7. What is glomerular filtration rate? What information would you require to calculate creatinine clearance rate?
8. Which clinical conditions require gastric function tests? How would you report gastric acidity?
9. What are the enzymes secreted by pancreas? Why is it necessary to make the duodenal content slightly alkaline before testing for trypsin?
10. Which enzyme is most useful in diagnosing myocardial infarction?
11. Why is urinary xylose excretion test diagnosis malabsorption syndrome?
12. Why are two standards selected for testing xylose excretion?
13. Define the following regarding gastric function test: basal acidity, maximal acidity, free acidity (HCl), total acidity, combined acidity.
14. What is the significance of D-xylose test? How is it done?

35

Clinical Toxicology and Therapeutic Drug Monitoring

Kaushik Kundu and Sanket Nayyar

Chapter Outline

- ◆ Role of Toxicology Laboratory
- ◆ Analytical Approach in Toxicology
  - Specimens
  - Microdiffusion analysis
    - ❑ General screening for ethanol and acetone
    - ❑ Chemical oxidation of ethanol (and acetone) with dichromate
  - Enzymatic oxidation method for ethanol
  - Acetone
  - Determination of carbon monoxide
  - Determination of cyanide
  - Determination of methanol, isopropanol and formaldehyde
- ◆ Drug Screening
  - Phenothiazine derivates
  - Acetaminophen
  - Chloral hydrate and halogenated hydrocarbons
  - Imipramine
  - Salicylates
  - Barbiturates
  - Cyclic antidepressants
  - Cannabinoids
  - Opioids
  - Cocaine
  - Sympathomimetic drugs
  - Date-rape and knockout drugs
- ◆ Heavy Metal Poisoning

- *Reinsch screening test*
- *Specific test for mercury*
- *Iron overdose*
- ◆ *Review Questions*

Clinical toxicology in laboratory medicine is defined as the analysis of poisonous substances in human biological fluids for the purpose of patient care. The **poisonous substances** are drugs that were taken beyond therapeutic limits, have been ingested accidentally or may be related to criminal or suicidal intent. Hence the technician must bear in mind that the investigation may have legal implications. Forensic medicine, however, goes into greater detail in order to identify the wrongdoer, while the goal of the biochemistry laboratory is to establish the cause in order to assist the clinician to resolve a diagnostic dilemma and indicate the prognosis of the poisoned patient. It is common incidence to find a patient in the emergency room in coma and the laboratory has to provide some kind of clue towards the possible identification of the toxicant so that appropriate measures can be taken.

Poisoned patients account for approximately 10% of all acute admissions to medical wards in hospitals. These include self-poisoning attempts, accidental poisoning or due to administration of illicit drugs. Many victims succumb to the poison before even reaching the hospital. Pregnant patients with a chemical dependency particularly that of cocaine, are at high risk for obstetric complications. **Urine** testing for drugs of abuse provides evidence for the diagnosis of drug dependency and subsequent monitoring of drug use during the course of the pregnancy. The majority of common drug interactions are known, and data should be available through hospital records.

In the case of therapeutic drug monitoring, the biochemistry laboratory carefully tracks the level of the drug in order to avoid overdose. The latter may lead to various side effects or may even threaten the life of the patient.

Toxicological investigations are not routinely performed in the biochemistry laboratory. In this chapter only a few common procedures will be discussed. Within the next few years, as the '**potently dangerous drugs**' are increasingly used for heart patients, patients under chemotherapy and for difficult-to-cure diseases, many of these procedures may become routine in the laboratory.

ROLE OF TOXICOLOGY LABORATORY

It is now accepted that a limited range of drug estimations should be available in all clinical biochemistry laboratories and that a wider range of assays, both screening and quantitative determinations should be available in a few selected centres. The average laboratory is not equipped to provide a comprehensive screening service in order to confirm or eliminate the presence of all drugs in common use, nor to provide quantitative assays for a large number of these compounds. A simple rule of thumb for the biochemist involved in clinical toxicology should not carry out quantitative analysis unless they are also able to interpret the result.

In the last few years, the wide spread abuse of illicit drugs has placed additional demands on the healthy-care system. Consequently, clinical toxicology laboratories have moved beyond their traditional activities and now are routinely perfoming urine testing of drugs of abuse for other clinical services such as obstertrics for pregnant drug abusers, pediatrics for their newborns and drug-dependency treatment programmes. Such testing usually focuses on a small panel of the most frequently abused drugs such as cocaine, cannabinoids and the benzodiazepines, rather than the broad-spectrum screening performed in emergency toxicology. In the following sections, we chose to discuss only the most important ones. Facilities for the analysis of drugs may not be available in peripheral laboratories but the technicians may be involved in specimen collection and the account presented here attempts to make them conscious of their crucial role.

ANALYTICAL APPROACH IN TOXICOLOGY

A drug screen is a compromise among rapid turnaround time, analytical specificity and sensitivity, and it may be a combination of qualitative and quantitative analyses. Following five methods for initial screening suit to the existing conditions of peripheral laboratories with limited facilities:
- Spot test with chromogenic reaction that can be done on paper or tile.
- Microdiffusion tests for volatile compounds.
- Quick chemical test in test tubes with visual observation.
- Colorimetric assay for chemical reactions that yields colour for quantitative assay.
- Immunoassays with agglutination or colour reaction as a result of immunologic reaction.

Reference laboratories have better capabilities to detect smaller quantities of the analytes as well as to their better identification for specific treatment. These analyses require sophisticated instuments such as TLC, Gas Chromatography (GC) and High Pressure Liquid Chromatography (HPLC). These techniques have been described in the Chemistry section of this book.

Specimens

The specimens most frequently submitted for analysis are urine, whole blood/plasma, clotted blood/serum and gastric juice. Drug screen in most clinical laboratories are performed on urine. The advantage of urine is that a large volume can be obtained, allowing analysis of drugs in low concentration. However, urine contains metabolites which may complicate identifidation. For those drugs tha are extensively metabolized, the parent drug may not be present. In addition, urine tests are qualitative, as drug concentrations in urine correlate poorly with clinical effects. Blood (serum and plasma) although limited by sample volume, is the specimen of choice for quantitative analyses of those drugs for which there is a correlation between drug level and toxicity. However, quantitative tests are usually more time consuming.

Blood is obtained by venipuncture and urine specimen is collected by 'random clean catch'. **Gastric aspirate** is obtained through **gastric lavage**. Gastric aspirate has advantages in that the unchanged drug or poison may be found in the aspirate, often in much higher concentrations than the blood or urine. The process of cleaning out the contents of the stomach by gastric lavage has been used for over 200 years as a means of eliminating poisons from the stomach. Such devices are normally used on a person who has ingested a poison or overdosed on a drug. Care should be taken to ensure that the gastric aspirate specimen is obtained before, not after washout. Gastric lavage is performed only by experienced nurse or by the physician.

Microdiffusion Analysis

For the routine laboratory, the microdiffusion technique is most helpful in the screening of volatile compounds. When this is supplemented with colorimetry, a wide range of drug-related investigations can be covered.

Microdiffusion analysis is a simple procedure and is used for the rapid isolation and detection of volatile poisons. A simple Conway microdiffusion dish (Fig. 35.1) is used which consists of two round, concentric chambers moulded into a porcelain or glass dish that can be sealed by a glass plate. The inner well has a lower wall than the outer rim of the dish so that the plate can be properly sealed. The outer well holds the sample (1–5 mL of blood or urine), and the inner well holds the 'absorbent' which traps the volatile substance. The absorbent is a reagent or solvent in which particular volatile substances will readily dissolve. The specimen and the trapping solution are in contact with the same atmosphere when the chamber is sealed. This allows the microdiffusion to occur. After the sample and absorbent are added to the proper well, the dish is sealed with a viscous sealant (stopcock grease or petrolatum jelly) material and a ground-glass cover plate. The substance to be separated, because of its vapour pressure, leaves the specimen and enters the atmosphere, from which it is absorbed by the trapping solution.

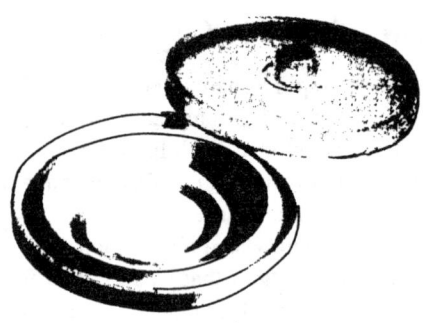

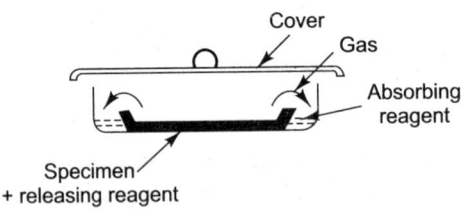

Fig. 35.1 *Conway microdiffusion dish.*

The microdiffusion process is usually carried out at room temperature for the desirable length of time as recommended in the procedure. The process of diffusion can be expedited by applying gentle heat. The process of gaseous diffusion continues until equilibrium is reached. The absorbent may show a colour change which is noted and this may help in the identification of the volatile substance under study. The microdiffusion procedure is applied in the analysis of carbon monoxide, cyanide and ethanol (Table 35.1).

Table 35.1 Summary for analysis of volatile substances by microdiffusion method

Toxic substance	Absorbing solution	Test (Colour change)
Volatile alcohols and acetone	Potassium dichromate	Orange colour to green orange
Carbon monoxide	Palladium chloride	Black film of palladium
Cyanide	Sodium hydroxide	Pyridine-barbituric acid: red

General screening for ethanol and acetone

Alcohol is undoubtedly the most commonly abused drug. During the past decade the consumption of alcohol in India has increased many-fold. This also includes 'country-made' alcohols. If the alcohol is contaminated with more harmful alcohols (e.g. methyl alcohol), which are unfit for consumption, it may lead to dangerous consequences on a mass scale.

Alcohol has a short half-life, thus most patients will show a fall in plasma concentrations between 2 and 5 mmol/L/h unless there is impairment of hepatic blood flow.

Specimen The commonly used specimens are blood and urine.

Chemical Oxidation of Ethanol (and Acetone) with Dichromate

Principle Alcohols, aldehydes and other volatile substances are released from the sample and absorbed in acid dichromate solution placed in the central well of a microdiffusion dish. The dichromate is reduced producing a colour change from orange to green-coloured chromic ion (for alcohol) or blue (for acetone). This colour change constitutes a rough qualitative indication of the presence of alcohol or acetone in the specimen (blood or urine). *Note:* The method is non-specific. The reaction occurs with other alcohols and paraldehyde.

Reagents
- **Potassium dichromate reagent:** Dissolve 1 g of potassium dichromate in 500 mL of water in a 2-L beaker with graduations. Dissolve by stirring with a glass rod. Add 0.1 g of silver nitrate to the solution. Then carefully and slowly add 500 mL of concentrated sulphuric acid. Add a little at a time and mix before adding more. Store the solution in a tightly capped dark bottle. This solution is stable for 1 year.
- Saturated potassium carbonate solution in water.
- **Control solution:** Add 1.8 mL of absolute alcohol to 1000 mL.

Procedure
1. Take two microdiffusion dishes and label them as 'T' (test) and 'C' (control).
2. Add 0.5 mL of potassium dichromate reagent to the centre well of each microdiffusion dish.
3. Place 1–2 mL of the specimen in the outer well of the plate marked 'T' and 1–2 mL of the control solution in the outer well of the plate marked 'C'.
4. Add 1 mL of saturated aqueous potassium carbonate solution in the wells containing the sample and control.
5. Place the covers on the dishes and heat at 50°C in an oven or on a hot plate (not more than 70°C).
6. Observe the colour change in the potassium dichromate solution.
7. A green colour developing In 30 min Indicates the presence of alcohols (methanol, isopropanol and aldehydes) or other reducing substances. The control should show a positive reaction.
8. A positive reaction may be due to methanol, isopropanol, aldehyde or acetone. Rule out methanol by its specific test described later in this chapter. Perform the acetone spot test with the urine specimen, as described here. If positive, presence of isopropanol may be suspected.

Note: **Acetone** is a metabolite of **isopropanol** and its presence in urine suggests the ingestion of isopropanol (an alcohol).

Enzymatic Oxidation Method for Ethanol It is a spectrophotometric method, which is specific to ethanol. The following chemical reaction is involved and can be carried out in any laboratory equipped with an **ultraviolet spectrophotometer**. Commercially available kits with clear instructions for the assay are available. The chosen specimen is serum.

$$C_2H_5OH + NAD^+ \xrightarrow{ADH} CH_3CHO + NADH + H^+$$

Acetone The method of detecting acetone in urine has been discussed in Chapter 25 in Vol. II. A quick spot test (Rothera test) is described here to detect the presence of ketone bodies in urine which include acetone, acetoacetic acid (diacetic acid) and beta-hydroxybutyric acid. Acetone and acetoacetic acid react with **sodium nitroprusside** in the presence of alkali to produce a purple colour.

Specimen Testing for ketone bodies should be done on fresh urine or the specimen kept at 4°C

Reagent
- Ammonium sulphate: Solid crystals.
- Sodium nitroprusside solution: 2% in water
- Concentrated ammonia solution (specific gravity 0.91)
- Timer
- Test tube (10 mL)

- Test tube rack
- Pipette
- Fume hood

Procedure
1. Place a test tube (10 mL) in the test tube rack.
2. Transfer 5 mL of fresh urine specimen into the test tube.
3. Add several crystals of ammonium sulphate into the tube and mix. Keep adding more until the crystals do not dissolve any more (saturated).
4. Add 10 drops of concentrated ammonia. *Caution*: Fumes of ammonia can be harmful. You may choose to work in a fume hood or in a well ventilated area.
5. Stand for 15 min.
6. Observation (semiquantitative):
   If acetone and diacetic acid are present, then a purple (permanganate calomel red) colour will form within 30–60 sec. The result can be graded from trace to 3+ based on the intensity of the colour formed, as detailed below.
   No change in colour: Negative
   Pinkish: +
   Red: ++
   Deep purple: +++
   Additional Note:
- If there is suspicion of a false positive test, heat the urine in a test tube on a Bunsen burner flame for 1 min, and allow cooling and repeating the Rothera's test. Heated urine will not give a positive Rothera's due to the absence of volatile ketone bodies.
- As a quality control measure, the reagent should be checked frequently using a positive control (1–2 drops of acetone is added to 5 mL of urine). The use of distilled water in place of urine for negative control is recommended

Determination of Carbon Monoxide

Carbon monoxide poisoning is caused by the inhalation of exhaust from automobiles and other vehicles using petrol. Because there is no governmental control maintaining the emission standard of automobiles driven in most developing countries, it is difficult to assess the damage done to the public and street dwellers. The affinity of carbon monoxide to haemoglobin is 210 times that of oxygen. The inhalation of carbon monoxide containing air readily leads to the formation of carboxyhaemoglobin (CO-Hb). This markedly reduces the oxygen-carrying capacity of blood.

Specimen
Anticoagulated whole blood is submitted to the laboratory for determining carbon monoxide poisoning. Fluoride and oxalate are used as anticoagulants for getting the whole blood specimen.

Principle
Whole blood is mixed with ferrlcyanide and lactic acid. This liberates carbon monoxide (a volatile gas) into the atmosphere of the microdiffusion chamber. This is then trapped on a palladium-chloride paper and thereby palladium ions are reduced to metallic form and appear as a black film. If the black film is visible, CO-Hb saturation greater than 30% is present.

Equipment
Microdlffusion dish (Fig. 35.1).

Reagent

- *Hydrochloric acid (0.01 N):* Dilute 0.85 mL of concentrated HC1 (11.6 N) to 1000 mL with water.
- *Palladium chloride solution:* Dissolve 220 mg of palladium chloride in 250 mL of 0.01 N HC1. The solution is stable. If protected from the carbon monoxide in the atmosphere.
- *Potassium ferricyanide solution (3.2%):* Dissolve $K_3Fe(CN)_6$ in 50 mL of water and make this up to 100 mL volume in a volumetric flask.
- *Lactic acid solution (0.1 M):* Dissolve 90 mL of lactic acid (85% pure) in water and make up to 1000 mL.
- *Haemolyslng solution*: Mix equal parts of potassium ferrocyanide solution with 0.1 M lactic acid solution.
- *Sealing compound*: either stopcock grease or petrolatum jelly can be used.

Procedure

1. Apply the sealant on the rim of the outer wall of the Conway microdiffusion dish (Fig. 35.1).
2. Pipette 2 mL of palladium chloride into the centre well of the dish.
3. Place 1 mL of whole blood on one side of the outer compartment. Place the cover over the dish, leaving an opening to permit the addition of haemolysing fluid opposite the blood.
4. Add 2 mL of haemolysing solution in the outer compartment (opposite the blood) and then slide the cover over the opening to seal the dish..
5. Carefully mix the contents of the outer well by swirling the Conway dish gently.
6. Allow the dish to stand at room temperature for 1 h the diffusion to occur.
7. In the presence of carbon monoxide, a mirror of metallic palladium will be noted on the surface of the palladium chloride solution in the inner compartment. A bright mirror covering the entire compartment is typical of the lethal level of carbon monoxide in the blood.

Determination of Cyanide

Cyanide poisoning frequently occurs through accidental ingestion of insecticides. Another common cause of cyanide poisoning is the inhalation of smoke from burning plastics. Identification and estimation of cyanide in blood may be carried out most simply by using the Conway diffusion method; however, retrospective analysis of thiocyanate in urine is a simple way of confirming cyanide intake.

Although cyanide is very toxic, levels up to 15 µg/dL blood can be found in adults without any symptoms. In case of death due to ingestion of an overdose of a cyanide salt, levels of 1.0 mg/dL or more may be found. A lethal level is about 100 µg/dL blood.

Inside the laboratory there are a number of reagents prepared from cyanide salts (e.g. potassium ferricyanide). These should be clearly labelled as **POISON**. None of the cyanide solution should be discarded in the open sink. If at all, it can be discarded in the sink which is inside the hood. Under no circumstances should you allow the cyanide reagent to get in contact with acid.

Specimen

Anticoagulated whole blood and urine samples are used for determining cyanide poisoning. Blood is anticoagulated with fluoride or oxalateas. Blood specimen should not be stored for a long period.

Principle

The microdiffusion method can be applied in screening as well for the quantitative analysis of cyanide in blood. Cyanide is liberated from the biological specimen by acidification. The hydrogen cyanide (HCN) evolved is trapped in dilute alkali and converted to cyanogen chloride; in subsequent steps it is converted to a coloured compound by reacting with appropriate chemicals.

Reagents

- *Sulphuric acid (3.6 N):* Dilute 10 rat, of concentrated sulphuric acid to 100 mL with water.
- *Sodium hydroxide (0.1 N):* Dissolve 4 g of sodium hydroxide (NaOH) in water and dilute to 1000 mL.
- *Monobasic sodium phosphate (1 M):* Dissolve 13.8 g of monobasic sodium phosphate in water and dilute to 100 mL.
- *Chloramine-T (0.25%):* Dissolve 0.25 g of chloramine-T in water and dilute to 100 mL. Store in a refrigerator.
- *Colour reagent* (pyridine-barbituric acid reagent): Add 15 mL of pyridine to 0.3 g of barbituric acid in a 25 mL volumetric flask; mix. Add 3.0 mL concentrated HCl; mix. Dilute to volume with distilled water. Mix thoroughly, since the ingredients dissolve slowly and it is a saturated solution. Let it stand for 30 min and filter if necessary. Prepare fresh as needed.
- *Cyanide standard*:
  (a) *Stock standard (100 mg/dL):* Dissolve 250 mg of potassium cyanide in approximately 50 mL water in a 100-mL volumetric flask. Add 2.0 mL of 0.5 N sodium hydroxide (20 g/L) and dilute to 100 mL. Store in a polyethylene container. Discard after three months.
  (b) *Working standard (200 µg/dL):* Dilute 0.1 mL of stock standard to 50 mL with water. Prepare this fresh before use.

Procedure

1. Place 4 mL of blood or urine into the outer compartment of a Conway diffusion dish.
2. Place 2 mL of 0.1 N NaOH in the centre compartment and prepare the cover with silicone grease for a tight seal.
3. Add three drops of 3.6 N sulphuric acid in the outer compartment, seal the top quickly and swirl gently to mix. Allow diffusion to proceed for 4 h at room temperature or 3 h at 37 °C.
4. After the diffusion period, transfer 1 mL of the absorbing solution (in the centre well) to a test tube. Label this as T (test).
5. Label a second tube as B (blank) and add to this 1 mL of 0.1 N NaOH.
6. To each tube add 2 mL of NaH_2PO_4 solution and 1 mL of Chloramine-T solution. Mix and wait for 3 min.
7. To each tube add 3 mL of pyridine-barbituric acid solution. Mix and allow standing for 10 min.
8. Observe the colour and make a semiquantitative report. A red colour is a positive test for cyanide in this procedure.
9. For a quantitative report, include the working standard (200 µg/dL) in the above series. Carry on the entire test procedure, including the diffusion step. Measure the absorbance of test (A_t) and standard (A_s) against the blank at 580 nm in a spectrophotometer.
10. *Calculation*:
    Concentration of cyanide (µg/dL) = $(A_t/A_s) \times 200$

Common Source of Error Chloramine-T can oxidize certain substances like glycine to produce cyanide. Thus care must be exercised to avoid mechanical contamination of the absorbing solution in the centre well by trace amounts of the specimen.

Determination of Methanol, Isopropanol and Formaldehyde

Methanol and **isopropanol** are important industrial chemicals that also are available as household items. Both these alcohols are absorbed readily following ingestion. Intoxication with methanol and isopropanol can be from accidental ingestion, industrial exposure, self-poisoning, or as substitute for ethanol. Isopropanol is metabolized to acetone which results in ketonuria. The method of choice for the identification and measurement of methanol and isopropanol is GC which is available only in reference laboratories.

Formaldehyde is closely related to methanol in its chemistry. It is frequently used in indoor household and occupational environments. Some of the other sources include automobile exhaust from cars without catalytic converters, food preservative, cigarettes and tobacco products. Inhalation of formaldehyde invokes an inflammatory response, including a variety of allergic signs and symptoms. Therefore, formaldehyde has been considered as the most prevalent cause of **sick building syndrome**, which has become a major social problem, especially in developing urban areas.

Specimen

Anticoagulated whole blood and clotted blood are both used as specimens. Use only oxalated or citrated blood for obtaining plasma. Do not use heparin or EDTA as an anticoagulant. These will give false positive results. 'Clean catch' urine sample is also collected simultaneously.

Reagents

- *Trichloroacetic acid* (20%) v/v in water. *Caution*: Use gloves while making the solution.
- *Potassium permanganate($KMnO_4$) reagent*:
  Dissolve 3 g of potassium permanganate in 15 mL of phosphoric acid. Add this potassium permanganate solution to 85 mL of distilled water.
- Sodium bisulphite
- Chromotropic acid (powder)
- Sulphuric acid (concentrated)
- *Positive control*: Add 1.8 mL methanol to 1000 mL water. This is approximately 150 mg/dL.

Procedure

1. Take two centrifuge tubes (#1 and #2) and add 2 mL serum in each. Mix with 4 mL of 20% TCA in each. Wait for 5 min.
2. Centrifuge at 2000 rpm for 5 min or filter through Whatman #1 filter paper. Save the supernatant or filtrate as #1 and #2 corresponding to their respective source.
3. Take 0.1 mL of supernatant (or filtrate) from each and add two drops of permanganate solution. Wait exactly for 2 min.
4. After 2 min, add a pinch of sodium bisulphite to decolorize the excess of permanganate in tube #1 (oxidized) but not in tube #2 (not oxidized).
5. Then add a pinch of chromotropic acid in each and mix.
6. Carefully underlay the solution with 3 mL of sulphuric acid in each tube.
7. A purple ring at the interface of the solutions in the tubes oxidized with permanganate solution (#1) is positive for methanol. A purple ring in tubes not oxidized (#2) is a positive test for formaldehyde. High concentrations of ethanol may produce a brown colour.
8. Mix and diffuse the purple colour. Let it stand for 20 min for the colour to develop. Spin for 5 min and then read the absorbances of the test solutions for a semi-qualitative report.
9. Run positive controls to check out the procedure.
   Note: The test described above is not specific to methanol. Other alcohols and aldehydes (formaldehyde) will also react. For the identification of the alcohol, other methods like GLC will be needed. Specific ethanol assay is presented earlier. By method of elimination, diagnosis of methanol poisoning may be concluded.

DRUG SCREENING

Drugs frequently encountered in overdose situations are classified as hypnotics, analgesics, sedatives, tranquillizers, antihistamines and those used for the treatment of psychiatric disorders. Overdose may lead to coma, violent reaction or death, depending on the drug taken. Therapeutic screening is important for effective treatment.

Specimen

Blood specimen and random specimen of urine are commonly submitted to the laboratory for diagnosis. Process the specimen as early as possible.

Principle

Presence of the drug is detected by colour reaction with an appropriate reagent. Intensity of the colour can be a rough index of the amount of drug taken. A colour test with a urine specimen is a handy tool for drug screening. The method can be easily adopted by routine laboratories in India. The colour reaction may detect a specific compound or it can be applied for a general group of compound. Only a few will be dealt with here and readers should refer to more advanced books on this topic.

Phenothiazine Derivates

Phenothiazine derivatives are used as tranquillizers and for their antihistamine effect. The primary use of phenothiazines is to treat psychoses, that is, conditions that include delusions and hallucinations.

Phenothiazines are **radioopaque**, and unabsorbed drug in the form of full or partial tablets may be visualized in the gastrointestinal tract by abdominal X-ray. These substances can be detected easily in urine by the use sf ferric-perchloric-nitric FPN (FPN) reagent. The method is sensitive enough to detect the drug at therapeutic levels (used as tranquillizers and antihistamines).

Reagents

- *Ferric chloride solution* (5% aqueous w/v): Not stable, use immediately to prepare FPN reagent.
- *Perchloric acid solution* (20% aqueous v/v, 2 N).
- *Nitric acid solution* (50% aqueous v/v, 7.5 N).
- *FPN (ferric chloride-perchloric acid-nitric acid) reagent*: Mix 5 mL of the ferric chloride, 45 mL of the perchloric acid and 50 mL of the nitric acid solutions. Store in a dark bottle. The reagent is stable without refrigeration for 1 year.
- Positive control: Dissolve 25 g of chlorpromazine hydrochloride in 100 mL water.

Procedure

1. Add 1 mL of FPN reagent to 1 mL of urine.
2. Note the colour change immediately.
3. Disregard all colours appearing after a delay of 10 sec or more.
4. *Observation and inference*: With a drug intake of 5–20 mg/day, the colour is light-orange, for 25–70 mg/day, the solution shows an increasing intensity of pink colour while it becomes deep purple at a 125 mg/day.
5. *Quality control*: Run the test with the positive and negative controls (using the standard and water instead of urine) in order to check out the test reaction.

Acetaminophen

This drug is usually used to reduce pain (analgesics) and as an antipyretic. About 2% of the drug is excreted unchanged. Accurate estimation of acetaminophen in the plasma is done in sophisticated laboratories using advanced analytic techniques (e.g. HPLC, gas liquid chromatography). Nevertheless, p-aminophenol test can be easily performed in laboratories where advanced instruments are not available.

Principle

Urinary metabolites are hydrolysed in acid solution to p-aminophenol, which is coupled with o-cresol to produce a distinctive indophenol blue colour.

Reagents

- *Saturated o-cresol reagent*: Shake 10 mL of o-cresol with 1000 mL of water. Allow to stand for 24 h before use
- *Ammonium hydroxide solution (4 N)*: Dilute 284 mL concentrated ammonia (15 N) to 1000 mL with water
- *Concentrated HCl (11.7 N)*
- *Positive control*: p-aminophenol solution

Procedure

1. Take 1 mL of the urine specimen in a test tube.
2. Add 1 mL of HCl and heat in a boiling water-bath for 10 min.
3. Transfer 0.1 mL of the above solution into another test tube and add 9.9 mL of o-cresol reagent and 2 mL of 4 N NH_4OH.
4. A blue colour indicates the presence of the drug acetaminophen.
5. Run a negative control (with water) and a positive control before reporting the result confidently.
   Note: Phenacetin may also give positive result for this test. The method is extremely sensitive, use good quality reagents.

Chloral Hydrate and Halogenated Hydrocarbons

These are hypnotic drugs. When heated with sodium hydroxide and pyridine, halogenated hydrocarbons produce an intense red colour.

Reagents

- Sodium hydroxide solution (20%, w/v, aqueous).
- Pyridine: Store in a dark, tightly closed bottle in a room free of halogenated hydrocarbons. Do not use the reagent if it appears cloudy.
- Positive control: Dissolve 500 mg chloral hydrate in 100 mL of ethanol. Store in a dark bottle in the refrigerator.

Procedure

1. Take 1 mL of the urine sample in a test tube.
2. Add 1 mL of 20% NaOH and 1 mL of pyridine.
3. Heat in a boiling water-bath for 1 min.
4. A pink red colour in the pyridine layer indicates the presence of chloral hydrate or other halogenated hydrocarbons.
5. *Caution*: There are numerous halogenated hydrocarbons used in the laboratory, which will give a positive reaction (chloroform, carbon tetra-chloride, ethylene dichloride and others). Do not run the test in the areas of the laboratory where halogenated compounds are in use as extracts.
6. Always run a positive and a negative control (with water) before finally reporting the result.

Imipramine

This is an antidepressant drug, strongly protein bound, and it never reaches very high levels in blood and serum.

Principle
Some of the metabolites of imipramine (tricyclic compounds) react with oxidizing agents leading to the formation of an intense blue colour.

Reagents
- Potassium dichromate (0.2%, w/v, aqueous).
- *Sulphuric acid (30%, v/v, aqueous)*: Add 30 mL of concentrated sulphuric acid in small portions to 100 mL of water in a heat-resistant beaker. Stir constantly while adding the acid. Follow the same procedure for all acids.
- *Perchloric acid (20%, v/v, aqueous)*: Dilute 20 mL of perchloric acid to 100 mL with water.
- *Nitric acid (50%, v/v, aqueous)*: Dilute 50 mL concentrated nitric acid to 100 mL with water.
- *Imipramine reagent*: Mix equal volumes of the above four reagents and store in an amber glass bottle.
- *Positive control*: Dissolve 25 mg imipramine hydrochloride in 100 mL.

Procedure
1. Take 1 mL of the urine sample in a test tube.
2. Add 1 mL of the imipramine reagent and shake gently.
3. Immediately observe if a green or blue colour is produced.
4. Always run a negative (with water) and a positive control in order to check out the system. *Note:* Chemically related drugs of imipramine (e.g. desipramine and trimi-pramine) will also give the same reaction.
5. *Observation*: Development of a purple colour may indicate the presence of phenothiazine drugs. The specific test for phenothiazine is given earlier. A positive test occurs only when the patient has taken an overdose of imipramine.

Salicylates

Salicylate, as one of the least expensive and most widely used drugs, has been the cause of many drug overdose cases, particularly in the very young and the elderly. Salicylate still ranks as the leading cause of childhood poisoning deaths and still is commonly used in self-poisoning by adults. If taken on an empty stomach, it may lead to perforation of the stomach and intestinal bleeding. Many derivatives of salicylic acid are available commercially; the most important is acetylsalicylic acid (aspirin), which is hydrolysed rapidly to salicylic acid, and circulates in the blood in the ionized form, salicylate.

Specimen
Whole blood, serum and urine are the common specimens submitted.

Principle
The procedure described here is for screening but it can be made quantitative after processing the standard solution in the same way as the test solution and comparing their absorbance against the reagent blank made with an equal amount of water as used for the standard or the test solution. The phenol group of **salicylate** forms a coloured complex with ferric iron. The test is not specific for salycylates but false negative results do not occur. The colour developing solution (Tinder's reagent) contains acid and mercuric ions to precipitate protein.

Reagent

- *Colour reagent*: Dissolve 40 g of mercuric chloride (AR) in 850 mL of water by heating. Cool and add 120 mL of 1 N HCl and 40 g of ferric nitrate [$Fe(NO_3)_3 \cdot 9\,H_2O$]. When all the ferric nitrate has dissolved, dilute the solution to 1000 mL. The reagent is stable indefinitely.
- *Salicylate standard*:
  (a) *Stock standard of salicylate* (200 mg/dL): Dissolve 580.0 mg of sodium salicylate (equivalent to 500 mg of salicylic acid) in water and dilute to 250 mL. Add a few drops of chloroform as a preservative. It is stable for about 6 months.
  (b) *Working standard* (20 mg/dL): Dilute 10 mL of stock salicylate solution to 100 mL in a volumetric flask. Add a few drops of chloroform as a preservative. Store in a refrigerator. It is stable for about 6 months.

Procedure

1. Take three centrifuge tubes (12 mL) and label them as 'T' (test), 'S' (standard) and 'B' (blank). If a clear urine specimen is subjected for assay, use ordinary test tubes, as centrifugation may not be needed. In case the urine specimen is turbid, treat it in the same way as the serum specimen.
2. Pipette 1 mL of serum (or urine) specimen in tube 'T', 1 mL of standard solution in tube 'S' and 1 mL of water in tube 'B'.
   Note: An additional sample blank for urine will be needed which is described later.
3. Add 5 mL of colour reagent in all. Mix well by shaking until the precipitate is finely dispersed. Precipitate will not form in case of clear urine.
4. Centrifuge for 2 min (2000 rpm).
   Note: The precipitate can also be removed by filtration, using Whatman No. 42 filter paper.
   This step can be skipped in case of a clear urine specimen.
5. Pour the supernatant of each tube into three separate cuvettes (matched) and read the absorbance of the test solution (A_t) and the standard (A_s) at 540 nm, against the blank ('B') which is used to set 100%T.
6. This step is followed for urine only; Prepare a sample blank ('SB') by mixing 1.0 mL urine, 5.0 mL of colour reagent and 0.1 mL phosphoric acid (specific gravity 1.75). Read the absorbance of sample blank (A_{sb}) against water blank ('B').

Calculation
  (a) Concentration of salicylic acid (mg/dL) in serum = $A_t/A_s \times 20$
  (b) Concentration of salicylic acid in urine = $(A_t - A_{sb})/A_s \times 20$

Additional information
- If the absorbance of the unknown is greater than 0.7, repeat the analysis using a diluted specimen. Multiply the result by the dilution factor.
- False positive reactions may be seen in diabetic patients due to the presence of acetoacetic acid. In this case boil the urine before subjecting it to analysis.
- Phenothiazines in high concentration may react with the colour reagent.
- Chlorpromazine and thioridazine react with the reagent and give pink and blue colours respectively.

Barbiturates

Barbiturates affect the central nervous system. It is commonly used for treating insomnia and convulsive disorders and as anesthaetic and preanesthaetic medications. It is, however, habit forming and can lead to **addiction** in case of prolonged use. Drug abusers get hooked to the feeling of high within a short time that stays until 6 h. Acute barbiturate intoxication is characteristically associated with coma and shock. Commercially available immunoassay kits can provide quick result from serum and urine specimens but identification of specific barbiturate will require more elaborate equipment.

Barbiturate poisoning has reduced in recent years because it has been replaced by the safer **benzodiazepines**. The benzodiazepines are among the most frequently prescribed drugs. They vary in their potency in hypnotic, muscle relaxant, anticonvulsant and anaesthetic effects. With the popularity of these drugs, overdose is a frequent occurrence, yet fatalities resulting from benzodiazepines alone are very rare. Commercial immunoassays for benzodiazepines in urine or serum are available and can be adopted by laboratories.

Cyclic Antidepressants

The cyclic antidepressants are a major cause of life-threatening drug overdose, and are responsible for more deaths than any other drug classes except the analgesics.

These drugs can be detected in urine and also identified for proper treatment. But it requires expanded facilities of referral laboratories with facilities for TLC, HPLC and others. For quick screening, enzyme immunoassays are available in the market.

Cannabinoids

The cannabinoids are a group of more than 60 compounds found in the plant *Cannabis sativa*. Marijuana belongs to this group. When smoked, the effects appear within minutes and seldom last longer than 2–3 h. Oral intake delays the onset of symptoms for 30 min to 2 h but the duration of drug action is longer. The drug brings a sense of euphoria, an altered perception of time, a keener sense of hearing and heightened vivid visual imagery. Both short term memory and task performance are impaired. Higher doses can induce frank hallucinations, delusions and paranoid feelings. The most consistent cardiovascular effects are in increase in pulse rate and conjunctive reddening.

Screening usually is done with immunoassays as they have high sensitivity. Other methods such as TLC and GC are available in reference laboratories.

Opioids

The **naturally occurring** opioids are morphine and codeine. They are found in poppy seeds. These opioid drugs could also be synthetic or semisynthetic. **Semisynthetic** ones include heroin, hydromorphine and others. Methadone, diphenoxylate and others are **synthetic opioids**. Opioids produce analgesic, respiratory depressant, euphoric and emetic effects. Heroin and methadone are the most frequently abused opioids. The preferred route of heroin administration is intravenous, although heroin of sufficient purity is now available and is smoked or administered intranasally. Most of these opioids metabolize to morphine and excreted through the urine.

Immunoassays are commonly used as preliminary tests for the opiates (morphine and codeine). Identification of drug comes from more adanced analytical techniques.

Cocaine

Cocaine is an alkaloid extracted from the leaves of Erythroxylon coca plant and purified as the hydrochloride salt (cocaine-hydrochloride). In recent years the illicit use of cocaine has increased rapidly. It is either snorted or administered intravenously. It is a powerful stimulant of central nervous system (CNS). It produces heightened alertness, self-confidence and an intense feeling of euphoria (rush). These stimulatory effects are followed by depression (crash).

Immunoassays are popular because they are fast and easy to perform. They are geared towards the use of urine specimen analysing the end products of their catabolism in the body. Various other advanced techniques (TLC, EIA and RIA) are available in reference laboratories.

Sympathomimetic Drugs

Sympathomimetic drugs mimic the actions of the endogenous neurotransmitters that stimulate the sympathetic nervous system. Many of the illegal street drugs belong to this group (e.g. amphetamines). These drugs can be detected by immunoassays which are available commercially. There are other kits, which are sold as reagent packs, that go with the automated instruments or single-use devices which are designed for 'near-patient testing' in the physician's office. Before referring the case to specialized laboratories, screeing test may save time and money. Some of the advanced techniques include TLC, GC and HPLC.

Date-rape and Knockout Drugs

The use of drugs to facilitate sexual assault is not new. Ethanol is the most frequently involved drug, being particularly effective when used together with other CNS depressants. These drugs impede the victim's ability to make rational decisions and lead to the loss of consciousness. Some of the street names for these drugs are rooflies, rochies, rocha, rophies and others. They dissolve readily in alcohol and are colourless, odourless and tasteless. Urine specimen is taken for the detection of the metabolites of these drugs. Many of the commercially available kits are able to provide sufficient information for quick diagnosis.

HEAVY METAL POISONING

The heavy metals that commonly bring toxicity are mercury, bismuth, arsenic, antimony and lead. The main role of the clinical laboratory is to determine whether these substances are present or absent. Therefore, qualitative screening procedures are needed to help make this decision. We will describe the **Reinsch test** for the screening of the aforesaid heavy metals except lead. Identification procedure for mercury will also be described. The only reliable test for lead is the use of atomic absorption spectrophotometer which is expensive and beyond the reach of most laboratories of developing countries.

Specimen

Specimens submitted for detecting heavy metal poisoning are urine and gastric content.

Reinsch Screening Test
Principle
Heavy metals, such as mercury, bismuth, arsenic and antimondy, react with copper in acid medium when subjected to a prolonged heating period (1 h). The surface of the copper metal takes different colours following the acid-heat treatment. The colour indicates the presence of specific heavy metal.

Reagents
- Nitric acid (concentrated)
- Alcohol (absolute)
- Ether
- *Hydrochloric acid*: (a) Concentrated (b) 10%, v/v
- *Copper wire*: From a 20-gauge copper wire make a spiral about 5 mm diameter and 1 cm long with the help of a glass tube. The wire is dipped into concentrated nitric acid for 1 sec, then rinsed with demineralized water, then alcohol and finally ether, and allowed to dry.

Procedure
1. Place 20 mL of urine or gastric contents into a 50 mL Erlenmeyer flask and add 4 mL concentrated hydrochloric acid. Mark the level of the acid and place a small funnel at the top to reduce evaporation.

2. Introduce a copper spiral and heat gently for 1 h on a steam bath.
   Note: A low-temperature hot plate (surface temperature of approximately 95 °C) can also be used.
3. Maintain the volume by adding 10% hydrochloric acid during the heating period.
4. After an hour, remove the copper spiral, rinse it thoroughly with water, and then dry it on a piece of absorbant filter paper.
5. Observe the colouration for presumptive identification of heavy metal:
   - *Dull black*: Arsenic (sensitivity as low as 10 µg).
   - *Shiny black*: Bismuth (sensitivity as low as 20 µg).
   - *Dark purple sheen*: Antimony (sensitivity as low as 20 µg).
   - *Silver sheet*: Mercury (sensitivity as low as 30 µg).
6. For further identification of suspected heavy metal perform specific tests. The specific test for mercury is described here.

Specific Test for Mercury

Principle

Mercury held on the surface of a copper wire reacts with cuprous iodide forming the pink coloured mercuric iodide compound.

Reagents

Cuprous iodide solution: Dissolve 5 g of copper sulphate and 3 g of ferrous sulphate in 10 mL water. While stirring constantly, add a solution of 7 g potassium iodide dissolved in 50 mL water. Filter the precipitate and wash with water. Suspend the precipitated cuprous iodide with the aid of a little water and transfer to a brown bottle.

Procedure

1. Place a small piece of filter paper on a watch glass and add 2 drops of cuprous iodide suspension.
2. Place the acid-treated copper spiral on the cuprous iodide spot and cover with a second watch glass.
3. If a rose to salmon-pink colour appears as a result of formation of mercuric iodide, mercury is present.

Iron overdose

Iron supplements in various forms of iron salts are readily available. Ferrous sulphate, the cheapest and most common iron salt, is involved frequently in overdose. There are several other over-the-counter iron pills, used as supplemental nutrients, but develop iron toxicity. Acute iron poisoning is particularly common in the paediatric population, with majority of the reported exposure occurring in children less than 6 years of age. In the worst scenario, the patient may develop systemic toxicity with cardiovascular collapse, seizure, coma and shock. Hepatic failure and GI tract obstruction alarms high level toxicity.

Serum (clotted blood) is the chosen specimen for determining iron toxicity. Both free iron and total iron binding capacity (TIBC) are determined in the chemistry laboratory. Simple colorimetric procedures are followed with the help of commercial kits. For more detail analysis, use of atomic absorption spectroscopy is recommended.

A heavy discharge of iron in urine is an indication of iron overdose. A new procedure is presented here which can be followed in small laboratories in order to diagnose iron toxicity.

Principle

The iron is reduced to ferrioxamine with sodium hydrosulphite (dithionite). The iron is determined after the addition of dipyridyl.

Reagents

Sodium hydrosulphite (dithionite) powder
  Sulphuric acid (0.05 N)
  Dipyridyl solution (1% w/v in 0.05 N sulphuric acid)
  Phosphate buffer 1/15 M, pH 7, according to Sorensen.
  Standards: 0, 10, 40 and 80 µg Fe/20 mL as solution of ferrous ammonium sulphate in iron-free water.

Procedure

1. Centrifuge the urine specimen.
2. Pipette 20 mL of urine into 50 mL volumetric flask.
3. Add 20 mL of phosphate buffer.
4. Add about 50 mg of dithionate with a small spatula.
5. Mix thoroughly.
6. Take 10 mL aliquots into each of two test tubes marked—T (test) and UB (urine blank).
7. Add to the first tube (marked as T) 0.2 mL of the dipyridyl solution.
8. To the other tube (marked UB) add 0.2 mL of 0.05 N sulphuric acid.
9. A reagent blank or RB (use iron-free water instead of urine) is prepared the same way as the 'Test'.
10. Allow the tubes to stand for 30 min.
11. Read colour against water (or the 0 standard) in a spectrophotometer (or colorimeter) at 510 mµ wavelength or with a suitable filter in a photometer.
12. Prepare a calibration curve with the standards (0–80 µgFe/20 mL). The calibration curve may not be linear for the entire range. Work in different ranges, 0–40 and 40–80 µgFe/20 mL.
13. *Calculation*: The optical density (OD) of the reagent blank (RB) and urine blank (UB) are subtracted from that of the sample (T).
14. Compare with the calibration curve and report.

Review Questions

1. Under what conditions specimens are referred to the toxicological laboratories? What are the commonly submitted specimens?
2. What is the role of toxicology laboratory?
3. What is microdiffusion technique? How does this technique help in the toxicological investigation?
4. Describe the screening tests for the following:
   Acetone, alcohol, heavy metal, acetaminophen and imipramine.
5. What is Reinsch test? How does this test help in diagnosing heavy metal poisoning?
6. Describe the microdiffusion test as applied in the diagnosis of toxicity due to carbon monoxide, halogenated hydrocarbons and cyanide.
7. How would you determine the toxicity caused by methanol and formaldehyde?
8. What is the clinical significance of the following drugs: phenothiazine derivates and acetaminophen? How would you recognize their overdose?

Section VIII
Histology and Cytology

36

Introduction to Histotechnology and Cytotechnology

Papreddy V. Kashireddy and Rohini Chakravarthy[*]

Chapter Outline

- *Introduction to Histology and Cytology Laboratories*
- *Basic Terminologies*
- *Specimen Handling*
- *Laboratory Equipment and Reagents*
  - Use and care of equipment
    - Microscope
    - Microtome
    - Paraffin oven
    - Tissue floating bath
    - Vacuum embedding oven
    - Slide warmer
  - Use and care of laboratory supplies
    - Microscope slides and cover slips
- *Preparation of Reagent Solutions*
- *Review Questions*

INTRODUCTION TO HISTOLOGY AND CYTOLOGY LABORATORIES

The histopathology laboratory prepares tissue sections for establishing a histopathological diagnosis. It is a science of studying the changes in the human body brought about by disease, identifying the disease and its cause, so that appropriate treatment can be given. Because of its convincing physical evidence, histotechnology has proved to be one of the most effective tools in diagnosing tissue abnormalities and cancerous conditions. In recent years, with the advent of freezing microtomy, the team work of the surgeon and the histopathologist has greatly contributed to the progress of medical science. Histotechnology is concerned with processing and preparation of the tissues of the body in such a manner as to enable a satisfactory study of the tissues and is an

---

[*] Calculations in preparation of reagents.

art by itself requiring skill and knowledge on the part of the histotechnologist as the final product can favourably or adversely influence the diagnosis.

The **specimens** submitted to the histopathology laboratory can be from the gastroenterologists in the form of small pieces of tissues, (biopsies), endoscopic sinus surgery specimen from an ENT surgeon, appendix, gallbladder for gallstones, enlarged lymphnode for lymphoma workup, amputated limb for diabetic gangrene, etc. from general surgeons and a resected whole kidney or liver for malignant tumours, radical mastectomy specimen in breast cancer, etc. and margins of a skin tumour for frozens from oncosurgeons. These specimens are submitted either fresh (unfixed) or immersed in a fixative fluid. As a histotechnician you are neither involved in the collection of the specimens nor in their laboratory evaluation. You are, however, responsible for the handling and preparation of the specimens to facilitate their gross and microscopic examinations which are done only by the histopathologist. With recent advances in histotechnology the histotechnologist apart from routine processing of the tissues should be aware of complicated procedures involving electron microscopy (EM), special stains, immunohistochemistry (IHC), immunofluorescence (IF), fluorescent *in situ* hibridization (FISH) techniques and also have a knowledge of using automated precessing and staining equipment. The basic steps of specimen processing include fixation, embedding, microtomy, staining and mounting. These will be discussed in the following sections. It is expected that the histotechnologist will be sufficiently trained to prepare the specimens according to the specifications, to recognize satisfactory preparation, identify and remedy the causes when unsatisfactory results are obtained.

Exfoliative cytology is different from histology. Here the specimens are constituted by the body fluids, secretions and excretions collected during physical examination of the patient. Laboratory techniques involve the preparation of smears, fixing, staining, mounting and microscopic examination. The cytopathologist evaluates the smears for exfoliated cells characteristic of not only cancerous and pre-cancerous conditions, but also of a variety of other alterations produced by Inflammatory and degenerative processes. Other than routine specimen processing the histotechnologist should have knowledge of fixation and staining of squash preparations, imprint/impression smears, fine needle aspiration cytology smears and frozen sections.

As soon as a specimen for surgical pathology or a fluid for cytology is received for analysis it is the responsibility of the technologist to accept only if the name on the **requisition form** and the details written on the specimen container label tallies correctly. Once this is done the specimen should be given a **surgical number** which should appear in all further subsequent steps till the slides are stained for reporting.

There are some inherent problems faced by the laboratory in preparing specimens for histological studies. As soon as a tissue is removed from the body for histological examination, it is cut off from its blood supply and begins to decompose (autolysis) and putrify. Autolysis is due to action of the enzymes which are liberated after cell death and putrifaction is caused by bacterial invasion and distruction of the tissue. This disintegration of the cell is prevented by either freezing or by adding certain chemical substances to the tissues/cells which are called fixatives. To preserve as nearly as possible the natural state of the tissue cells, it is essential to check the autolysis with a minimum of delay. This process is known as **fixing**. Based on the chemical action fixatives are further classified. **Aldehydes**: formaldehyde (10% formalin used in routine histology) and gluteraldehyde used in EM. **Oxidising agents**: Osmium tetroxide, potassium permanganate and potassium dichromate. **Protein denaturing agents**: methyl alcohol, ethyl alcohol and acetic acid.

Large specimens are cut into slices of 1–2 cm thick and fixed in adequate formalin for fixation before submitting 1–2 cm^2 and 3–4-mm-thick sections from the specimens for histology. To enhance the speed of fixation and processing floor model microwave processors are being used lately.

Tissues are either too soft or too hard and calcified, which makes them difficult to cut into microscopic sections. Thus the procedures of decalcification, dehydration and embedding precede microtomy and staining.

The process of **embedding** involves the infiltration of paraffin wax into the tissues, which provides the necessary hardness to cut sections. Since the tissues contain water, and paraffin wax is insoluble in water, the removal of water (**dehydration**) is the first step of tissue preparation for embedding. This is accomplished by using increasing gradients of ethyl alcohol until the tissues are finally bathed in 100% (absolute) alcohol. The dehydration is followed by infiltrating a **clearing agent** such as xylene or chloroform into the tissue. The clearing agent also acts as a solvent for paraffin wax. Finally, the paraffin is impregnated into the tissues in a molten state while the infiltrated xylene diffuses out into the paraffin bath. When the paraffin is solidified, the tissue is ready to be made into blocks and cut into thin slices or sections. The thin sections are then prepared for staining. Most stains are soluble in water, however, and cannot cross the paraffin barrier to react with the tissue constituents. Hence the thin sections are first **rehydrated** or 'taken to water' prior to staining.

To rehydrate the sections, they are first floated onto a microscope slide. The sections are then bonded to the slides by heating them above the melting point of the paraffin in an oven or on a warming plate. The sections are then de-waxed by immersing in xylene, followed by dipping in ethyl alcohol in decreasing gradients. The rehydrated sections are then stained and again subjected to **dehydration** before they are permanently mounted. The sections will fog with time if not dehydrated properly. Staining is usually done with multiple stains in order to differentiate between various cells, tissues and cell constituents by their differential staining properties.

The study of exfoliated cells in body fluids does not involve the cutting of sections, but the cells may need to be concentrated by centrifugation. A smear is made from the fluid or the sediment on a microscope slide, fixed and then stained. The techniques of cytotechnology closely resemble those of histotechnology except in the preparation of specimens prior to staining.

BASIC TERMINOLOGY

Although a glossary of technical terms used in various clinical laboratories has been presented in Chapter 39 in this Volume, some of the terms commonly used in histotechnology and cytology are presented here.

Adhesion: The process of placing the section on the slide so that it is not washed away during dehydration, staining or other treatments. Egg albumin and gelatin are popular adhesives

Autolysis: Self digestion and decomposition of tissues.

Biopsy: A fragment of tissue taken out of an organ from a living person and examined. The literal meaning of the word is 'to see for oneself'.

Block: Portion of specimen properly cut and trimmed for processing. *Cryostat:* A cold box containing the microtome used to cut frozen sections which are fresh specimens mostly margins of a malignant tumour. The temperature of the box is kept well below freezing, in the −20 to −30°C range.

Fixation: A process by which the specimen is preserved in its original condition. Formaldehyde (10% buffered formalin) is a commonly used fixative.

Clearing agent: A substance that makes tissues more transparent for microscopic examination. Xylene and chloroform are the commonly used clearing agents.

Decalcification: A process to remove calcium from bone and other mineralized hard tissues in order to facilitate the process of cutting thin sections. Decalcification is done after fixation and before dehydration and paraffin infiltration. Nitric acid, formic acid and hydrochloric acid are commonly used to decalcify hard tissues.

Dehydration: The process of removing water from tissues. The common procedure is to treat the specimen blocks with increasing gradients of alcohol followed by treatment with the clearing agent.

Exfoltative cytology: Entails the microscopic examination and interpretation of cells which are shed (exfoliated) spontaneously from epithelial surfaces of the body, or which may be removed from such surfaces or membranes by physical means. Common specimens include cervical and vaginal smears, buccal smears, bronchial brushings, bladder washings and various body fluids (pleural effusion, pericardial effusion, ascitic fluid, joint effusions and cerebrospinal fluid) and secretions.

Freezing microtomy: Preparations of sections from frozen tissues.

Histology: Study of stained sections of tissues under the microscope.

Infiltration: A process by which the clearing agent is eliminated from the tissue making room for the impregnation of the embedding medium (paraffin wax).

Impregnation: A process that allows the embedding material to enter the tissue while the clearing agent is diffused out.

Microtome: An instrument used for preparing thin sections (4–5 μm) of tissue. The most common types are rocking microtome and rotary microtome. Microtomy is the process of section cutting.

Mounting: The arrangement of specimens on slides for microscopic study.

Rehydration: Commonly referred to as 'taking the section to water'. The goal is to replace the water insoluble paraffin wax with water prior to staining with water soluble stains.

Staining: The process of colouring of tissues in order to facilitate their identification under the microscope.

Smear: Specimen spread on a slide surface to facilitate microscopic observation. This is the standard method of specimen preparation in exfoliative cytology.

LABORATORY REAGENTS AND EQUIPMENT

Most histotechnology laboratories will require the following equipment and supplies: some of these are shown in Fig. 36.1.

- Microscope
- Microtome
- Microtome knife (disposable), or razor
- Timer
- Oven, Bunsen burner, forceps, scalpel, dissecting set
- Constant temperature water-bath, flotation bath, paraffin bath
- Equipment for embedding and vacuum infiltration
- Containers (bottles) for holding specimens
- General glassware as any other laboratory (pipettes, beakers, etc.)
- Microscope slides and cover-slips
- Slide carrier
- Slide trays for storage
- Coplin staining dish or staining jar: Vertical and horizontal
- *Accessories*: Labels, diamond pencil for marking glass slides.
- Plastic disposable cassettes for embedding.
- Automatic tissue processor (for advanced laboratories)
- Automatic stainer (for advanced laboratories)

Reagents

A great number of histologic procedures in use call for a variety of chemicals and reagents. These include fixatives, decalcifying solutions, embedding materials, stains, solvents, clearing reagents, mounting media and a large number of miscellaneous solutions. In preparing various reagents, one should first read the label on the bottle for care and storage instructions and precisely follow the directions given in the method of their preparation. Some of the basic rules of preparing solutions are given later in this section. The boiling point of solvents is important if certain limits; are stated. Many of them are highly flammable and should not be inhaled. All instructions from the Material safety data sheets (MSDS) of all chemicals should be read and

precautions taken accordingly. All reagents and stains should be tested for proper reactivity before being put into regular use.
- *Embedding material:* paraffin wax (melting point 50–55°C)
- *Fixative*: formaldehyde
- Ethyl alcohol, xylene (or xylol)

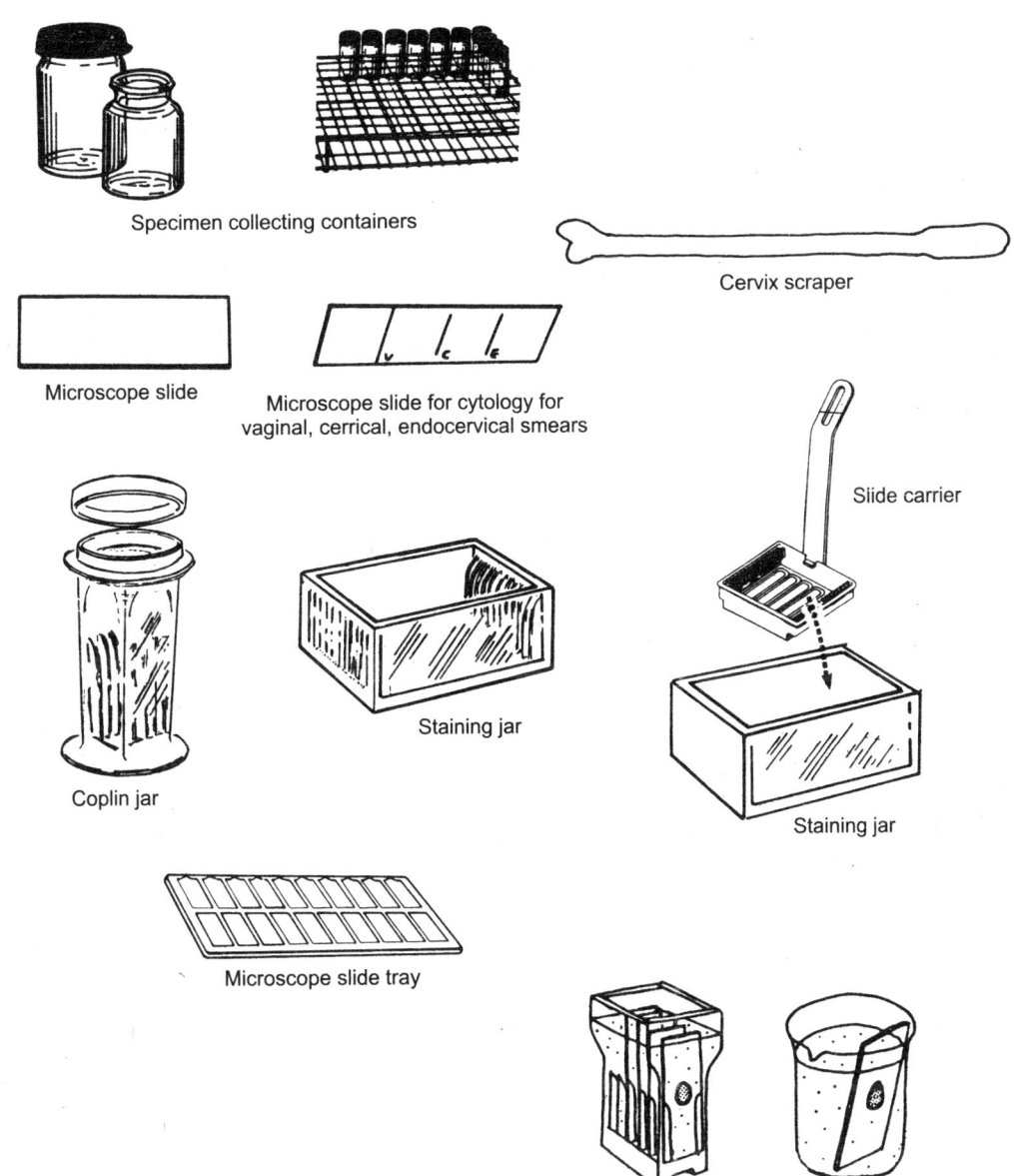

Fig. 36.1 *Materials commonly used in histological and cytological studies.*

- *Mounting medium*: DPX, Permount
- Egg albumin
- Glacial acetic acid, mercuric oxide, ammonium aluminium sulphate
- *Decalcifiers*: formic acid, nitric acid, hydrochloric acid
- *Stains*: haematoxylin, erythrosin B, eosin, fast green FCF, alizarin red S, rose Bengal, aniline blue, fuchsln, auramine 0, safranin 0, azure dyes, Giemsa stain, light green, Sudan III, malachite green, indigo carmine, brilliant green, sudan black B, methyl green, thionin, carmine, Wright stain, methyl orange, carbol fuchsin, Congo red, gentian violet, neutral red, iodine solution, Gram crystal violet, methylene blue, orange-G, Papanicolaou stain, phloxine, safranin solution and periodic acid Schiff reagent

Commonly Used Equipment

The microtome and the microscope are the two most important pieces of equipment in a histology laboratory. Other equipment include a paraffin oven, vacuum embedding oven, and tissue floating bath. The technician must know their proper use and care so that this equipment can give many years of service. Some of the other equipment used in the histology laboratory such as the refrigerator, balance, incubator, magnetic stirrer and others have been discussed in Chapter 4 in Vol. I.

Microscope

The microscope is used to examine thin sections cut by the microtome. It is an integral part of most of the clinical laboratories except chemistry. The backbone of histotechnology lies with the use of various types of microscopes—light microscope, polarizing microscope, dark-field microscope and fluorescence microscope. The uses of phase-contrast microscope and electron microscope are rather limited in the histology laboratories of developing countries.

Of the various types of microscopes used in the laboratory, the **light microscope** is used routinely. Detailed description of the use and care of **light microscope** has been presented in Chapter 4 in Vol. I. For examining objects under the light microscope staining is done with differently coloured dyes in order to create contrast.

Fluorescence is essentially an optical phenomenon in which light of one wavelength is absorbed by a substance and almost instantly re-emitted as light of longer wavelength. In **fluorescence microscopy**, the substance is bombarded with short-wavelength light in the ultraviolet (UV), violet or blue range, and visible light is emitted. The source of illumination is high intensity ultraviolet rays (mercury vapour lamp). The object (antigen) is stained with a fluorescent dye, conjugated to the corresponding antibody, through immunological reaction (Chapter 24 in Vol. II). The antigen—antibody complex glows with the availability of ultraviolet light and thus the object (antigen) is located. Its use in the identification of spirochetes through IF techniques is explained in Chapter 20 in Vol. II.

The **polarizing microscope** is finding increased use as a diagnostic tool in histopathology primarily for the identification of crystals. In the case of patients with gouturate crystals are sought under polarized microscope. It also is used to make the identification of amyloid stained with Congo red more specific. The use of polarizing microscope in exhibiting double refraction, anisotropism, birefringence has helped in many diagnostic situations. The light microscope can be converted easily to a polarizing microscope for its wider use.

Dark field microscopy excludes the directly transmitted light and uses only the scattered or oblique light during viewing. The light reflected from the microscopic object like stars with a dark background of the sky at night. This type of microscopy is used primarily for the study of unstained microorganisms and is rarely used in routine histopathology.

Embedding equipment

The embedding centre provides a supply of melted paraffin, warm storage for embedding molds, small warming and chilling plates for orientation during embedding, and a large chilling plate. Some centres include magnifying glasses to aid in specimen orientation. The paraffin is kept 2–4°C above the melting point of the paraffin used. If the temperature of the embedding paraffin is allowed to go too high, the nature of the paraffin and the resultant sectioning qualities will be affected

The **paraffin oven** (Fig. 36.2) maintains a temperature between 50 and 60°C which can be accurately adjusted according to need. The drier oven described above can be shared. The oven should be large enough to have space for melting and storing molten paraffin, infiltration of paraffin in sections, drying of slides and warming of solutions during the preparation of reagents. **Vacuum embedding** saves time and is the method of choice because it allows for a more thorough impregnation of paraffin into the tissue (Fig. 36.2). It is specifically recommended for those tissues which are likely to become overhardened during the usual 2–3 h of immersion in hot paraffin. The temperature of the bath is kept at 56–58°C and the vacuum is created by a suction pump.

Microtome

The use of microtomes is in section cutting. Two basic types of microtomes are commonly encountered—rocking, rotary and sliding. Routine histological sections are cut after embedding.

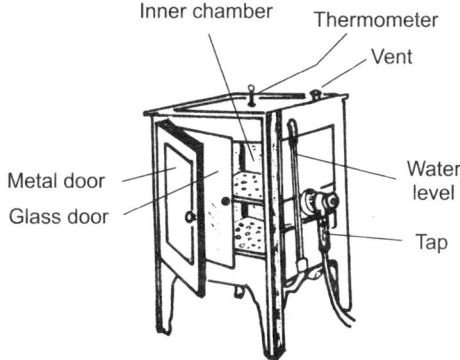

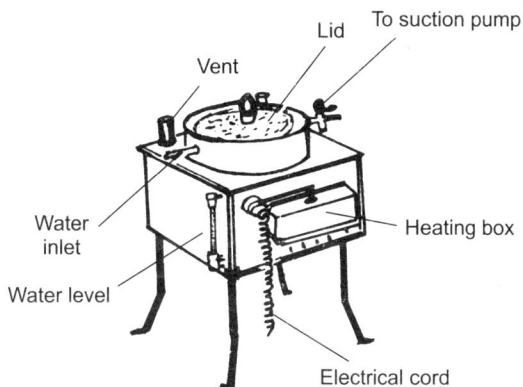

Fig. 36.2 *Components of paraffin embedding oven (a) and vacuum paraffin embedding bath (b).*

Use of the **rocking microtome** (Cambridge model, Fig. 36.3) is common in the histology laboratories of developing countries. It is relatively inexpensive, simple to operate, is practically maintenance free and it has the ability to produce sections of high quality. For getting serial sections, the **rotary microtome** is preferred (Fig. 36.3). It is a delicate machine and designed to cut extremely thin sections. This is slowly replacing the rocking microtome. Rotary microtome is found in most laboratories where routine paraffin and frozen sections are the sole requirements. Most rotary microtomes operate with a screw feed; the block moves up and down, and either the knife or the block advances a preset number of micrometers with each revolution of the wheel. This type of microtome is found in most cryostats and is the type most commonly used for sectioning paraffin-embedded material. Celloidin-embedded sections are cut by the **sliding microtome**. Sliding microtome holds the block, and the knife is moved along a horizontal plane past the block face. As the knife is returned to the starting position, it completes each section cycle and a screw feed causes the block to be raised toward the knife at a predetermined thickness. This type of microtome is used for sectioning celloidin and large paraffin blocks; it is not used in routine histopathology.

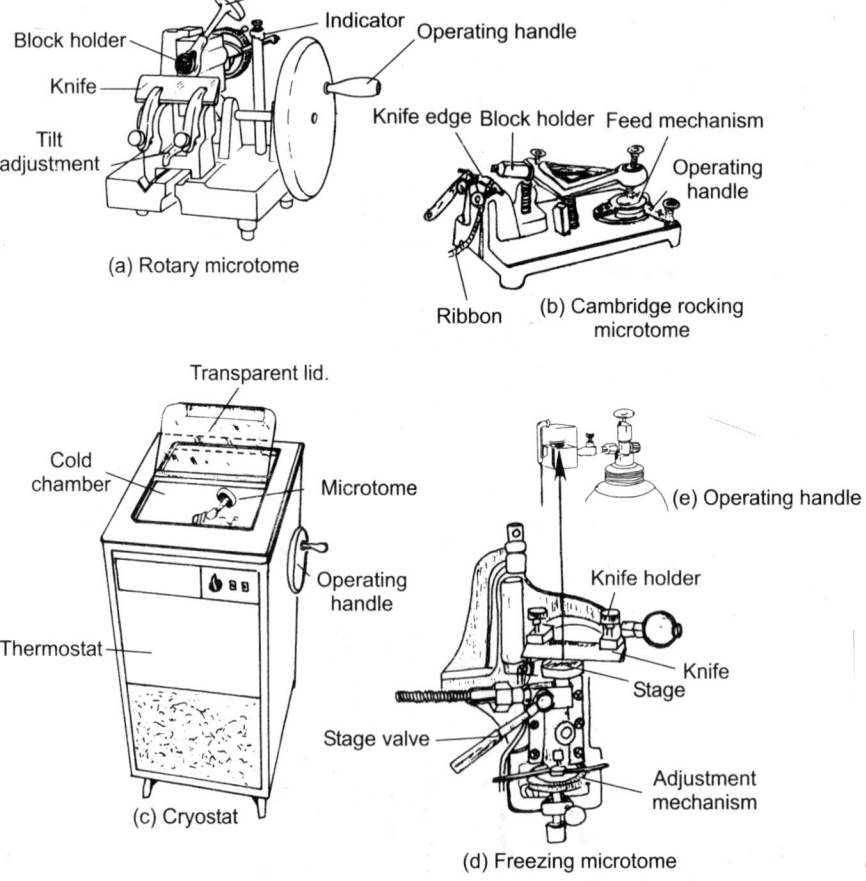

Fig. 36.3 *Commonly used microtome in the histology laboratory. (a) Rotary microtome, (b) Cambridge rocking microtome, (c) cryostat and (d) freezing microtome. Note the carbon dioxide quick freezing chamber with gas cylinder (e).*

Microtomy of frozen sections plays a vital role in modern histology laboratories. Frozen sections do not need to be embedded. Soft specimens are cut in frozen condition which gives the necessary rigidity for the section cutting. This method is useful for rapid diagnosis during an operation or to examine the sections for a substance (e.g. fat) or structure that would otherwise be destroyed by preparing the sections in the routine way.

The **clinical freezing microtome** (Fig. 36.3), used in cutting frozen sections is relatively portable and can be fixed on the table top. A chuck with an attached supply of carbon dioxide allows for horizontal freezing of the tissue section. The knife is kept cold. Section must be removed from the knife edge and floated in a dish of distilled water. The clinical freezing microtome has been replaced to a great degree by **cryostat** (Fig. 36.3). Cryostat is a refrigerated chamber containing a microtome, usually of the rotary type. It is cooled by a mechanical refrigeration unit. Although a cryostat is easy to operate, practice and skill are needed to obtain good frozen sections. The microtome knife of the cryostat must be very sharp and the edge must be free of defects. The knife stays warm in the freezing microtome. After sectioning the tissues it should not be stored unprotected. It should be wrapped carefully to exclude air and then stored in a $-70°C$ freezer. Cut sections are stained in the same manner as the embedded sections.

All good microtomes are correctly adjusted by the manufacturer. If lubricated and cleaned, they should stay that way for a long time. The instructions from the manufacturer should be carefully read and reviewed periodically so that all subsequent adjustments and maintenance will be exactly as the manufacturer recommends. Since the repairing of instruments is difficult under the existing conditions of the developing countries, especially when foreign equipment is imported, the technician must get fully acquainted with the manufacturer's instructions for use, maintenance and trouble shooting. Dust is probably the single most important enemy of most equipment. The basic care of the microtome includes regular removal of dust.

All microtomes have three major parts:
- The block holder: in which the tissue is held in position.
- The knife carrier and the knife.
- The adjustment screws and rachet device that line up the tissue in proper relation to the knife and feed the proper thickness of tissue for successive sections. The microtome feeding mechanism is graduated in microns (µm).

With all types of microtomes, the **micrometer** setting is very important. This setting is only approximate and is not an exact determinant of section thickness; the actual thickness is determined by the condition of the microtome and the quality of knife edge as well as the skill of the technologist.

Care of Microtome Maintenance of the microtome is crucial for its proper functioning. Keep the moving parts well lubricated and clean. Put a cover on the microtome when not in use to prevent dust accumulation. Do not permit rust, dust or paraffin to accumulate between the bearing surfaces of the knife holder, brackets, etc. The surfaces should be cleaned frequently, and then wiped with good neutral oil (e.g. coconut oil); this will prevent rust formation.

After cutting sections on the microtome, all accumulated paraffin and tissue should be removed with a soft brush. Metal parts are cleaned with xylene (do not use xylene too frequently; it will remove the painted finish). All moving parts of the microtome must be kept lubricated with a light lubrication oil (e.g. sewing machine oil), and kept free from paraffin. Xylene (or petroleum ether) helps to remove the paraffin. The rigidity of the knife-holder and the knife are important but never adjust any screws so tightly that they may cause binding. The instrument should be tight only to the point of smooth, firm operation.

Efficiency and the results of microtomy are largely dependent on the proper preparation of the specimen prior to section cutting, and the use of a sharp knife in good condition. This is discussed separately under 'cutting of sections' (Chapter 37 in this Volume).

Knife sharpener

One of the key points of getting good section is to use a sharp knife. The abrasive surface of the **knife sharpener** helps to keep the knife sharp. The abrasive surface is provided by glass, copper or iron plates. The amount of abrasive used for knife sharpening is very important. Use of excessive amount (common tendency) defies the purpose. Follow manufacturer's instructions with necessary modifications to get the optimum edge. If more than one sharpener is available, it is a good idea to assign certain knives to a specific sharpener. One critical step common to most sharpeners is that the knife should be placed in the holder the same way each time, otherwise sharpening may not duplicate the established cutting facets. Plates must be kept flat, with one plate used for the coarse abrasive and one plate used for the fine abrasive. Make sure that the plates are not mixed up. Whenever plates lose flatness or become too smooth and knife edge. If more than one sharpener is available, it is good idea to assign certain knives to a specific sharpener. The knife should be cleaned of abrasive and carefully dried (always wipe and never across the edge) after sharpening. In areas of high humidity, the knife should be lightly oiled for storage, and then cleaned to remove the oil before using.

Flotation bath

Flotation baths is used to float and facilitate separation of paraffin embedded tissue ribbons while mounting the section on the slide (Fig. 36.4). It is basically a temperature controlled water bath that is kept at 5–10 °C below the melting point of the paraffin used for embedding. Ideally, the bath should have a dull black interior to optimize the visibility of the floating translucent paraffin ribbons. After using the bath, pour off the water while warm and wipe thoroughly to remove adherent bits of paraffin while they are still soft. *Note:* If it is an electric bath, pour the water over the rim opposite the electrical element. If water gets into the electrical element, it may be a source of electrical hazard. One should be careful in using the flotation bath. If the bath is too hot, the ribbons get overstretched. If the ribbon is allowed to float for too long period artefacts may develop and mimic many pathological conditions like edema. Ribbons must be stretched gently as they are placed on the flotation bath, and then small wrinkles and folds should be quickly but cautiously teased out of the sections. Air bubbles may get trapped under the section which can be drawn to one side by blunt dissecting needle that has been bent at an angle to reach under the ribbon. Care should be exercised so that the ribbon is not pierced or torn. Sections may be removed from the knife and transferred to the flotation bath with the fingers, forceps, a brush, or a wooden application stick. The applicator stick attached to one end of the ribbon will aid in stretching the ribbon and will float on the bath in tact without getting detached from the ribbon. The preparation of slides to pick up the paraffin section is discussed in the tissue processing section.

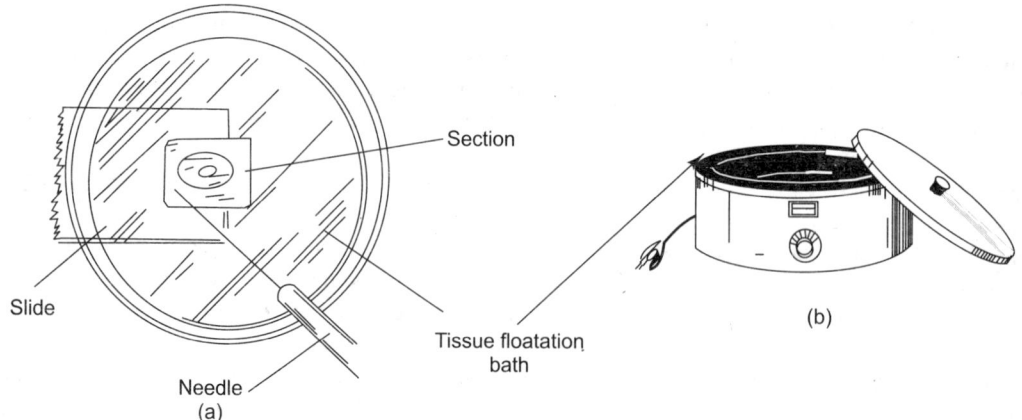

Fig. 36.4 *Method of guiding section: (a) on to a slide and (b) on a tissue floatation bath.*

Dryer oven and slide warmer

In the preparation for staining, paraffin has to be removed. In order to remove paraffin (deparaffinization) the slides need to be warmed which can either be done in the paraffin oven or on the **slide warmer** (Fig. 36.5). The latter is handy and can be placed adjacent to the staining area. The slides must be completely dry before they are deparaffinised, because water left on the slides will not mix with xylene (clearing agent) and will cause incomplete removal of paraffin. This is indicated by white spots that can be seen in tissue as the slides are removed from xylene. This artefact is difficult to correct as they stain more intensely later. These slides should be treated with absolute alcohol to remove any residual water and then placed back in xylene to remove any remaining paraffin. The slides should then be taken through absolute and 95% alcohols to water and stained as desired. Incomplete drying can also cause sections to wash off during staining. Overheating of the sections during drying also can create artefacts.

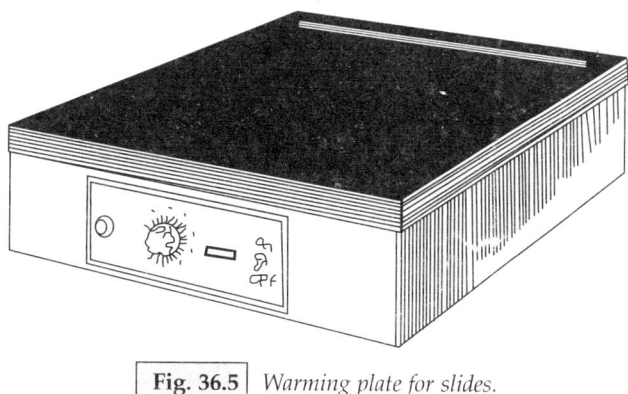

Fig. 36.5 *Warming plate for slides.*

The temperature of the dryers and hot plates are usually kept at 60°C which is just above the melting point of paraffin. Forced-air slide dryers take 7–10 min while hot oven requires 1 h, ensuring complete drying.

Automated tissue processor and stainer

Manual staining is done in smaller laboratories. Use of staining dishes, like the coplin jars (that holds 5–10 slides) is common and a timer is used for determining the duration in different reagents. The results are, however, not always reliable. Hence many laboratories in urban areas of developing countries are now switching to automated tissue processor. This equipment automatically fixes, dehydrates, clears, and infiltrates tissues and makes them ready for embedding. The two major types of tissue processor include the open type and the closed type. In the open type, tissues are transported from one solution to the next, and in the closed system the tissues stay stationary while the solutions are changed. The processor must be kept clean and a routine reagent rotation and/or change cycle determined by usage must be established and rigidly adhered to. The temperature of the paraffin must be carefully adjusted to no more that 2–4°C above the melting point of the paraffin in use, or the tissue will be brittle and over hardened. The temperature must be monitored and recorded daily, with adjustments made in the paraffin bath temperature when indicated by improper temperature readings.

The machine consists of a time clock, a circular superstructure that contains the basket carrier, a receptacle basket and receptacles (stainless steel or plastic capsules), and a circular deck which holds the reagent beakers and paraffin baths. Small blocks of tissue are enclosed in the perforated capsules. These capsules are placed in the basket, which in turn is attached to one of 12 yokes in the superstructure while it is in the raised position. The entire superstructure descends, immersing the basket in the first solution and sealing the other reagent beakers to prevent evaporation. To move the basket from one reagent to the next in the processing sequence, the entire superstructure ascends and descends at scheduled intervals controlled by the time clock. During immersion in the fluids, the basket oscillates up and down in a reciprocal motion to keep, the tissue and reagents in a state of controlled agitation, which significantly increases the speed of penetration. After the prescribed amount of time in the last paraffin bath, the tissue remains there until removed manually.

It takes about 16 h for routine processing. Hence the machine is set in the afternoon and the processed material is taken out on the following morning for embedding.

The solutions must be changed at regular intervals (twice a week). If any of the solutions is cloudy, changing should be done more frequently. If there are several beakers of the same solution, discard only the first beaker and move the others up in place by decanting the reagent from one to the other beaker and then add the fresh one at the end. If the solution has evaporated, replace the lost fluid. Clean the beakers with detergent (do not use acid). If the paraffin is sticking to the rim of the beaker containing paraffin, remove it carefully or it may come in the way of the moving parts of the automatic processor.

Automatic stainers perform routine staining that saves time and yields consistent reliable results. Slides are placed in staining troughs with separate baskets that enable up to 20 slides to be stained at the same time. There are three types of automatic stainers—linear, revolving and robotic. In linear stainers slides are transferred from one container (vat) to the next with same time allowed in each container. The time in each different solution can be changed only by varying the number of containers holding that particular reagent. Revolving stainers operates on the same principle as the open tissue processor, and the time allowed in each solution may be varied. Robotic stainers are computerized and the timing in each solution is programmed.

In the following chapter (Chapter 37 in this volume), automatic tissue processors will be rediscussed along with the procedure.

Incubators

Some special stains require incubation which is done either in a water bath or in an incubator. The incubator maintains temperature of 37°C.

Freezers and refrigerators

Freezers and refrigerators are used for storing many of the reagents. Freezers maintain a temperature of –20°C while the refrigerators are kept at 4°C.

LABORATORY SUPPLIES

Microscope Slides and Cover-slips

Microscope slides and cover-slips are most frequently used in the histology laboratory and hence a short discussion of their cleaning and storage is in order. Procedures for the labelling of slides and storage of specimens will also be mentioned in the following discussion.

In recent years special microscope slides are introduced into the market, which bear a permanent positive charge. They electrostatically attract tissue sections and cytology preparations, binding them to the slide. These slides form a bridge so that covalent bonds develop between sections and the glass. Tissue sections and cytological preparations adhere better to these glass slides without the need for special adhesives or protein coatings.

Cleaning of slides and cover-slips

Reagent Acid alcohol (1% HCl in 70% alcohol)
    70% ethyl alcohol   1000 mL
    HCl (concentrated)   10 mL

Procedure Clean the used slides and cover slips in acid alcohol, rinse in water, and then place in 95% alcohol. Finally, take out from the alcohol, polish and dry each one with lintless cloth (e.g. surgical gauze). Cleaned slides and cover-slips should be stored in clean covered boxes or in dishes with lids. For routine work, dip new slides and cover-slips in 95% alcohol and polish. Slides and cover-slips to be used in fluorescent microscopy must be thoroughly cleaned with acid alcohol.

Labelling of slides

If the slides have frosted ends, glass-marking ink can be used (India ink can also be used). If the slides are not frosted, the slides are etched with a diamond marking pencil. Some laboratories use etching for temporary marking of the slides and then at the final stage (after mounting) use a special label that is attached to the slide. Do not use a wax pencil in marking the slides.

Another safe way is to write (or type) the identification number on a piece of paper which is placed on the slide next to the section. The mounting reagent is then applied, and the cover slip placed in position. The number remains permanently sealed with the section.

Containers for slides

Cardboard trays are the most convenient. Wooden or plastic boxes or metal filing cabinets are more expensive.

Containers for Specimens

The use of plastic bags to store specimens with preserving solutions is becoming more popular. Only thick plastic bags should be used. The specimen can be kept initially in a wide-mouthed bottle; after fixation, the fixative is poured out and the specimen is kept in a heat-sealed plastic bag.

Paraffin blocks with embedded specimens should be stored with embedded identification tags. These are then stored in wooden or plastic boxes. Cardboard boxes can also be used, but these must be protected from rodents and insects. It is important to store the paraffin blocks in a cool place.

Mounting Media

Stained sections need to be mounted on an appropriate mounting media and then covered with the cover slip before the sections can be examined under a microscope. There are two basic mounting media—aqueous and resinous.

Aqueous mounting media

These are used when dehydrating and clearing will adversely affect the stain. Gelatine–glycerine mixture is non-hazardous water-based, mounting media which are ideal for mounting immunohistochemical stained tissues. These tissues can be damaged by the organic solvents, such as xylene or toluene. Hence, tissue sections stained with organic chromagens are best preserved using aqueous mounting media.

Resinous mounting media

Some mounting media oxidize rapidly upon exposure to air making the slides unsuitable to examine after long storage. This is why use of Canada-balsam has now become obsolete. It is replaced by resinous mounting media. These include DPX, Parmount and Biomount. The resinous media consists of solid resin dissolved in an appropriate solvent; the viscosity of the medium should be such that the solution will enter the tissue spaces and flow readily between slide and cover glass. Air bubbles should be displaced quickly. Most resinous media are dissolved in toluene or xylene. Many laboratories prefer xylene as the solvent because the slides are usually mounted after xylene (clearing) treatment. All of the resinous mounting media will cause a gradual fading. The two most commonly used resin-based mounting media are DPX, Permount and Biomount. They will now be discussed here.

DPX mountant is a mixture of distyrene, a plasticizer and xylene. It is a colourless synthetic resin mounting media that replaced Xylene-balsam in modern laboratories. It preserves the stain and dries quickly. **Permount (Fisher-Scientific)** is a toluene-based synthetic resin mounting medium. Many laboratories consider its use as the right choice for both rapid mounting and long term storage of slides. Its low viscosity allows for a thinner mounting layer offering better optical quality and bubble-free preparations. It has a refractive index near that of a fixed protein which helps to keep images free of distortion. It is deal for mounting cover slips to slides with thick or thin specimens Permount preserves most biological stains with little or no fading when the slides are stored in darkness. It contains an anti-oxidant to prevent the formation of annular rings. **Biomount** is a specially formulated mounting medium that reduces fading of some stains. It is suitable for resins as well as wax embedded sections of tissue.

PREPARATION OF REAGENT SOLUTIONS

While working in the histology and cytology laboratories the technician will have to prepare a number of reagent solutions. It is essential to be familiar with the expressions of the strength of solutions to be made (Chapter 6 in Vol. I). Most laboratories keep stock solutions which are diluted to working solutions when needed. Stock solutions have a better shelf life and take up less storage space. The technician must be very careful in preparing reagent solutions. An error made at this stage may cause considerable aggravation. A solution has two components, the solvent and the solute. The strength of the solution is most often expressed in the weight/volume ratio or volume/volume ratio. Water is the most common solvent into which pre-weighed solutes are dissolved and made up to the desired volume. The use of tap water is discouraged because it contains a considerable number of impurities. Distilled water is the ideal solvent, but deionized water is both cheaper and easier to obtain and is adequate for most purposes. It is important to check the efficiency of the deionizer column frequently to make certain that the electrolytes are totally removed (Chapter 4 in Vol. I).

The presence of chloride as an impurity in the solvent can create problems with the solutions made for histological studies. A simple way to test the presence of chloride in water is by adding a drop of silver nitrate solution (2%, w/v, aqueous) in an aliquot of water. If the water becomes cloudy, chloride is present. Re-purify the water before use. Occasionally, boiled, cooled and decanted water may be free of chloride and can be used in places where distillation or deionization facilities are pot available.

Dilutions from Stock Solutions

If a series of working solutions are needed with varying strengths, the technician should be able to figure out the mathematical relationship (Chapter 6 in Vol. I). As varying strengths of alcohols are needed in processing specimens for histological examination, we will use two examples in order to show the calculation steps. *Note:* Only 95% alcohol is commercially available unless one treats 95% alcohol with calcium chloride or some such dehydrant to remove the water (5%). This is not necessary.

Example 1: Prepare 1000 mL of a 70% alcohol (#1, working solution) from 95% alcohol (#2, stock solution).
Solution
    Formula: $S_1 V_1 = S_2 V_2$,
    where S_1 and S_2 are strengths of solutions #1 and #2, respectively.
    Note: All the strengths are expressed in the same unit (%).
$$S_1 = 95 \text{ (initial) and } S_2 = 70 \text{ (final)}$$
    V_1 and V_2 are the volumes of the solutions 1 and 2, respectively.
    Consider $V_1 = x$ mL when the final volume $V_2 = 1000$ mL
    Then the above formula will be written as
$$90 \times x = 75 \times 1000$$
$$\text{Or, } x = (75 \times 1000)/90 = 736.8 \text{ mL.}$$

Thus, if 736.8 mL of 90% alcohol is made to (qs) 1000 mL with distilled water, the strength of the resulting solution will be 70% alcohol.

Example 2: Prepare 500 mL of 5% ferric chloride solution (working solution) from 29% ferric chloride solution (stock solution)
Solution

$$S_1 V_1 = S_2 V_2$$
$$29 \times x = 5 \times 500$$
$$x = 86.2$$

Take 86.2 mL of 29% ferric chloride and make it to 500 ml. The final solution will be of 5% strengths.

Example 3: Prepare a 1000 mL solution of 80% alcohol from 95% and 50% alcohol solutions.
Solution

The following formula is the elaboration of the same principle of strength/volume relationship. Here, however, we are involved in two initial solutions which when mixed, gives a third solution of different strength.

$$(S_1 \times V_1) + (S_2 \times V_2) = S_3 \times V_3$$

The strengths (all in the same % units) of initial solutions are, respectively, S_1 (95) and S_2 (50) while the final strength S_3 is 80.

Now consider the volume of V_1 (95%) = x, then V_2 will be 1000 – x because the final volume is 1000 mL. If you put the values in the above formula, it looks like this

$$(95 \times x) + [50 \times (1000 - x) = 80 \times 1000$$
$$\text{or, } 95 x + 50,000 - 50 x = 80\,000$$
$$\text{or, } 45 x = 30\,000$$
$$x = 666.7 \text{ mL}.$$

Thus, if you take 666.7 of the 95% alcohol and make it to 1000 mL with the 50% alcohol, you will have 1000 mL of 80% alcohol.

Review Questions

1. What are the functional differences between histotechnology and cytotechnology?
2. What is autolysis? How can this be prevented?
3. What is the significance of the following in the preparation of histological specimens: fixation, embedding, dehydration and rehydration?
4. What is the use of a microtome? What are the different types of microtomes? How would you maintain a microtome in order to give many years of efficient service?
5. Why is the vacuum embedding oven superior over the ordinary embedding oven?
6. What is the temperature maintained by the paraffin oven and tissue floating bath?
7. How are the microscope slides and cover-slips cleaned and stored?
8. How would you prepare a 500 mL of 70% alcohol from 95% alcohol?
9. How much ferric chloride would you weigh in preparing 1000 mL of 29% solution?
10. What volume of 30% ferric chloride would you need, which, when diluted with water, will make 100 mL of 5% ferric chloride?
11. What are the steps involved in preparing sections for staining?
12. What is the most commonly used stain for histological sections? What are its advantages and disadvantages?
13. What is freezing microtomy? State its significance.
14. How would you maintain the microtome knife for its best performance?

15. What are the uses of the following stains and techniques?
    (a) Weigert–van Gieson stain
    (b) Masson's trichrome stain
    (c) Verhoeff's stain
    (d) Weigert's resorcin-fuchsin stain
    (e) Periodic acid-Schiff stain
    (f) Prussian blue stain
    (g) Von Kossa's technique
    (h) Silver impregnation technique
16. What is the recommended procedure for staining?
    (a) Reticulum fibres
    (b) Amyloid
    (c) Systemic fungi
17. What do you understand by metactyromic stain? Give example.
18. Make a list of possible problems in cutting sections. How will you resolve them?

37

Laboratory Techniques in Histology

◆

Venk Mani

Chapter Outline

- *Logging in of Specimens*
- *Preparation of Tissues*
  - *Fixation*
  - *Preparation of fixatives*
    - *Routine fixatives*
    - *Special fixatives*
    - *Decalcification*
      - *Acid method*
      - *Chelating method*
      - *Combination method*
      - *Detecting the end point of decalcification*
- *Processing of Tissues*
  - *Dehydration*
  - *Clearing*
  - *Infiltration (impregnation)*
  - *Manual and automatic tissue processing*
  - *Embedding*
- *Preparation of Sections*
  - *Section cutting*
    - *Attaching section to microscope slide*
    - *Storage of paraffin blocks*
    - *Problems in section cutting*
- *Routine Staining Procedure in Histology*

- *Basic information*
- *Pre-staining treatments*
- *Staining*
- *Post-staining processes*
- *Routine haematoxylin and eosin staining (H&E)*
- *Special Stains and Staining Techniques*
  - *Connective tissue stains*
    - *Collagen and collagen fibres*
      - *Reticulin*
      - *Elastic fibres*
- *Stains for Particular Substances*
  - *Carbohydrate*
  - *Amyloids*
  - *Lipids*
  - *Pigments and minerals*
- *Stains for Microorganisms*
  - *General purpose*
  - *Bacteria*
    - *Gram staining*
    - *Acid fast staining*
    - *Demonstration of Helicobacter*
  - *Fungi*
  - *Tissue parasite*
- *Frozen Section Technique*
  - *Staining of frozen sections*
- *Handling and Embedding of Small Tissue Fragments*
- *Review Questions*

A specimen brought to the histology laboratory must first be logged, identified and then subjected to specimen preparation prior to tissue processing. Processed tissues are then cut into thin sections, stained and mounted for microscopic examination. These steps can be broadly divided as follows:
- Preparation of tissues which includes fixation and decalcification.
- Processing of tissues, which includes dehydrating, clearing and embedding?
- Preparation of sections, which includes the process of microtomy, attaching section to slides (adhesion) and removal of pigments and precipitates.
- Staining and mounting procedures: dewaxing, staining, dehydrating, clearing and mounting.

In the following sections, we will discuss the techniques involved in processing the specimens until they are ready for microscopic examination.

LOGGING IN OF SPECIMENS

The routine histology laboratory receives specimens in the form of biopsies or whole organs. The strictest attention must be paid to specimen identification. Tragedy may happen if the specimens are interchanged in the laboratory. For example, a normal patient may be diagnosed as having the disease, say cancer, and treated for a disease that he does not have, whereas, the diseased person may not be treated and may die from the disease.

In most hospitals, small specimens are placed in fixative solution by the operating room personnel following biopsy. This protects the specimen from drying. Large surgical specimens may arrive unfixed in the laboratory but they must be put in plastic bags or wrapped in saline moistened towels and should be kept in the refrigerator until examined by the pathologist. This slows down autolysis and the plastic bag with the saline moistened towel protects the specimen from drying. If the specimens are mailed outside, they must always be fixed prior to mailing and larger specimens should be opened so that the fixative can reach inside. It is best if the fixation of large specimens is done under the direction of a pathologist, to ensure significant tissue is not lost or destroyed.

The laboratory must maintain a log book wherein each specimen is entered when first received in the laboratory. From the log book the specimen receives an identification number. Usually the numbers are given as the specimens arrive rather than grouping them. The interposing of dissimilar specimens helps to avoid possible errors between similar specimens.

The pathologist assistant first examines the specimens. The morphological description of the fixed tissue is narrated by the pathologist and typed by the secretary. This becomes the permanent record of the patient, much as the hospital chart. Following the gross external and internal examination of the tissue, a portion of the tissue is trimmed (called a block) by the pathologist and given to the histotechnician for laboratory processing. It is important that one of the technicians receive the block so that any special problems of orientation of specimens and the need for special stains can be discussed.

After receiving the block, the technician copies the identification number (same as entered in the log book), with a soft lead pencil on a tag that is always kept attached to the specimen. The technician now enters a record of the specimen's identification number into a laboratory register and the locations of the tissue block taken. In addition, a sketch of the large specimen is drawn in a separate column on the laboratory register that provides a general outline of the tissue as it looks.

The specimens with identification tags are then transferred into small plastic cassettes with fresh fixative or directly into the cassettes as described later. When using an automatic tissue processor, further processing begins in the late afternoon. If the tissues are in containers, they are first taken into perforated cassettes, properly wrapped with the identification tag. Several slices from the same specimen may be placed in the same cassettes. These cassettes then go through the subsequent steps of tissue processing prior to microtomy. In the case of bone and calcified tissues, specimens should be cut into small blocks with a saw before fixation. These will need decalcification before they are lined up with the soft tissues for dehydration and embedding.

PREPARATION OF TISSUES

Fixation

Fixation of tissues (Fig. 37.1) is necessary to prevent subsequent changes (autolysis). When the tissue is dropped in a fixative it is immediately killed and enzymatic digestive processes are inhibited thus preserving the normal structure. Hence, this must be done promptly. The other purpose of fixing the tissues is to harden them. This should be done to such a degree that the tissue components and architecture will be little affected by any subsequent procedures.

The process of fixing is carried out twice. First is at the operation theatre as initial fixation, where a large amount of tissue or organ may be involved. The re-fixing is done in the histology laboratory after cutting bits or blocks of tissues submitted for histological diagnosis. The blocks should be thin enough (3–5 mm thick) in order to facilitate penetration of the fixing fluid into the tissue within a reasonably short time (3–5 h). The volume of the fixative should be at two times the volume of the tissue block. Specimens must be securely held in a holder along with the identification number. Mini specimens should be wrapped in lens or cigarette paper or placed in a special fine mesh capsule before immersing in the fixative. If these steps are not taken, the small segments of tissue (biopsy specimens) may migrate through the perforations in the capsule and be lost in processing.

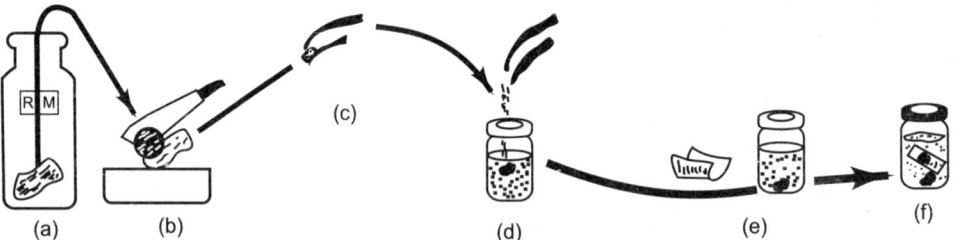

Fig. 37.1 *Specimen preparation in histology (a) Following surgical procedure, specimens are sent to the histology laboratory in containers with formalin (b) A portion of the specimen is removed and (c and d) transferred to a smaller container for further processing (e and f). It is important that the specimen bears the identification tag.*

From the practical point of view, fixatives are classified as routine or special. The most widely used fixative is 10% formalin (*Note:* formaldehyde gas dissolved in water yields formalin). It is relatively inexpensive, readily available, easy to prepare, compatible with most stains and penetrates the tissues well. It, however, has an unpleasant vapour which is irritating to the eyes. It may cause an allergic reaction on the skin and hence one should wear rubber gloves while handling formalin and work inside a hood while preparing the solution.

Formalin is slightly acidic which interferes in some staining procedures. In such cases, neutral formalin is preferred. Formalin is neutralized with calcium carbonate. The routine laboratory should have other fixative solutions available for special purposes (**Zenker's fluid**, **Bouin's fluid**, Helly's fluid and Carnoy's fluid).

Preparation of Fixatives

Fixatives affect the staining reaction. An ideal fixative should be rapid in action, permit a broad range of staining techniques, and be suitable for a wide variety of tissues processed collectively. Formalin does not necessarily meet all the requirements discussed earlier. Formalin occasionally creates a problem in some staining reactions. In these cases deformalinization of the tissue sections prior to staining will usually rectify the problem. Formalin can cause the appearance of dark spots, but these can be removed. Under special conditions, other fixatives are used. For example, fats will dissolve in fixatives with organic solvents (alcohol, acetone) while water-soluble materials (e.g. carbohydrate) will be preserved.

Routine fixatives

Formalin (10%) is the most commonly used routine fixative. The commercially available formalin (formaldehyde in solution) has 40% formaldehyde gas dissolved in water. Hence it is diluted to obtain 10% formalin fixative.

- *10% formalin*
    - Commercial formalin (full strength)   100 mL
    - Distilled water   900 mL
- *Neutral formalin*
    - 10% formalin solution   1000 mL

  Add excess amount of calcium carbonate.

Storage of specimen in formalin: 10% formalin is most frequently used for wet storage of tissue. The tissues are preserved for future use.

Removal of formalin from formalin-fixed tissues: After the tissue is fixed with the primary fixative (formalin), the excess fixative is removed by washing briefly in water followed by placing in 70% alcohol. Formalin is extracted more rapidly in 70% alcohol than in unchanged water.

Problems with formalin fixative: Formalin sometimes produces a fine dark-brown or black crystalline precipitate (perhaps due to lake of haemoglobin). This precipitate is recognized when the sections are examined under the microscope. To remove the precipitate, first deparaffinize the sections to water (xylene–alcohol–water) and then place in the following solution:

Ammonium hydroxide (58%)	2 mL
Alcohol (70%)	100 mL

Place the section in this solution for about 1 h, then wash thoroughly in tap water to remove excess ammonia and proceed to stain. This procedure may not be necessary if the formalin is of good quality.

Deformalinization and secondary fixation

Occasionally it is desirable to re-fix formalin-fixed sections in some other fixative (e.g. Zenker's, Helly's or Bouin's) in order to produce a more brilliant stain. The secondary fixation is done in the following way:

Deparaffinize and take the section to water. Then treat it with ammonia water (30 drops of 58% ammonium hydroxide in 100 mL of water) for 1 h followed by washing in running water.

Following deformalinization, re-fix in Zenker's or Helly's fluid for 1 h and wash for 15 min in running water. Residual mercuric chloride is then removed by the procedure described later. This is called mordanting.

For Bouin's mordanting, deformalinize and refix with Bouin's fluid (or in saturated picric acid) for 1 h. Remove excess fixative by washing in running water for 30 min (Fig. 37.2); rinse with distilled water and proceed for staining.

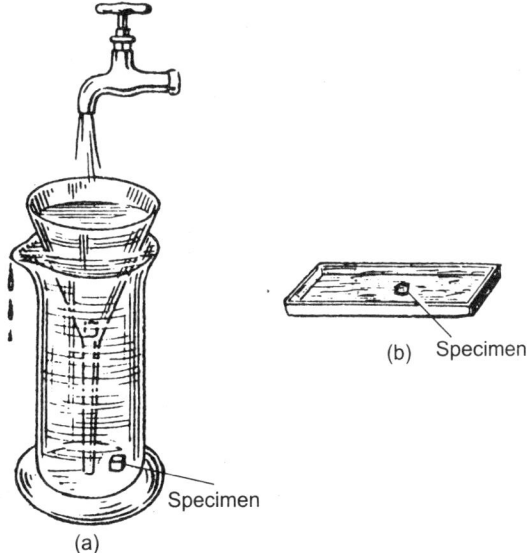

Fig. 37.2 *Washing of fixed specimen. (a) Washing for a prolonged period. (b) Quick washing of section can be done in a porcelain dish.*

Zenker's Fluid Zenker's fluid is a commonly used secondary fixative. Tissues preserved by this method stain well with many techniques provided the tissues are thoroughly washed in running tap water for several hours after fixation. The penetration power of the fixative is, however, poor and the tissues should not exceed

5 mm thickness. A longer time may be required for Zenker-fixed tissues to take the haematoxylin stain. Many workers prefer this fluid for fixing bone marrow aspirate as the acid present will decalcify bone spicules that may be in the specimen. Others have recommended Zenker's fluid for small pieces of tissues such as spleen and liver. The fixative permits excellent staining of nuclei and of connective tissue fibres. It is recommended particularly for tissues which are to be stained by one of the trichrome techniques.

- *Stock solution*:

Mercuric chloride	60 g
Potassium dichromate	25 g
Sodium sulphate	10 g
Distilled water	1000 mL

    Dissolve the ingredients by gentle heating or stirring at room temperature.

- *Working solution*:
    Add 5 mL of glacial acetic acid to 95 mL of Zenker's fluid just before use. The solution does not keep well after the addition of acetic acid.

Helly's Fluid Here the glacial acetic acid is replaced with formaldehyde, which is added to 95 mL of the mixture at the time of use.

- *Stock solution:*

Mercuric chloride	5 g
Potassium dichromate	5 g
Sodium sulphate	10 g
Distilled water	1000 mL

- *Working solution:*
    Add 5 mL of formalin (37–40%) to 95 mL of stock solution.

Fixation with either of these chromate fixatives (Zenker's or Helly's fluid) produces greater cytologic detail than with ordinary formalin. The major disadvantage in the use of these fixatives is the necessity of washing overnight in running tap water after fixation in order to remove the yellow-staining dichromate. In addition, the mercury precipitates in the tissue as fine granules, which must be removed from the sections before they are stained.

Removal of mercuric chloride deposits

Zenker's and Helly's fluids contain mercuric chloride which should be removed prior to staining. The method is described here.

Deparaffinize the slide with xylene followed by treatment with absolute alcohol and 95% alcohol. Then place the slide in alcoholic iodine solution (0.5% iodine in 80% alcohol) for 5–10 min. This will remove the deposits. Following the iodine treatment, wash in running water (Fig. 37.2), then place the section in 5% sodium thiosulphate solution (hypo) for 2–5 min. This will bleach out the iodine. Finally wash the slide in running tap water to remove the hypo and then proceed for staining.

Bouin's Fluid Bouin's fluid is recommended for general purposes and for special study of haematological and lymphoid tissues.

Picric acid, 1.22% (Saturated aqueous solution)	750 mL
Formalin, full strength (37–40% formaldehyde)	250 mL
Acetic acid, glacial	50 mL

Fix tissues for 4–18 h, depending on the size and density of the tissue. Following fixation wash in several changes of 50% and 70% alcohol for 4–8 h. Residual picric acid (yellow coloured) interferes in the staining reaction. If a yellow colour is seen in the section, deparaffinise, re-wash and re-stain.

Carnoy's Fluid Carnoy's fluid is a penetrating and quick acting fixative. It is suitable for cytological specimens and small pieces of tissues (biopsy specimens). It is recommended for glycogen since aqueous solutions are to be avoided, but it readily removes fats.

Absolute alcohol	60 mL
Chloroform	30 mL
Acetic acid, glacial	10 mL

Tissues are fixed for 12–18 h in the refrigerator (recommended) or 1–3 h at room temperature. Tissues fixed in Carnoy's fluid do not require washing. Dehydration of the tissue is already achieved during fixation.

Decalcification

When preparing sections of bone, and other calcified tissues, decalcification is necessary in order to facilitate cutting. Only on special circumstances undecalcified bones are requested. In diagnostic pathology, most evaluations are made on decalcified sections; undecalcified bone sections are examined primarily for the diagnosis of metabolic bone disease.

The calcified hard tissues should be first cut into small pieces (2–6 mm) with a thin blade hacksaw or sharp knife in order to minimize the tearing of surrounding tissues. This is followed by fixation in neutral or buffered formalin. Unless a decalcifying agent combined with a fixative is used, tissue must be thoroughly fixed and washed before it is submitted for decalcification or the tissue morphology can be affected. Thorough removal of the fixative by washing is necessary.

There are basically only two method of decalcification—acid method and chelating method. Decalcifying reagents are commercially available

Acid Method of Decalcification Acid method of decalcification is most widely used. The acid present in the decalcifying fluid removes the calcium salt present in the tissue (which gives the tissue its hardness), thereby renders the tissue soft enough for sectioning. The acids are used as simple dilute aqueous solutions or mixed with other chemicals (fixatives).

Out of the many acids the best results are probably obtained with nitric and formic acids.

Reagents

- *Nitric acid (5%, v/v, aqueous):* add few milligrams of urea to each 100 mL.
  Dilute nitric acid solution is probably used most often as it decalcifies rapidly and is reliable in that it will complete the decalcification. Because of its rapid action, nitric acid is ideal for urgent bone biopsies. Unfortunately, if tissue is left too long in nitric acid considerable damage to the tissue will occur; this damage will become apparent after 2 days or if in concentrations of acid above 8%. After decalcification the tissue is washed well in 70% alcohol before being processed to paraffin wax.
- *Formic acid (10%, v/v, aqueous)*
  Dilute formic acid solution is a good routine decalcifying agent; it is slower in its action than nitric acid, but causes less damage to the tissue by over-exposure. Decalcification for a piece of cancellous bone 4 mm thick should be complete in 48 h, while for dense bone two weeks or longer may be required. It is recommended that the formic acid is changed every two days. The staining results obtained after formic acid is superior to those using nitric acid.

Special Note:
With simple acid methods, calcium ions are allowed to migrate out of the tissue into the surrounding solution. The solution around the tissue may become saturated with calcium ions, almost forming a barrier to further decalcification. For this reason, the solution should be changed frequently, and agitation may also be beneficial. Vacuum at the initial stage of decalcification will aid in infiltrating the specimen with decalcifying fluid and will draw off carbon dioxide bubbles that form on specimen surfaces. Suspension of the specimen in an

embedding bag will expose all surfaces to the action of decalcifying fluid, and will allow any precipitated calcium salts to sink to the bottom of the container. Heat should never be used to speed up decalcification with acid as heat also increases the effects of decalcifying fluids on other tissue components and swelling and maceration will most likely result.

Chelating Method of Decalcification Chelating agents are organic compounds that have the property of binding certain metals. Ethylenediaminetetraacetic acid (EDTA) will bind calcium ions. Satisfactory results are obtained if EDTA is used in a solution with a pH between 5.0 and 7.2., but a slightly acidic pH is preferred.

Reagents
- *Ethylenediaminetetraacetic acid (EDTA, 15%, w/v, aqueous), pH 7.2*

Procedure
1. Immerse the representative portion of bone in decalcification solution, twice its volume, for 24–72 h (or longer) in order the remove the calcium out of the tissue. This makes the tissue soft enough for sectioning.
2. The tissue may be mechanically tested for adequate decalcification. Bending or piercing with a very sharp needle is often adopted by an experienced histotechnician, but these procedures may damage the cells and ruin the specimen for histological examination if done too roughly.
3. Wash the decalcified specimen in running water for 24–48 h. Every trace of decalcifying solution must be removed before dehydration and embedding. Some laboratories neutralize the decalcifying acid by treating the block with 10% formalin to which an excess of calcium or magnesium carbonate has been added. The tissue is now ready for dehydration, clearing and embedding.

Special Note:
Little damage occurs to the tissue although it may be in EDTA for several months before decalcification is complete. The speed with which the calcium is removed can be accelerated by heating to between 37 and 42°C, without causing tissue damage. Staining is of an acceptable standard after using this chelating agent and good differential results can be obtained.

Combination Method of Decalcification This combination method, using both acid and chelating agent, is recommended by many laboratories that helps to expedite the decalcification process.

Reagent

EDTA	700 mg
Potassium sodium tartrate	8 mg
Sodium tartrate	140 mg
Conc. Hydrochloric acid	99.2 mL
Distilled water (qs)	1000 mL

Procedure
Follow the standard procedure of decalcification described before.
Note: The tissue should not be left in this solution for no longer than 36 h (one and a half days).

Detecting the End Point of Decalcification It is important that when decalcification is complete the tissue should be removed from the decalcifying fluid immediately. Under decalcified tissues will be hard to section and over calcified tissues will have problem in staining. There are three ways to determine the end point of decalcification—mechanical (or physical), chemical and radiographic (X-ray).

Mechanical methods involve testing the flexibility of the specimen, probing the specimen with a needle or pin, and scraping the section surfaces. They are the least desirable for determining the end point because of their inaccuracy and the likelihood of creating histological artefacts.

Chemical methods depend on the precipitation of calcium oxalate when a sample of the used decalcifying fluid is mixed with a solution containing ammonium hydroxide and ammonium oxalate. Approximately 5 mL of the used decalcifying fluid is made neutral to litmus paper with concentrated ammonium hydroxide, and then approximately 5 mL of saturated ammonium oxalate solution is added. The resulting solution is mixed well and allowed to stand for 30 min; a persistent turbidity of calcium oxalate indicates the presence of calcium. The decalcifying fluid must be changed after each chemical check. Once the decalcifying fluid is free of calcium ion, decalcification process is complete. Chemical test is most suitable for the developing countries.

Radiographic method is the most accurate method, and the small X-ray units available in many histology laboratories are easy to use. This method yields visual evidence that demineralization is complete. Radiography methods cannot be used with metallic-fixed tissue, such as Zenker's solution (contains mercuric compound).

After decalcification is complete, the specimen should be washed well with running water to remove any excess acid. Some laboratories use an alkaline solution, such as lithium carbonate, to **neutralize** any remaining acid before processing the specimen routinely.

Summary
For routine use: Cancellous bone: 5% nitric acid (aqueous, with added urea), 1–2 days
For non-urgent material: EDTA, 15%, 2 weeks to 3 months.
For urgent material: Warm (37 °C), 5% nitric acid, 5–12 h or combination (acid-EDTA), 36 h.

PROCESSING OF TISSUES

Following fixation and decalcification (in the case of bone and calcified tissues) the tissue-blocks are processed in preparation for the paraffin embedding. Paraffin embedding gives the tissue the necessary hardness for microtomy. Since paraffin is not miscible or soluble in water, the water must be removed from the specimen to allow the paraffin to infiltrate into the tissue. The four major steps of tissue processing that come under the 'paraffin wax technique' are:

- Dehydration
- Clearing
- Infiltration
- Embedding

Manual tissue processing procedures and their timings are shown in Table 37.1. Except remote laboratories, automated tissue processing has become a part of any average or advanced laboratory. Apart from saving time, it yields reliable results. Many local companies have also learnt how to fix them. Computerization has also added to their life with less reported breakdowns.

Table 37.1 Manual paraffin wax technique (10 h)

Steps	*Processing step*	*Treatment*	*Time (h)*
1–2	Dehydration	80% alcohol (2 times)	1 + 1
3	Dehydration	90% alcohol	1
4–6	Dehydration	100% alcohol (3 times)	1 + 1 + 1
7–8	Clearing	Xylol (2 times)	1 + 1
9–10	Infiltration-impregnation	Paraffin (2 times)	1 + 1*

*Proceed for embedding

Dehydration

Dehydration means the removal of water, a process necessary in two major areas of histotechnology: in preparation of tissue for embedding and sectioning, and in the preparation of stained tissue sections for permanent mounting. Dehydration is necessary in the preparation of tissue blocks for embedding in a non-aqueous medium; paraffin, celloidin and some plastics will not infiltrate tissue that contains water. Before attempting infiltration with the embedding medium, the free, rather than the molecularly bound, water in the tissue must be removed. If dehydration is incomplete, the clearing agent will not act properly and soft, mushy blocks will be the result. There two ways in which the dehydrating agents act to remove water. Some reagents are hydrophilic (water-loving) and attract water from the tissue, while others dehydrate by repeated dilution of the aqueous tissue fluids. **Ethyl alcohol** (ethanol) is commonly used as the dehydrating reagents. It is hydrophilic and mixes with water, as well as many organic solvents, in all proportions. It is probably the best dehydrant but because it is also a drinking alcohol, it is strictly controlled by the federal government and troublesome record keeping is required if the alcohol is purchased tax-free. Many laboratories use **denatured alcohol** (methanol added) which makes it unfit for human consumption. If time permits, ethyl alcohol should be used in a sequence of solutions that **gradually increase in concentration**; this gradual increase probably reduces some of the tissue shrinkage that occurs in the process of dehydration. To save time, the dehydration process frequently begins with 95% ethanol followed by absolute alcohol. But some laboratories prefer to start from 60% followed by two changes each of 95% and absolute alcohol.

Clearing

Clearing agents are used to remove the alcohol used in dehydration and make the tissue receptive to the infiltration medium. Clearing agents must be miscible with both the dehydrating agent and the infiltration medium, which is most frequently paraffin. Remember, inadequate clearing will be followed by inadequate infiltration of tissue and, as with dehydration; it will result in soft, mushy tissue unfit for sectioning. On the other hand, prolonged periods in many of the clearing agents will produce hard, brittle tissues. **Xylene** is the most widely used clearing agent. It is used both in tissue processing and staining procedures. Caution: Xylene is flammable reagent and is considered as a hazardous substance. So, waste solutions must be either recycled or disposed of in an approved manner. Xylene should not be poured down the sink, as it will not mix with even small quantities of water. Xylene turns cloudy in the presence of water. Hence, if the xylene on the tissue processor is ever noted to be cloudy, the reagent should be changed immediately. There are other substances used as clearing agents—toluene, benzene, chloroform, acetone and volatile essential oils of natural origin. Most common of these is the clove oil and cedarwood oil. Since past decade **limonene** or lime oil has become popular. It has an overpowering citrus odour.

Infiltration (Impregnation)

Infiltration or **impregnation** is done after dehydration and clearing. Tissue must be infiltrated with the supporting medium. This medium generally referred to as an embedding medium, will hold the cells and intercellular structures in their proper relationship while thin sections are cut. Paraffin wax remains the most popular medium because large numbers of tissue blocks may be processed in a comparatively short time, serial sections are easily obtained, and routine and most special staining can be done easily. Paraffin is a fairly inert mixture of hydrocarbons produced by the cracking of petroleum. Inadequate impregnation leads to drying and shrinking of embedded tissues. In addition, during section cutting, cracks and crumbles develop if the tissues are inadequately supported by wax. On the other hand, excessive exposure of the tissues to high temperature of the wax beyond the optimal point will overharden the tissues and will not yield good sections.

Manual and automated tissue processing

In modern laboratories dehydration, clearing and infiltration are all carried out by the **automated tissue processor** (Fig. 37.3). Individually identified cassettes containing tissue/biopsy specimens are processed automatically yielding reliable and reproducible results. It can also perform in an **accelerated mode** (taking shorter time period) by subjecting it to vacuum and heat (40°C). Smaller laboratories in developing countries, however, still perform these tasks manually. In the hands of a good technician, the manual procedure is in no way inferior to automated tissue processing but the former is tedious and requires constant attention. The tissue processor is an excellent device and should be available to technicians if the conditions are favourable. Interruptions in the supply of electricity, however, can create serious problem in the use of an automatic tissue processor. In addition, the lack of service support is a nightmare for most technicians.

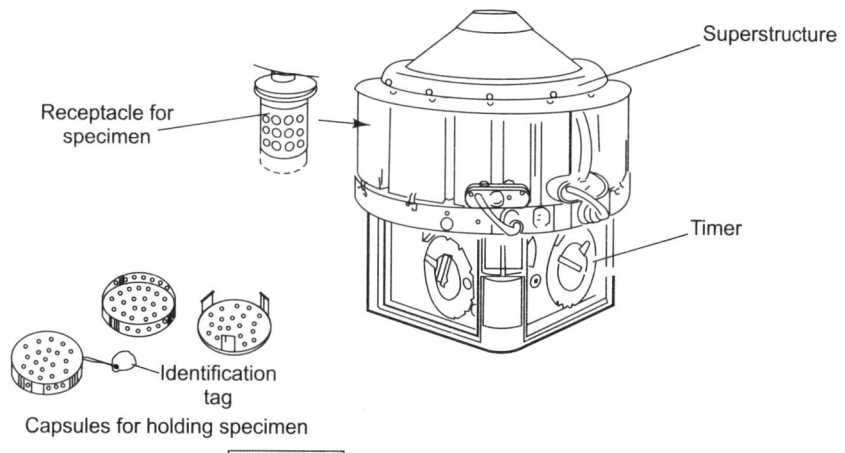

Fig. 37.3 *Automatic tissue processor.*

These automatic tissue processors are essentially a series of vats, arranged in a circle with a timing device (Fig. 37.4). These containers hold reagents and paraffin wax. The transfer arm changes the position of the basket through the processing reagents. An attempt is made to complete the tissue processing during the night (Table 37.2). To achieve this schedule, the timing disc is cut, screwed on the plate so as to be held in place by the disc-holder frame. With the timing lever set at zero, the machine is started at about 4.30 p.m. (Fig. 37.5). The basket with the cassettes automatically changes position and takes a bath in different reagents kept in beakers in order to accomplish dehydration, clearing and infiltration. The final dip is in the warm paraffin wax until the technician arrives in the morning. The cassettes are then opened and the tissues are embedded.

Table 37.2 Commonly followed schedule of tissue processing

Step	Timing	Solution	Period (h)
1.	Starting point	80% alcohol	0
2.	4.30–6.30 p.m.	80% alcohol	2
3.	6.30–7.30 p.m.	95% alcohol	1
4.	7.30–8.30 p.m.	95% alcohol	1
5.	8.30–9.30 p.m.	100% alcohol	1
6.	9.30–10.30 p.m.	100% alcohol	1
7.	10.30–11.30 p.m.	100% alcohol	1
8.	11.30 p.m.–12.30 a.m.	Xylol	1
9.	12.30–2.30 a.m.	Xylol	2
10.	2.30–4.30 a.m.	Paraffin	2
11.	4.30–6.30 a.m.	Paraffin	2
12.	6.30–8.30 a.m.	Paraffin	2

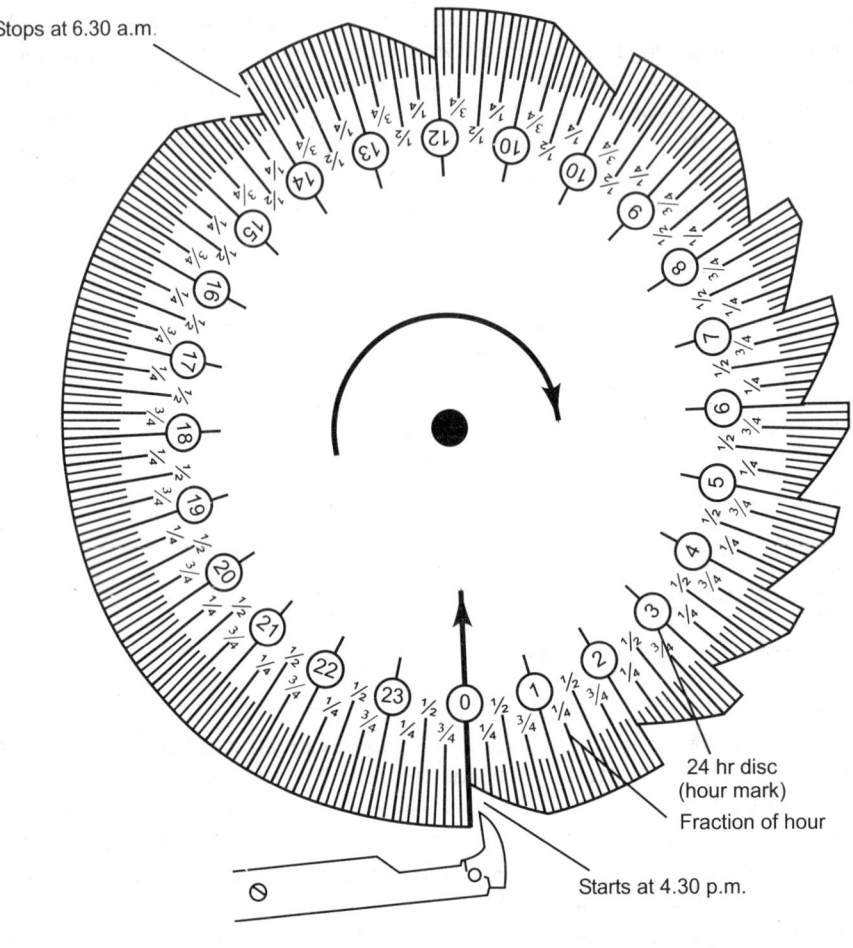

Fig. 37.4 *Timer disc for automatic tissue processor.*

Changing of solutions

The fluids used in complete dehydration and clearing tend to become contaminated with fluid carried over from the previous vat by the tissue. Hence more than one are kept in a series, for example, 100% alcohol three times, and xylene two times. After using them for 2–3 days, the last solutions in the series are replaced by fresh solutions of 100% alcohol and xylene and the previously used ones are moved forward while the first one is discarded. Other solutions are changed once a week or earlier with an average work load. It is far better to change the solution a day or two earlier than to have a precious surgical specimen improperly infiltrated.

Embedding

Embedding is the method of placing the infiltrated-impregnated tissue in warm liquid paraffin (embedding medium) that solidifies into a firm block when it cools down to room temperature. This is also known as casting or blocking. The process of embedding enables the tissue to be cut on a microtome. During this process the tissue samples are placed into moulds along with liquid embedding material which is then hardened.

This is achieved by cooling in the case of paraffin wax and heating in the case of the epoxy resins (curing). The acrylic resins are polymerized by heat, ultraviolet light or chemical catalysts. The hardened blocks containing the tissue samples are then ready to be sectioned. Embedding can also be accomplished using frozen, non-fixed tissue in a water-based medium. Pre-frozen tissues are placed into moulds with the liquid embedding material, usually a water-based glycol or resin, which is then frozen to form hardened blocks.

Paraffin wax with a higher melting point (56–58°C) is used for routine embedding. Commercially available paraffin wax should be filtered before being used for embedding. This will protect the knife edge. The cakes and trimmings from blocks are put in a clean enamel pitcher and kept in the oven. The molten paraffin is filtered inside the oven through a coarse filter paper into another container, which is used in embedding. Embedding centres (Fig. 36.2) are available nowadays for dispensing the hot paraffin into the metal moulds that hold the tissue specimen and cool the tissue blocks.

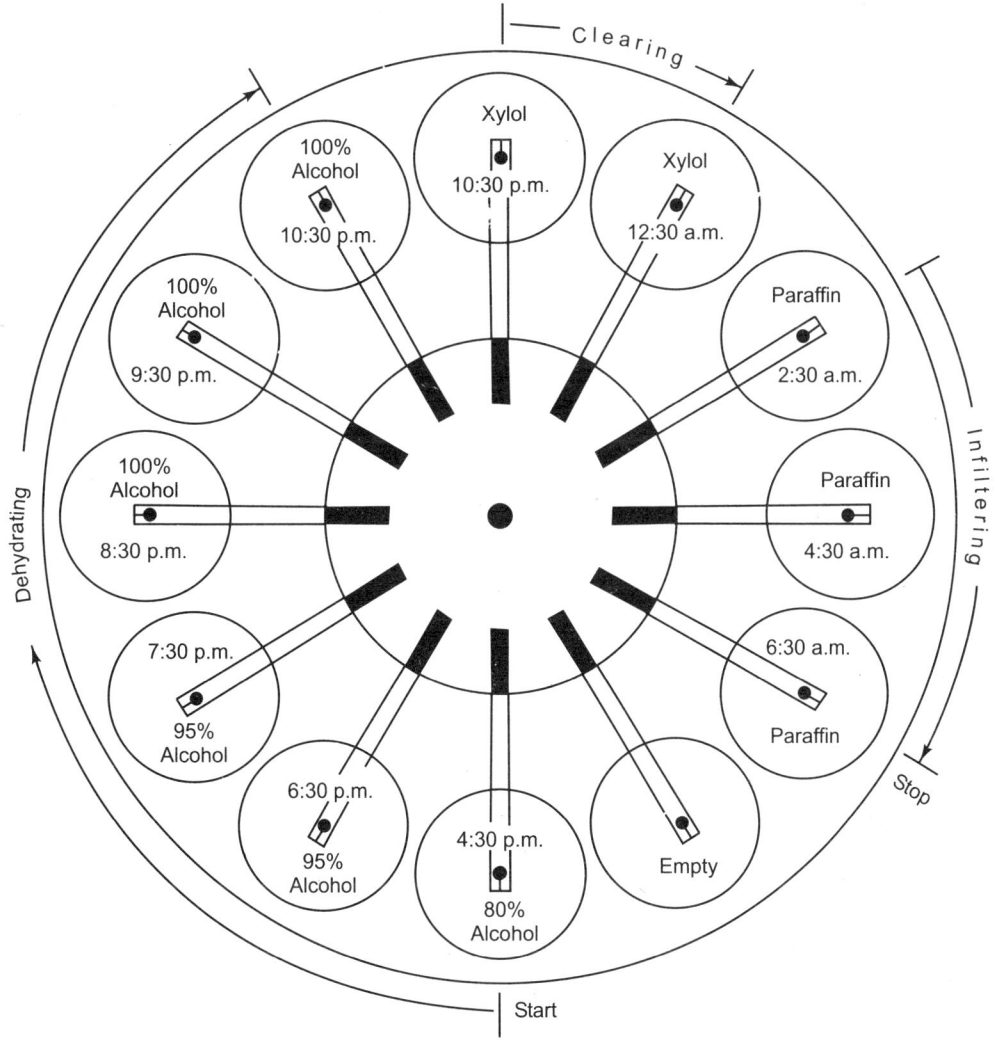

Fig. 37.5 *Timings in various baths for automatic tissue processing.*

The inexpensive plastic moulds, however, are replacing other types of embedding containers (Fig. 37.6). These plastic moulds support the block while it is being sectioned, and are designed to fit the microtome vise, eliminating the step of mounting the specimen on a block holder.

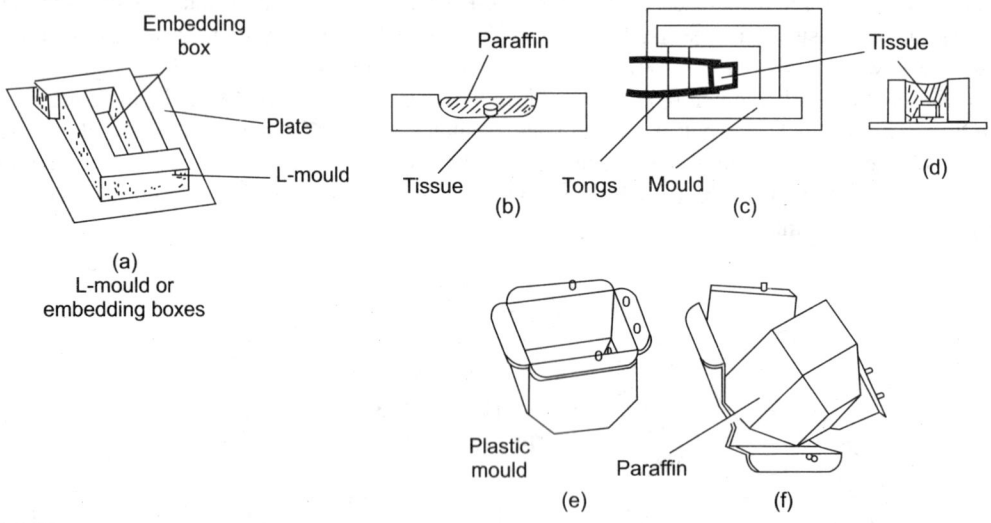

Fig. 37.6 *Paraffin embedding: L-moulds or embedding box (a). The process of tissue embedding in L-mould (b–d). Plastic mould (e) and paraffin block (f).*

During the embedding, it is important to orient the tissue in a way that will provide the best information to the pathologist. Ideally, this is done at the time the pathologist is taking out the 'bit' or biopsy from the gross specimen. The pathologist may notch with a scalpel or mark with India ink the side of the tissue opposite that is to be cut. If the type of tissue is marked on the identification label (e.g. 'S' for skin), it may help to orient the specimen accordingly. Plastic moulds are identified with the pathology numbers written on the frame with graphite pencil or by placing barcode sticker.

One of the ways of, orienting the specimen (Fig. 37.7) is to place the mould on a chilled enamel tray (keep several trays in the refrigerator); use warm blunt forceps to anchor the tissue firmly in place; hold it flat with the forceps until it retains its position. Quickly pour the remainder of the paraffin up to the top of the mould. Run the warm forceps around the tissue to ensure that any wax, which may have solidified during the transferring from the paraffin bath to the mould, is melted. Make sure that there is no air bubble around the tissue. When the tray is filled with moulds, transfer to a cold plate or to an ice tray to complete hardening of the paraffin. This will take about 15–30 min.

Proper identification of the specimen is extremely important. The identification label, bearing the accession number, is previously typed (or written with graphite pencil) and it accompanies the specimen through all steps of tissue processing. Remember that if the accession number is not clear or is lost during processing, the tissue cannot be properly identified. In addition, if the number is applied to the wrong tissue, a grave error in diagnosis may result.

Frozen sections do not need any embedding medium. The water in the tissue is frozen and as ice produces a firm block of tissue, the ice acts as the embedding medium.

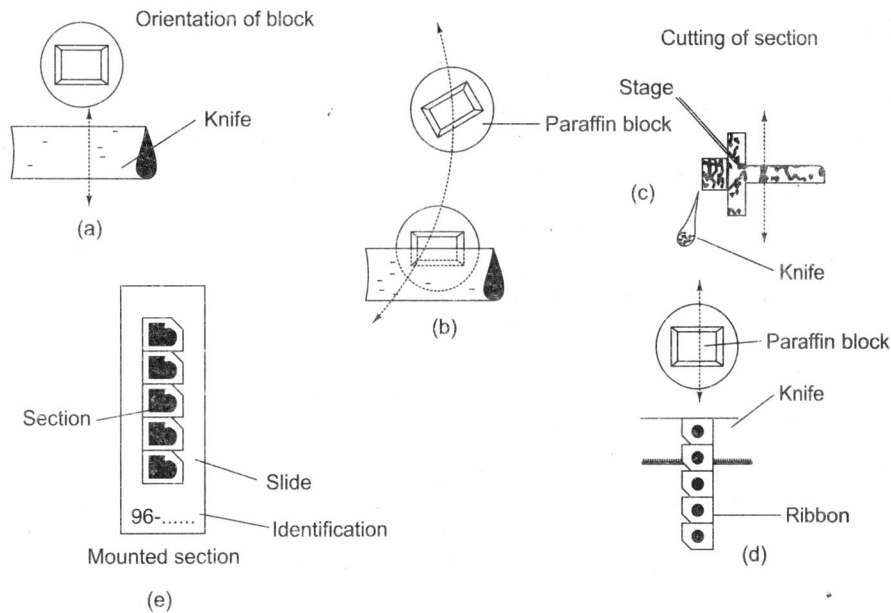

Fig. 37.7 *(a) Orientation of paraffin block with knife. (b) Section cutting and (c) formation of ribbon during section cutting. Note: Arrow indicates movement of block over the knife. (d) A microscope slide with mounted sections.*

PREPARATION OF SECTIONS

The embedded tissues are now taken for section cutting. This involves the technique of microtomy which yields thin sections of the tissue for microscopic examination of the internal structure.

The ability to cut paraffin sections of excellent quality can only be acquired with practice. We will only be able to point out some of the basic problems and their possible solutions. The skills can only be acquired with diligent practice and an appreciation of the necessity for a quality product.

We have described earlier the basic instrument used for cutting paraffin sections. Rocking microtome is no longer in use in most histology laboratories. It is replaced by rotary microtome. The rotary microtome can cut sections of 2–10 μ thick. Since the results produced by histologic technique depend greatly upon the knives used to cut the sections, disposable sharp knives are currently use in all modern laboratories. It is imperative that the technician should know how to care for his knife as well as how to use it.

Special razor blades are now available in the market which is used in conjunction with a special holder to cut paraffin sections. The use of a razor blade eliminates the tedious job of sharpening since it is discarded when dulled or nicked. The blade is convenient for cutting bone sections (after softening), but the cutting edge of razor blade is short. Hence standard microtome knife is occasionally used, interchangeably on the same microtome, when readjustment of the angle setting will be necessary.

Cutting of a hard object like bone without softening will ruin the microtome knife. Hence, decalcification of bone and treatment of warts (epithelial tissues) with alkali solution (1 N NaOH) aim to soften the tissue before cutting.

Section Cutting

Trim the paraffin block with a hand razor or sharp knife. In the case of multiple embedding, separate out the blocks so that one block contains only one tissue. The block face, however, is finally trimmed with the microtome knife. The sides of the block must be parallel and the tissue should be 1–3 mm from the edge on all sides. Return the shavings to the wax oven and use again. The labelled trimmed blocks are stored in cardboard boxes.

Attaching the paraffin block to the microtome

The paraffin block has to be attached to the microtome head before it is ready for cutting. To do this, the knife is first fixed in a clamp and the tissue block is drawn across the knife edge and is mechanically advanced. Positioning the knife edge helps in orienting the paraffin block.

When using a rotary microtome, the paraffin block (known as 'chuck') should be clamped into the head. The block will crumble if clamped too tightly. The chuck can be clamped firmly into the microtome without fear of crumbling the block.

Orienting the Block The technician must be aware of the nature of the tissue he is cutting so that he can orient the tissue block appropriately before beginning to cut the block. Screws are provided in the rotary type microtome to change the position of the paraffin block as needed.

The correct orientation of the paraffin block before cutting a section is important (Fig. 37.7). If the pathologist has given any specific instructions at the time the block of tissue was given to the technician, they can be taken care of at this point. The orientation should be such that the top and the bottom of the block are parallel and horizontal to the edge of the knife at the moment of impact. Check the orientation with the position of the knife already in place. Tighten the screws, if necessary. The block face should be as small as possible and at least 1 mm of paraffin should be present on all sides beyond the tissue. In the beginning set the gauge controlling the thickness of the sections to 15 mm. Use the extreme end of the knife to trim the block, when the whole surface is being cut. The block is now ready for sectioning.

Cutting the Sections Trim the block with the knife before beginning to cut the section. In a properly trimmed block face, the top and bottom edges will be parallel, the block face touching the knife. All of the tissue desired on the slide should be exposed on the face and no scratch marks should be visible on the surface. If scratch marks are visible on the block face, the knife must be moved laterally to use a new portion of the knife edge and the face trimmed again (Fig. 37.8).

When the block face is trimmed and the microtome advance is set at the desired thickness for the sections, usually 5 µm, the cutting begins. The centre of the blade is the most desirable place to cut. It is a good practice to check the position of the knife and then screw back the feed mechanism. Many technicians will cool the block face with an ice cube for a moment or so at this time. As the microtome head moves with the block, a section is cut from the block and will lie on the knife. Maintain a regular cutting rhythm at a rate that is comfortable to you. The rate will vary with the size of the block, the nature of the tissue and the type of microtome used. Each time the block hits the knife it leaves behind a cut section which will slide onto the knife, pushing the previous one ahead. Thus a 'ribbon' of sections is produced. A ribbon will form if the upper and lower edges of the block face are parallel to the edge of the knife. Should the top and bottom edges of the block not be parallel, then the ribbon would not be straight but would curve. When the ribbon is about 5 cm long, grasp the first section with a pair of fine forceps held in the left hand. A small camel-hair paint brush held in the right hand can be used to brush away the last section from the knife, and with both hands the ribbon can be transferred to the water bath. The ribbon can be manipulated easily if static electricity and drafts are kept to a minimum.

There are numerous technical errors that will lead to poor section quality. These will be dealt with separately. The cut sections should now be attached to the microscope slide before they are further processed.

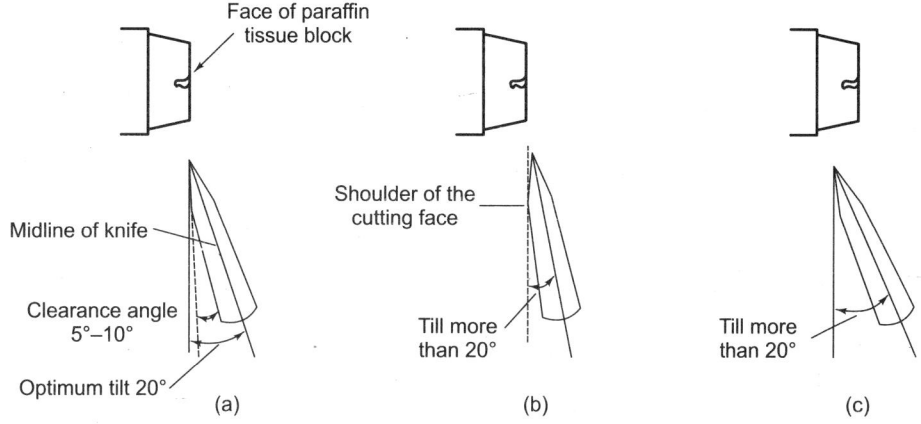

Fig. 37.8 *Setting the tilt of the knife for best section cutting. Optimal angle of the tilt is (a) 20°, which if decreased (b) or increased (c), will yield undesirable sections.*

Attaching section to microscope slide

A thin, flat section of a tissue will usually adhere to a clean glass surface and stay in place through the common preparative procedures of staining, washing, dehydration and clearing. The adhesion may be largely due to the close contact between two flat surfaces. Ionic attractions between the sections (protein) and the clean surface of the slides (silica) also help to hold them together. Unfortunately, not all sections are perfectly flat and not all slides are perfectly clean. Even when these conditions are met, there are some staining techniques that are harsh enough to remove the flattest section from the cleanest slide. There are two ways to prevent or reduce the loss of sections subjected to harsh treatments: (a) by using an adhesive and (b) by inclusion in a permeable protective film. One can also use special slides described in Chapter 36 in this Volume.

Preparation of Slide   Microscope slides are first prepared before attaching the section on the slide. Since the subsequent manipulation of the slide involves many movements of the slide in and out of various fluids and stains, an adhesive must be used to keep the section firmly fixed to the slide. Otherwise the section may wash away.

For a large number of sections the following procedure is recommended. The slides can be prepared en masse in advance. Prepare a 0.2% (w/v, aqueous) solution of gelatine to which a few crystals of thymol have been added to discourage bacterial growth. Allow to dissolve at 56°C (30 min will suffice). Dip clean microscope slides into the gelatine solution when cool, agitating for several seconds. Take out the slides, drain thoroughly and allow to dry on edge (for maximum drainage) at room temperature. It is useful if slide racks are used; place these on clean cloth to obviate the collection of gelatine solution at the bottom edge of the slides. Dry the coated slides for 1 h at 56°C. Allow to cool and store until required in suitable containers. Sections may be subsequently mounted in the usual way from the floating-out bath, followed by conventional drying treatment.

Procedure of Attaching the Section to the Slide   The sections tend to crease slightly on cutting; therefore, they are first flattened before they are attached to the slide. To do this they are first floated on warm water in a shallow water bath (Fig. 36.4) maintained at a temperature of about 46°C (10°C below the melting point of wax). The cut section or short ribbon of section is gently lowered by means of a camel-hair paint brush or fine forceps on to the surface of warm water in the water bath. The tissue ribbon will float and the wrinkling of the tissue should flatten out. Gently pulling on the opposite ends of the ribbon can help to flatten out the sections. The technician then closely inspects the sections and picks one which is flat and fully expanded, without scratches or cracks and with no recognizable distortion when compared with the tissue in the block face. A pre-coated slide is dipped obliquely into the water as close to the section as possible. If the water in the water bath contains adhesive, an uncoated clean slide can be used. Slowly withdraw the slide allowing its surface to touch the edge of the section. Completely remove the slide with the attached section from water. Adjust the section to a suitable position on the slide with a mounted needle. Drain off the excess water and lay the slide flat on the table. Then inscribe the identification number of the tissue-block as recorded in the laboratory register. The number must correspond with the original number given by the reception desk and recorded in the log-book for the specimen received. Do not put the number on the slide at any other time; it should be inscribed immediately after attaching the section to the slide to avoid any mix up. Then transfer the slide to an incubator or warming plate (40–50°C) for at least 1 h to ensure that the section is thoroughly dried (Fig. 36.5). When all the sections are dried, they are ready for staining.

Transference of Sections The transfer of a section from one glass slide to another is effectively achieved by covering the section with a plastic resin film, which when hardened can be soaked off with the section. For a successful result, it is important that the solution be of the right consistency and that hardening of the film be complete. If the film is too thin it will fail to attach to the section, conversely if the film is too thick problems will be encountered when cover slipping.

Reagent

DPX[*] mountant — 1 part
Butyl acetate — 6 parts

This is conventionally done in a glass test-tube and requires thorough mixing by repeated inversion.

Storage of Paraffin Blocks

Paraffin blocks are stored in an orderly fashion by serial number, in cool dry storage place for future re-sectioning if needed.

Problems in Section Cutting

1. *Failure of block to form ribbons*: This may be caused by overly hard paraffin, a knife tilted too far towards the block, too thick sections, a dull knife, or a knife not parallel to the block. The following are recommendations for getting a good ribbon: unroll the first section with a fine camel-hair paint brush and hold it down lightly against the knife. The ribbon will form and follow. If not, try to chill the face of the block with an ice cube and try again. A paint brush is recommended rather than forceps or dissecting needle. The latter may nick the edge of the microtome blade.
2. *Crooked and uneven ribbons*: This is commonly caused by wedge-shaped or round blocks, a knife not parallel to the block, an irregular knife edge or non-homogeneous or impure paraffin.
3. *Compressed, wrinkled or jammed sections*: This may result from a dull knife, too vertical a knife tilt, coating of paraffin on the knife edge or loose screws of the clamp holding the knife.
4. *Crumbling of sections:* This may be caused by improper tissue processing.
5. *Split ribbon or lengthwise scratches:* These are caused by nicks on the knife edge, a dirty knife edge, too great a knife tilt, or microcalcifications in the tissue.
6. *Lifting of sections from the knife on the upstroke:* This may be caused by too vertical a knife tilt, too soft paraffin, too warm an environment or a dull knife.
7. *Adherence of sections to the knife:* This is caused by a dirty knife edge, a dull knife or too vertical a knife tilt.

---

[*]DPX is a colourless synthetic resin mounting medium that has replaced xylene—Balsam mountant. It preservers the stain and dries quickly. The alternative mountant is Permount, which is a toluene-based synthetic resin.

8. *Varying thickness of sections*: This problem is caused by insufficient tilt of the knife to clear bevel (with resulting compression of tissue), a loose clamp or improper adjustment of the microtome.
9. *Accumulation of air bubbles under the ribbon after it is spread on the water-bath*: Remove the bubbles with a smooth teasing needle bent at a right angle.
10. *Caution*: Be gentle with the section and do not tear it by rough handling. Bubbles may also be removed by pulling the ribbon very gently across the long edge of a glass slide held below the section in the water bath. After the section is mounted on the slide, bubbles in the tissue may be removed by gently brushing with a fine camel-hair paint brush.

ROUTINE STAINING PROCEDURE IN HISTOTECHNOLOGY

Unstained sections are of very little use for studying the internal structure of tissues as the cellular components cannot be clearly differentiated. Dyeing or staining of the sections enables one to study the physical characteristics and relationships of tissues and of their constituent cells. These biological stains are prepared from dyes which are either natural or synthetic. The mechanism by which these dyes attach to the different components of cells is beyond the scope of this book. In the routine histology laboratory, haematoxylin–eosin (H&E) is the standard stain. In the vast majority of cases this is the only stain necessary for diagnosis. References to other common stains will also be made in order to familiarize technicians with their uses under special conditions.

Basic Information

Pre-staining treatments under special conditions

If the tissue is fixed in a fixative containing chromate, the precipitate must be removed with iodine in solution, followed by sodium thiosulphate to remove the residual iodine. An iodine solution in alcohol (tincture of iodine) can be used.

Reagents
- Tincture of iodine solution:
    - Iodine crystal — 1 g
    - Alcohol, 95% — 100 mL
- Sodium thiosulphate (hypo) solution:
    - Sodium thiosulphate — 5 g
    - Water — 100 mL

Procedure
1. Remove the dry section from the oven.
2. Deparaffinize the sections through two changes of xylene.
3. Dehydrate with down graded alcohol: Absolute alcohol, 90%, 80%, 70%, 1 min in each, with agitation.
4. Treat with iodine (for fixatives with chromate) for 10 min.
5. Treat with 5% sodium thiosulphate for 5 min.
6. Thoroughly wash with tap water and proceed for staining.

Formalin-produced precipitate Occasionally fine black granules develop in tissues fixed in formaldehyde. This artefact is troublesome and must be removed before staining. One of the ways to avoid this is to use a large volume of fixative as compared with the amount of tissue. If the tissue is in excess, acidity develops in the fixative which causes the formation of precipitate. As an alternative, use buffered formaldehyde as the fixative. The artefactitious precipitate must be removed before staining. The following methods can be adopted.

Treatment with saturated alcoholic picric acid
1. Deparaffinize the sections through two changes each of xylene, absolute alcohol and 95% alcohol.
2. Rinse well in distilled water.
3. Let it stand in saturated alcoholic picric acid solution for 1–3 h.
4. Wash well in running tap water before taking for staining.

Note: This picric acid solution will not bleach malarial pigment.

Preparation for Staining

Prior to most staining procedures the paraffin must be removed from the section on the slide. Very few staining techniques do not require the removal of paraffin because most stains do not penetrate paraffinized tissue very well. The following steps are involved in the process which is commonly referred as 'taking the sections to water':

- **Drying:** Carefully check that the slide is completely dry in the oven at 55°C or on the ward plate before proceeding for de-waxing or removal of the paraffin. Rushing the sections by bringing them out of the oven before they are completely dry may result in the sections floating off the slides during the staining, a very frustrating experience for the technician and pathologist alike.
- **Deparaffiinnizing:** To remove the paraffin from the sections, take the warm slide from the oven and allow it to cool to room temperature. Use of warming plate is more convenient (Fig. 36.5). Place the slide in xylene for 5 min and then for an additional 5 min in a second xylene bath. This will adequately remove the paraffin from the sections. Dissolving of the paraffin is aided by agitation of the slide in xylene. If the xylene is old, discard the first xylene, move forward the second xylene bath (marking it as 1) and replace the second xylene bath with fresh xylene fluid.
- **Hydration:** To complete the hydration of the sections (or 'taking to water') pass them through decreasing grades of alcohols (absolute, 90%, 80% and 70%), and finally wash in distilled water. The last few steps can be done quite rapidly, especially if the slides are agitated while soaked in the reagent. Many laboratories prefer to treat the sections with xylene–alcohol mixture (1 : 1) before switching the sections directly from xylene to absolute alcohol.

Staining

Various stains are used in the histotechnology laboratory. Some are routine while others are applied under special circumstances. Two basic **principles of staining** are—direct and indirect. These are shown in Fig. 37.9. In the direct procedure, the stain directly react with the section while in the indirect, a mordant is needed that stands in between the section and the stain. Automated stainers closely operate like the tissue processor.

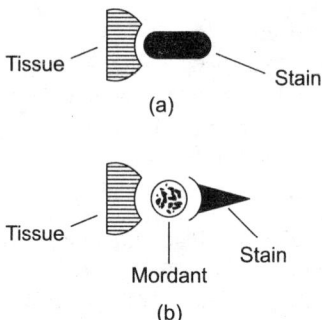

Fig. 37.9 *Principles of staining: (a) direct staining and (b) indirect staining with the mediation of the mordant.*

Automatic stainers perform routine staining that saves time and yields consistent reliable results. Slides are placed in staining troughs with separate baskets that enable up to 20 slides to be stained at the same time. There are three types of automatic stainers—linear, revolving and robotic. In linear stainers slides are transferred from one container (vat) to the next with same time allowed in each container. The time in each different solution can be changed only by varying the number of containers holding that particular reagent. Revolving stainers operates on the same principle as the open tissue processor, and the time allowed in each solution may be varied. Robotic stainers are computerized and the timing in each solution is programmed.

Manual staining is done in smaller laboratories. Use of staining dishes, like the coplin jars (that holds 5–10 slides) is common (see Chapter 36 in this Volume) and a timer with alarm is used for determining the duration in different reagents.

Post-staining Processes

Following staining, the sections are dehydrated (opposite of 'taking to water'), cleared, and mounted on a slide before examining the section under the microscope. 'Mounting' is a two step procedure. In the first step, the section is transferred to a mounting medium and then a cover-slip is placed over the medium. It is accomplished in different ways and some of them are being shown in Fig. 37.10.

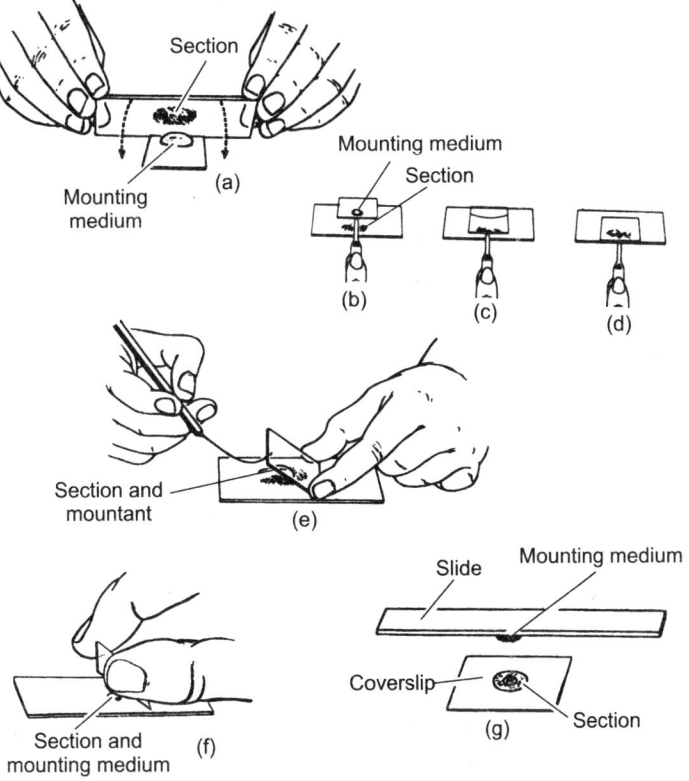

Fig. 37.10 *Techniques of mounting section. (a) Place the slide with stained section on the cover slip with mounting medium. (b–d) Mounting medium on the cover slip, which is gently placed over the section. (e and f) Mounting medium on the slide with stained section, cover slip gently placed over it like wet mounting. (g) If the cover slip holds the section, the slide with the mounting medium is laid over it.*

Mounting of stained sections

Sections are normally examined after mounting. Mounting involves placing a mounting medium on which the cover slip is laid down. There are two types of mounting media—aqueous and resinous. Choose the medium as per instruction in the procedure. The choice of various mounting media has been presented in Chapter 36 in this Volume. Various procedures of mounting are shown in Fig. 37.10.

Routine Haematoxylin and Eosin Staining (H&E)

Haematoxylin, a natural dye, is undoubtedly the most valuable staining reagent used in histological work. It is the principal stain for demonstrating the nucleus and the cytoplasmic inclusions. It works in conjunction with alum, which acts as a **mordant** (iron is used in other methods). Alum containing haematoxylin stains the nucleus a light transparent blue which rapidly turns red in the presence of acid (**accelerator**). In addition, the stain picked up by the cytoplasm will be removed more rapidly than from the nuclei when the section is treated with the acid solution. This step is called **differentiation** since during this step the stain differentiates nuclei from cytoplasm. The **oxidizing agent** (mercuric oxide) converts haematoxylin to haematin. In some preparations (Carazzi's haematoxylin solution) glycerol is added to slow down the oxidation process that improves the keeping properties. The counterstain used is **eosin** which is picked up by all tissues revealing the general structure.

Reagents

- *Harris's haematoxylin solution*

Haematoxylin crystals	5 g
Ethyl alcohol	50 mL
Ammonium or potassium alum	100 g
Distilled water	950 mL
Mercuric oxide	2.5 g
Glacial acetic acid	40 mL

    Preparation
    1. Dissolve the haematoxylin in ethyl alcohol using gentle heat (56°C oven or in water bath).
    2. Dissolve the alum in distilled water using heat (Bunsen) with frequent stirring.
    3. Mix haematoxylin solution (step 1) with alum solution (step 2) while the latter is hot.
    4. Bring to the boil as quickly as possible, stirring frequently.
    5. Turn off the Bunsen burner just before adding the mercuric oxide in the next step.
    6. Add mercuric oxide. Carefully watch the effervescence which may cause spillage.
    7. The solution at once assumes a dark purple colour. As soon as this occurs, remove from the flame and cool rapidly in ice-cold water or under running tap water.
    8. Add acetic acid and filter.
    9. When cool, the solution is ready for use but will need re-filtering.
    10. Transfer to a suitable storage bottle, record the date and label (the technician who prepared the solution should put his initials). The solution stays stable for years. Keep in the refrigerator.

    Commercially prepared ready to use haematoxylin solution is now available in the market.

- *Eosin solution (1% aqueous)*

    Eosin is used as the counterstain that stains the cytoplasm rose-coloured. The intensity of the eosin staining desired in the final sections is a matter of individual\preference. The most widely used eosin is **eosin Y**. The 'Y' stands for yellowish. It is available in either water soluble or alcohol soluble form. Most laboratories use the water soluble form of eosin Y in an alcohol-water solution which is described here.

Eosin Y (water soluble)	1 g
Distilled water	100 mL

Add a crystal of phenol or thymol to the prepared solution of eosin to inhibit mould.

- *Dilute hydrochloric acid (1% in 70% alcohol)*: Differentiator

Conc. hydrochloric acid	1 mL
70% alcohol	99 mL

- *Aqueous sodium carbonate (Bluing agent)*

Sodium bicarbonate	2 g
Distilled water	100 mL

Procedure

1. Sections to water through down graded alcohol baths (100%–90%–70%–water). Drain well.
2. Stain with Harris haematoxylin for 3–5 min (or longer, depending on the age of the stain, and to some extent the fixative). The time factor for each batch of stain must be determined by trial in order to obtain proper nuclear staining. Drain well.
3. Wash briefly in water and differentiate in acid–alcohol by a quick dip.
4. Wash well in water and blue for 10–30 sec. Check microscopically—the nuclei should be deep blue in colour with the vesicular nuclei showing a well-marked chromatin pattern (dark purple). The background should show only weak residual haematoxylin coloration, very pale.
5. Keep the slide wet during checking. If the nuclei are not dark enough, rinse in distilled water and repeat the staining.
6. Wash briefly in water and stain with eosin solution for 1–5 min. The time in eosin solution depends on the staining intensity desired and the age of the stain. Drain the stain before going to the next step.
7. Wash quickly in water, differentiate and dehydrate in alcohol.
8. Clear in xylene, two changes (30–60 sec each). Drain off the excess.
9. Mount on Permount (Fisher Scientific). This mounting medium is a toluene-based synthetic resin. It is the right choice for both rapid mounting and long term storage of slides.

Additional Information

- Every second correspond to one dip; hence timing can be regulated by the number of dips.
- Change the alcohol when they appear to be saturated or diluted due to carry over of the reagents. Change the xylene as needed by the work load; usually twice a week.
- Decalcified tissues may take 15 min to stain with Harris haematoxylin.
- The intensity of the routine stain should be checked with the pathologist for proper staining so that the routine staining can be standardized.
- It remains the responsibility of the technician to produce the very best possible H&E staining. The slides should be differentiated microscopically and not left to the capricious effect of 'dips' and time intervals, which are actually only baseline guides.

Note: Automated staining machines are now available in the market which helps for a consistent result of staining.

Result

Nuclei, some calcium salts, urates, bacteria—blue
Muscle, keratin, coarse elastic fibres, fibrin—bright red
Collagen, reticulin, connective tissue, amyloid and cytoplasm—varying shades of pink
Red blood cells—orange
The morphology of some of the important types of cells is shown in Fig. 37.11.

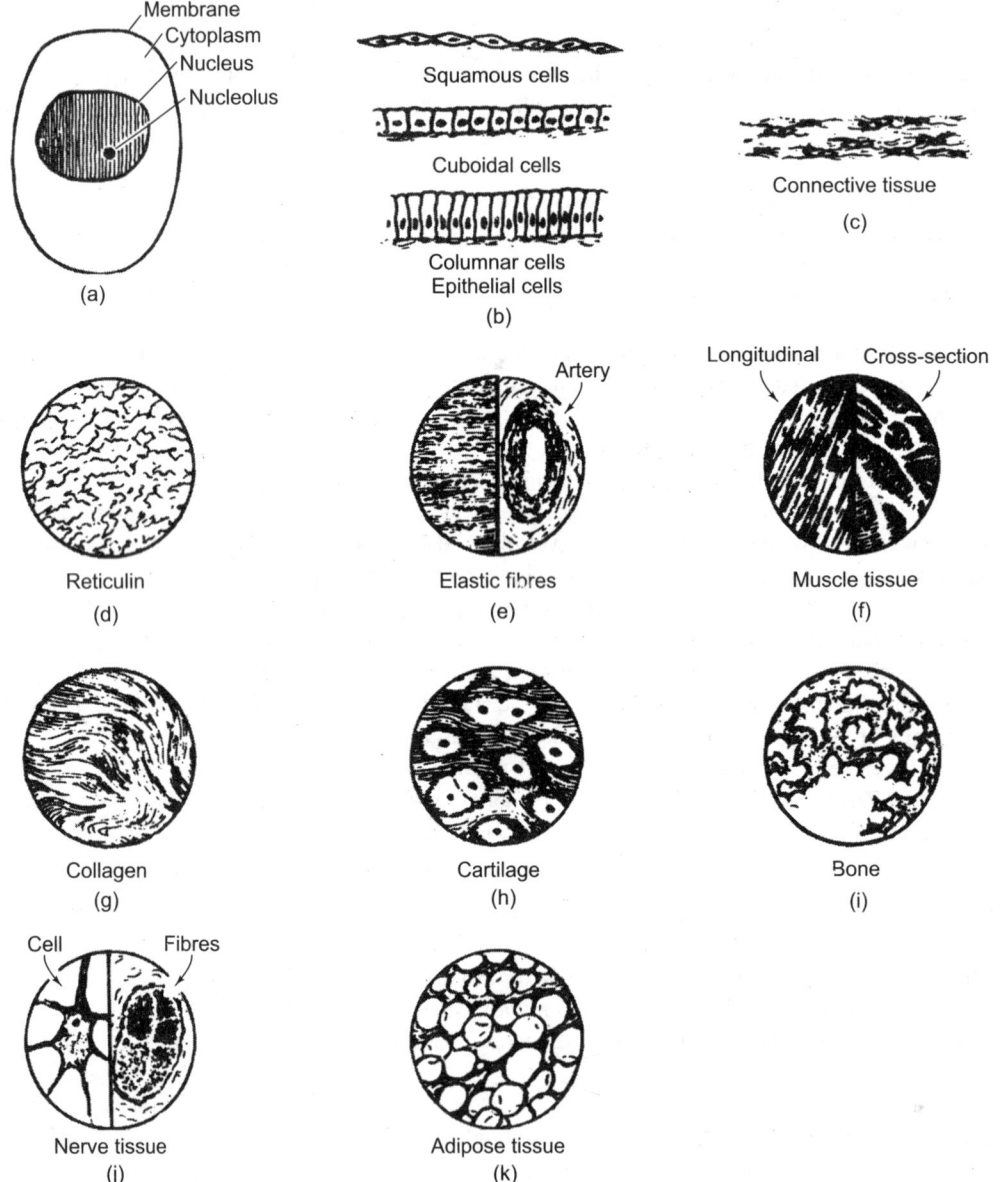

Fig. 37.11 *Morphology of some of the important types of cells: (a) basic cellular components, (b) epithelial cells, (c) connective tissue, (d) reticulin, (e) elastic fibres, (f) muscle tissue, (g) collagen, (h) cartilage, (i) bone, (j) nerve tissue and (k) adipose tissue.*

SPECIAL STAINS AND STAINING TECHNIQUES

The histology laboratory spends most of its time doing the routine haematoxylin staining, but it should also be prepared to do special stains. Technicians must be aware of these stains and perform them upon special request.

The special stains and techniques (which do not involve a stain) can be divided into three major types:
- Stains used for particular parts of tissues, usually components of connective /tissues not readily seen or well stained by the haematoxylin stain.
- Stains for particular substances, such as iron and mucin, which do not pick up the haematoxylin stain.
- Stains for micro-organisms such as fungi and bacteria.

Connective Tissues

The term connective tissue is used here in a broad sense to include fibrillar connective tissue, and tissues that are histologically associated, including muscle. Two chief components of connective tissue are dealt here—collagen fibres and reticulin. Cartilage, with its high mucin content, is dealt with under carbohydrates,

Collagen and collagen fibres

Collagen is a fibrous insoluble protein found in the connective tissue. These fibres are formed by fibroblasts and may be arranged in either fine or coarse bundles.

There are several pathologic conditions that cause cellular changes in connective tissue. Histological diagnosis of collagen diseases is based on the study of the sections of various connective tissues. Other laboratory tests are also available which will be discussed in their appropriate places.

Zenker's fluid or formalin-fixed tissues may be used, but in the case of the latter, the tissue sections will require mordanting prior to staining (iodine treatment).

In a routine stain, the elastic fibres, collagen, and smooth muscle are eosinophilic (pink or reddish in colour). In the following sections, we will try to focus on two commonly used staining procedures—van Gieson's technique and Masson's trichome technique. Use of phosphotungstic acid haematoxylin stain is less common.

van Gieson's Stain van Gieson's technique is probably the most successful single histological technique devised; over a hundred years after it inception it is still in regular use in histological laboratories. Its success is due to the specific staining of collagen with clear colour distinction from other tissues. The potential flaw, however, is the non-staining of young collagen fibres; for their demonstration use a trichrome stain (discussed further).

Reagents
- *Weigert's iron haematoxylin*
  This is stored as two solutions and mixed in equal proportions immediately prior to use. It has been shown that the working solution retains its staining avidity for up to 60 days if stored at 4°C.
  Solution A:

Haematoxylin	1 g
Absolute alcohol	100 mL

  Solution B:

30% aqueous ferric chloride	4 mL
Hydrochloric (concentrated)	1 mL
Distilled water	100 mL

  Working solution
  Mix equal parts of solution A and solution B before use. Put solution A first in the beaker and then solution B. The staining solution should look violet black.
- *van Gieson's solution*

1% aqueous acid fuchsin	10 mL
Saturated aqueous picric acid	100 mL

  Boil for 3 min, cool and filter.

Procedure

1. Take the section to water.
2. Stain with Weigert's haematoxylin for 15–30 min.
3. Wash in tap water.
4. Differentiate with acid alcohol. Wash and blue.
5. Check microscopically; the nuclei should be dark-black and the background a paler blue-black colour.
6. Rinse well in distilled water.
7. Counterstain in van Gieson's solution for 5 min.
8. Rinse in distilled water or drain, rinse in alcohol.
9. Dehydrate, clear and mount in DPX or Permount.

Result

Nuclei—brown-black
Mature collagen—bright red
Elastic fibres—dark (often black)
Other tissue elements (smooth muscle and red blood cells)—yellow
Some bile pigments—green

Masson's Trichrome Stain This is a connective tissue stain, comparable with the van Gieson's stain that uses phosphomolybdic and phosphotungstic acids as mordant along with a haematoxylin stain (Weigert's iron haematoxylin). The trichrome stains are of particular value for demonstrating fibrin or young collagen fibres and for differentiating muscle from connective tissue. Formalin fixative can lead to indifferent results that may be partly overcome by pre-mordanting sections in Helly's fixative for at least 5 h. Bouin's (or Zenker's) fluid can also be used. Sections of formalin-fixed (10% formalin) should be pre-mordanted in Bouin's fluid for 1 h at 56°C or overnight at room temperature.

The success of this method depends on the degree of differentiation of the ponceau acid fuchsin by phosphomolybdic acid. It is important to prolong differentiation until the connective tissue is almost unstained. This may be expedited at 56°C.

Reagents

- *Weigert's iron haematoxylin stain* (described before)
- *Acetic acid solutions:* Make 1% and 2% solutions acetic acid by mixing appropriate amounts of glacial acetic acid and distilled water.
- *Ponceau-acid fuchsin solution:*
  Equal volumes of 0.5% aqueous solution of ponceau 2R and 0.5% acid fuchsin in 1% acetic acid.
- *Phosphomolybdic acid solution*:
  1% aqueous phosphomolybdic acid
- *Aniline blue solution*:
  Boil 97.5 mL of distilled water and add 2 g aniline blue (water soluble). While still hot, add 2.5 mL glacial acetic acid. Cool and filter.
- *Light green solution (2%)*:
  This can be used in place of aniline blue. 2% light green in 2% acetic acid; dilute with distilled water prior to use.

Procedure

1. Take the section to water.
2. Stain nuclei with Weigert's iron haematoxylin solution for 15–30 min.
3. Differentiate to blue.

4. Rinse in distilled water (do not use tap water).
5. Treat with the ponceau-acid fuchsin solution for 2–3 min.
6. Rinse in distilled water.
7. Differentiate in the phosphomolybdic acid solution (usually for between 5 and 15 min at room temperature).
8. Wash well in water.
9. Counterstain either with aniline blue for 5 min or the light green solution for 1 min.
10. Wash, dehydrate, clear and mount as desired.

Results
Nuclei—blue-black
Muscle, red blood cells, fibrin—red
Connective tissue—blue or green according to the counterstain used

Reticulin

The reticulin fibres (collagen type III) consist of a fibrillary extracellular framework in the connective tissue. These fine branching fibres are difficult to see in haematoxylin–eosin (H&E) preparations and need other techniques to be properly visualized.

The pattern of the deposited reticulum in a tumour is sometimes characteristic enough so that the origin of the tumour can be identified on the basis of the way the reticulum is arranged in the tumour. Therefore, a reticulum stain will occasionally be requested when a tumour of uncertain origin is encountered. In addition, mild degrees of fibrosis in organs can be recognized by the reticulum stain.

Silver impregnation methods are widely used for studying the microscopic structures of reticulin and collagen. Reticulum fibres have an affinity for silver (argyrophilia) where the silver metal gets deposited on the fibres in ammoniacal solution. This is subsequently converted to reduced (black) silver by suitable reducing agents, allowing visualization of the fibres. Most silver techniques for reticulum are preceded by a permanganate oxidation step; this prevents the normal affinity for silver stains of structures like nerve fibres. The final step in silver methods is to remove any remaining unreduced silver by treating with sodium thiosulphate ('hypo'). This prevents subsequent background precipitation due to light reduction, but does not appear to be strictly necessary in reticulum methods.

Formalin is the recommended fixative for the silver impregnation method, but other fixatives can also be used. The sections tend to get detached from the slide due to the high alkalinity of the silver solution. Use special slides or use an albumenized slide with thorough drying.

The silver impregnation method is notoriously capricious. Consistent results can only come from scrupulous technique. This includes the following:
- Always use well washed glassware (wash with 10% nitric acid) and rinse well with distilled water. This is particularly true for the containers and baths holding silver solutions.
- Do not use metallic forceps; use plastic ones.
- Avoid dust, since it (and not light) is the greatest single factor in the deterioration and precipitation of silver solutions.
- Do not use glass rods without careful washing between solutions. *Note:* Improper procedure will lead to non-specific precipitation of silver on the slide and tissue.

Silver Impregnation Method (Gordon and Sweets)
This is a popular and reliable method. The ammoniacal silver solution may be kept without deterioration for many weeks, even when stored at room temperature in a clear container. The formalin is best diluted with tap water, maintaining a better and more even reduction of the silver solution. This is partly a result of the dissolved chlorides, which give a more intense reduction, and partly the higher pH of tap water.

Reagents

- *Oxalic acid (5%, w/v, aqueous).*
- *Ferric ammonium sulphate—iron alum (2%, w/v, aqueous)*
- *Formalin (10%, v/v, aqueous).*
- *Neutral red (1%, w/v, aqueous)*—counter stain.
- *Acidified potassium permanganate solution:*

0.25% aqueous potassium permanganate	47.5 mL
3% aqueous sulphuric acid	2.5 mL

  These can be conveniently kept as stock solutions; the composite solution will keep for several weeks.
- *Ammoniacal silver nitrate solution*:

10% aqueous silver nitrate	5 mL

  Add concentrated ammonia drop by drop with frequent mixing until the formed precipitate just redissolves. Add 5 mL of 3.1% aqueous sodium hydroxide and mix. A precipitate will form that gradually dissolves upon the addition of ammonia, drop by drop as before. Stop when there are only a few precipitate granules remaining. Make up the final volume to 50 mL with distilled water.

Procedure

1. Section to water.
2. Treat with acidified potassium permanganate solution for 5 min.
3. Wash off in water for about 2 min.
4. Bleach with oxalic acid solution for approximately 1 min or until colourless.
5. Wash well in water and rinse in distilled water.
6. Treat with iron alum solution for 5 min.
7. Wash well in several changes of distilled water.
8. Treat with ammoniacal silver solution for 4–5 sec with agitation of the slide.
9. Wash well in several changes of distilled water.
10. Reduce in 10% formalin in tap water for about 30–60 sec with agitation of slide.
11. Wash in tap water and then rinse with distilled water.
12. Treat with 5% sodium thiosulphate solution for 5 min.
13. Wash in distilled water.
14. Counterstain, if desired, in 1% aqueous neutral red for 5 min.
15. Dehydrate, clear and mount as desired.

Result

Reticulum fibres—black (some pigments like melanin are also impregnated).
Collagen—yellow-brown
Background—clear if not counterstained, red if counter stained.

Elastic fibres

Elastic fibres are branching fibres of varying size and diameter that consist of the protein elasticin and glycoprotein microfibrils. They are easily seen in tissue sites such as dermis of skin, lung, heart and blood vessel walls. Elastic fibres may be increased because of a stromal reaction to the presence of tumour cells, as in breast cancer, or secretion of tumour cells, as in the rare elastoma dorsi.

Specific staining is required to identify changes in the elastic laminae of blood vessel walls that may be increased due to hypertension or lost because of a degenerative process. The finer elastic fibbers are not easily delineated in H&E preparation unless special stains are used. Celloidinization of sections prior to staining, particularly of skin and blood vessels, is desirable as they may detach from the slide.

Wiegert's Resorcin—Fuchsin Stain There are several variations of the technique described here. The rationale of these variations is obscure. Most of these methods, however, show a remarkable selectivity for elastic fibres and give the best demonstration of fine fibres. The techniques tend to be slow and the solutions are time-consuming to prepare. These solutions stain well at room temperature and may be used repeatedly. Some variations in staining avidity will be found with different dye batches so a variation in staining times will occur. Staining at room temperature for longer periods gives better results than a shorter time at 56°C. Pretreatment with an acidified permanganate-oxalic acid solution sequence gives a clearer background. Fixation is not critical. Any well-fixed tissue can be used.

Reagents

- *Oxalic acid solution (5%, aqueous)*
- *Acidified potassium permanganate solution:*
    0.3% aqueous potassium permanganate
    3% Sulphuric acid

  Mix equal parts immediately prior to use. These can be conveniently kept as stock solutions.
- *Acid alcohol*—Differentiator

Conc. hydrochloric acid	1 mL
70% alcohol	99 mL

- *Ammonia water (2%, aqueous).*
- *Neutral red (1%, w/v, aqueous)*—counter stain.
- *Weigert's resorcinol fuchsin solution*

Basic fuchsin	2 g
Resorcinol	4 g
Distilled water	200 mL
Ferric chloride, 30% (w/v, aqueous)	25 mL
95% alcohol	200 mL
Conc. hydrochloric acid	4 mL

Dissolve the basic fuchsin and resorcin in the distilled water, bringing to the boil in an evaporating dish. While boiling, slowly add the aqueous anhydrous ferric chloride solution, stirring continuously. Continue for approximately 5 min. Cool and filter into a conical flask taking care that all the precipitate is collected. Discard the filtrate, dry the flask, and add the dried filter paper containing the precipitate to the flask. Add the alcohol and heat gently on a hot plate until the precipitate is dissolved. Remove the filter paper, add the concentrated hydrochloric acid, cool and filter. Make up the final volume to 200 mL by pouring fresh 95% alcohol through the used filter paper. Filter before use. This solution keeps well for several months. The purified basic fuchsin commonly used for Schiff's reagent gives inferior results.

Procedure

1. Take the sections to water.
2. Treat with acidified potassium permanganate solution for 5 min.
3. Wash in water and bleach with 5% oxalic acid for approximately 1 min.
4. Wash well for in water, rinse in alcohol.
5. Stain in resorcin—fuchsin solution for 1–3 h at room temperature. The time will vary according to batch and type of solution. Check with the microscope and stain until elastic fibres are black. Save solution. If overstained, rinse in ammonia water for 3 min. This will remove excess stain.
6. Differentiate in acid–alcohol until the background is clear of stain.
7. Wash well in tap water.

8. Counterstain as required with neutral red stain (or eosin or van Gieson). Save solution. If overstained, water will remove excess stain.
9. Dehydrate, clear and mount as desired.

Result

Elastic fibres—blue-black
Background—Red (or according to the colour of the counterstain used)

Verhoeff's Stain   This is a rapid method for staining elastic fibres a strong black colour. The disadvantage is that some expertise is necessary to stain the finer elastic fibres and obtain a well-differentiated background. The principle of the technique is rather obscure. Both iodine and ferric chloride, with which the haematoxylin is combined, are oxidizing agents and it is this property that probably accounts for the production of a black dye with cationic properties (nuclei are also stained), rather than a simple dye-mordant tissue mechanism. Any well fixed tissue can be used.

Reagents

- *Verhoeff's solution*:
  For best results, make up solutions the same day they are to be used. Freshly prepared solutions give stronger staining results.
  Solution A:

Haematoxylin	5 g
Absolute alcohol	100 mL

  Dissolve with the aid of heat. Cool and filter.
  Solution B:

Ferric chloride	10 g
Distilled water	100 mL

  Solution C (Lugol's iodine solution):

Iodine	1 g
Potassium iodide	2 g
Distilled water	100 mL

  Add 8 mL of solution B into 20 mL of solution A and to that add 8 mL of solution C.
  Note: Follow the sequence as given.
- *Ferric chloride solution (2%)*

Procedure

1. Take sections to alcohol.
2. Stain with freshly made Verhoeff's solution until the sections are black (15–45 min).
3. Wash in distilled water.
4. Differentiate in 2% ferric chloride with agitation, only for a few minutes. Check differentiation by rinsing in distilled water and examining under the low power of the microscope. Discontinue when elastic fibres and nuclei are black and other tissues are grey or weakly stained. Should the section be overdifferentiated, it may be returned to Verhoeff's solution for further staining.
5. Wash in water and then in alcohol for approximately 5 min to remove the iodine colouration of the background.
6. Wash in water and counterstain in van Gieson's stain for 1–2 min.
7. Dehydrate, clear and mount as desired.

Results

Elastic fibres—black
Nuclei—grey to black
Background—according to counterstain

STAINS FOR PARTICULAR SUBSTANCES

Staining of carbohydrates, amyloids, pigments and minerals (iron and calcium) and micro-organisms is occasionally done in the histopathology laboratory for the diagnosis of specific pathologic conditions. Staining of fat is done with frozen sections. This is discussed separately under the frozen section technique.

Carbohydrates

A simple carbohydrate molecule is a monosaccharide such as glucose that plays a central role in nutrition but is difficult to demonstrate within tissues. Glycogen, on the other hand, is a polysaccharide, with long chain sugar molecules. It is stored in liver and in muscle and available to the body in times of its need. Shorter and more complex chains of sugar molecules may be covalently linked to protein and lipid molecules forming glycoproteins and glycolipids, respectively. The carbohydrate component modifies the function of the main protein or lipid molecules. Mucin, present in the connective tissue is an amino sugar. Mucopolysaccharides are group of compounds composed of protein and complex sugars (polysaccharides), The staining and identification of the various types of carbohydrates (polysaccharides and mucopolysaccharides) have contributed greatly to our understanding of tissue structures such as liver (glycogen), heart, striated muscle, gastrointestinal tract glands, respiratory lining cells and others. The periodic acid-Schiff stain is generally presumed to be for a demonstration of carbohydrate but the stain is rather non-specific.

Periodic acid-schiff (PAS) stain

Periodic acid is a strong oxidizing agent and under the controlled conditions of the staining reaction, it reacts with the aldehyde group of the carbohydrates without allowing over-oxidation. Schiff reagent then reacts with the product. A red or purple-red colour indicates a positive PAS reaction. PAS positive substances include a host of organic compounds (amyloid, cerebrosides, glycogen, etc.), micro-organisms (amoebae, Mycobacterium, fungi, etc.), body tissues and cells.

The use of post-Schiff sulphite rinses to reduce background colouration is not necessary, provided washing in running water is thorough and that the alkalinity of the tap water is not too high.

Reagents

- *Periodic acid solution (1%, w/v, aqueous)*:
  - Periodic acid crystals — 1 g
  - Distilled water — 100 mL
- *Schiff's reagent*:
  - Basic fuchsin — 1 g
  - Distilled water — 200 mL
  - Potassium or sodium metabisulphite — 2 g
  - Conc. hydrochloric acid (Analar grade) — 2 mL
  - Decolourizing charcoal — 2 g
- *Harris's haematoxylin solution*: Preparation of this reagent is described earlier (see routine).
- *Light green counterstain*
  - Light green — 100 mg
  - Acetic acid (0.1%) — 100 mL

Procedure

1. Sections to distilled water.
2. Treat with periodic acid solution for 5 min (longer time, 10 min, for basement membranes).
3. Rinse well in distilled water.
4. Treat with Schiff's reagent for 15 min.
5. Wash in running tap water for 5–10 min. This intensifies the colour reaction.
6. Stain nuclei with Harris's haematoxylin solution as counter stain or light green.
7. Differentiate and blue.
8. Dehydrate, clear and mount as desired.

Result

PAS-positive materials[†]—magenta (rose to purple red).
Nuclei—blue or blue-black

Amyloids

Amyloid is a starch-like material, principally a glycoprotein, formed by the combination of carbohydrate with protein. In various pathologic conditions abnormal quantities of glycoprotein may occur in organs and tissues, leading to amyloidosis with pathologic lesions. Some of the commonly used dyes to stain amyloid are Congo red, toluidine blue and crystal violet. These stains show metachromasia. In other words, the colour that appears in the section following these stains is different from the dominant colour of these stains. Hence, to avoid confusion, these stains must be used without a counterstain. In a section stained with toluidine blue, the metachromatic areas will be red-purple and the remaining tissue various shades of blue. These stains tend to fade and therefore the sections should be examined soon after they are stained. Stained sections should be examined immediately as many mounting media reverse the metachromasia. Another disadvantage of these stains is that they are not truly specific towards amyloid.

Congo red stain

Congo red, an anionic dye, is commonly used for the staining and demonstration amyloid or glycoprotein in microscopic tissue section. Bennhold's Congo red stain is simple and reliable and the stained sections can be kept indefinitely, since it is dehydrated and mounted in a permanent mounting medium.

An important feature of Congo red staining is the red to green birefringence seen when using polarized light, although this is not very specific. Hence a weak birefringence may require other confirmatory techniques.

Carnoy's fluid or absolute alcohol is used as the fixative. Ten percent formalin or Zenker-formal may be used.

Alkaline congo red technique

This is a progressive method, requiring no differentiation step. Salts act as ionic competitors for the dye, and background (polar) staining is eliminated; only the non-polar binding of Congo red occurs. The main disadvantages of the method lie in its complexity and the short bench-life of the solutions used.

Reagents

- *Harris's alum haematoxylin solution*: Described earlier
- *Sodium hydroxide solution (1%, w/v, aqueous)*:
  Keep in air-tight plastic bottle. Discard the solution when turbid.

[†]These include glycogen, mucin, hyaluronic acid, reticulin, fibrin of thrombi, colloid droplets, hyaline of arteriosclerosis, hyaline deposits in glomeruli, most basement membranes, colloid pituitary stalk and thyroid, amyloid infiltration and other elements. If light green is used as the counterstain, the section will have a pale background of the counterstain.

- *Stock alcoholic sodium chloride*:
  Saturated sodium chloride in 80% alcohol. This is a stock stable solution that keeps well
- *Working solution*:

Stock solution	50 mL
1% aqueous sodium hydroxide	0.5 mL

  Mix and filter, use within 15 min.
- *Congo red alkaline solution*
  A. *Stock solution*:
  Saturated Congo red in 80% alcohol saturated with sodium chloride. Filter and keep in a tightly stoppered container. The stock solution will be stable for several months.
  B. *Working solution*:

Stock solution (Congo red)	50 mL
1% aqueous sodium hydroxide	0.5 mL

Procedure

1. Section to water.
2. Stain the nuclei with an alum haematoxylin.
3. Differentiate and blue.
4. Treat with the alcoholic sodium chloride-hydroxide solution for 20 min. Drain.
5. Stain with the Congo red solutions for 20 min.
6. Rinse with alcohol.
7. Dehydrate, clear and mount as desired.

Result

Amyloid—orange-red
Nuclei—blue
Background—clear

Toluidine blue stain

Toluidine blue is a basic dye which has been reported to stain many tissue components—including amyloids—an orthochromatic blue colour. Under polarized light, amyloid is distinguished by its striking dark red birefringence. Occasional amyloid deposits, especially those of endocrine origin, are negative with this method and minimal deposits are sometimes difficult to visualize.

Reagents

- *Isopropanol (50%, v/v, aqueous)*.
- *Toluidine blue solution*: 1% solution in 50% isopropanol.

Procedure

1. Well-paraffinized sections to water, removing fixation pigment, where necessary.
2. Stain in toluidine blue solution for 30 min at 37°C.
3. Blot section carefully then place in absolute isopropanol for 1 min.
4. Clear and mount as desired.

Result Amyloid and many other tissue components stain an orthochromatic blue colour, but when examined under polarized light amyloid gives a dark red birefringence.

Lipids

Lipids can be defined as substances that are insoluble in water and may be extracted from the tissues by organic solvents. Lipids are normal constituents of tissues, found in adipose tissue as stored lipid for energy production, or as specialist lipid structure such as myelin. Lipids are rarely found in a pure state in tissue sections; they are usually in combination with carbohydrates in glycolipids or with proteins in lipoproteins. The demonstration of lipid in the routine laboratory is infrequently called for and, unless dealing with a suspected lipid storage disorder, is unlikely to require precise identification of the type present. The accumulation of fat in some tissues may be diagnostic of certain pathologic conditions. Fat embolism (obstruction of a blood vessel) is not uncommon in bone injuries and fractures. Extraneous examples of conditions requiring lipid staining include aortic atheroma and lipid pneumonia of the lungs (due to aspiration of fatty material from the oral cavity). Certain tumours, too, contain significant quantities of fat and this can sometimes be used to advantage in their recognition.

Fat is soluble in alcohol. Thus, it is not possible to use sections cut from ordinary paraffin-embedded blocks to demonstrate fat, as the fat will have been dissolved by the alcohols used in the embedding procedures. **For the examination of histological specimens, the frozen section technique is most often used**. In addition, there is no really good fixative for lipids. Formalin fixes only a minority of lipids. It is inert towards simple lipids and allows appreciable diffusion and loss of phospholipids. Cryostat sections of fresh unfixed tissue involve the least loss of lipids. Lipids (broadly includes both simple fats and conjugated fats) may be demonstrated histochemically by a variety of techniques. Of all the methods, the use of oil soluble colourants is most popular. This includes oil red O and Sudan black stain. These will be described here. Counterstaining present problems as most dyes diffuse or are bleached by aqueous mountants. For the red lipid dyes haematoxylin is used, but it tends to fade in time.

Oil red O stain

The deep red staining of lipids by this method makes it one of the most popular techniques for the identification of fat in the tissue sections. Always use a covered container and ample amounts of solution when staining and use care in washing. Of the various alternative staining solutions, the isopropanol variant is more commonly chosen, which is described here.

Reagents

- *Isopropyl alcohol (absolute and 60%, v/v, aqueous)*
- *Acetic acid (1%, v/v, aqueous).*
- *Ammonia water (2%), v/v, aqueous).*
- *Oil red O stain*:

Dissolve 0.5 g of oil red O dye in 200 mL of isopropyl alcohol. Warm the solution in a long-necked container (2-L volumetric flask) in a 56°C water bath for 1 h. Cool. The working solution is prepared prior to use by adding four parts of distilled water to six parts of stock solution. Mix and stand for 10 min. Filter through a fine filter paper (Whatman No. 42). This working dilution should be used within 2–4 h. Such saturated staining solutions must be kept in air-tight staining vessels to avoid precipitation of the dye because of the evaporation of the solvent.

- *Counterstain*: Harris's haematoxylin or light green.
- *Glycerine jelly (mounting medium)*:

Gelatine	10 g
Distilled water	60 mL
Heat until gelatine is dissolved then add:	
Glycerine	70 mL
Phenol	1 mL

Procedure

1. Rinse frozen sections in water.
2. Rinse in 60% isopropyl alcohol.
3. Stain in oil red O for 10 min.
4. Wash briefly in 60% isopropyl alcohol.
5. Wash gently in tap water.
6. Counterstain in Harris's haematoxylin for 1–2 min.
7. Wash in water.
8. Blue in ammonia water: If sections are too dark when removed from the haematoxylin, they may be differentiated in 1% acetic water for a few seconds, and then blued in ammonia water.
9. Wash in water and mount in an aqueous mountant (glycerine jelly)

Result

Fat—orange to bright red
Phospholipids—pink
Nuclei—blue
Other tissues—pale brown

Sudan black stain

Sudan black is the most sensitive lipid stain known. In fact, it is too sensitive as a general fat stain. Valid objections, however, exist to the use of acetone and ethanol as vehicles for these dyes in that these solvents remove a significant portion of the lipids. As a result, small fat droplets are likely to be dissolved out and escape detection. Isopropyl alcohol, propylene or ethylene glycol is less objectionable.

Reagents

- *Sudan black solution*: Saturated solution of Sudan black in 70% alcohol.
- *2% carmalum solution*:

Carminic acid	2 g
5% aqueous ammonium alum	100 mL
Salicylic acid or thymol	0.2 g

    Add the carminic acid to the ammonium alum solution and dissolve by boiling for 1 h. Cool and restore to original volume with distilled water. Add fungicidal agent (salicylic acid or thymol) and mix thoroughly. Filter and use. The solution keeps quite well if stored at 4°C.
- *Glycerine jelly (aqueous mountant)*: Described earlier.

Procedure

1. Mount the sections on to slides and allow to dry
2. Rinse in 70% ethanol.
3. Stain in a saturated solution of Sudan black in 70% ethanol for 15 min. Filter before use.
4. Remove excess stain in 70% ethanol.
5. Stain nuclei with the carmalum solution for 5–30 min.
6. Wash well in water and mount in an aqueous mountant (glycerine jelly).

Result

Fat—blue-black
Nuclei—pale red

Pigments and Minerals

The pigments seen in the sections are broadly classified as artefact, endogenous and exogenous. Artefacts originate from fixation materials such as formalin, mercury and chromate. Endogenous pigments are those produced within the tissue while exogenous pigments are those which are gaining access to the tissues—mainly minerals. Fixation pigments (artefacts) are not clinically important but they should be recognized in order to avoid improper diagnosis. Many histochemical pathologists have paid considerable attention to endogenous tissue pigments. The chemistry of these substances seems less important and less known. Nevertheless, the presence of haemosiderin and melanin in tissues are of diagnostic significance. The deposition of haemosiderin in excessive amounts inside the tissue (**haemosiderosis, haemochromatosis**) may indicate red blood cell related disorders, or a haemorrhagic condition or iron overload. Melanin is a black pigment normally present in certain tissues but some malignant tumours (**melanomas**) produce this pigment and their diagnosis is often based on the histochemical identification of melanin in tissues. Haemosiderin contains active ferric iron which combines with potassium ferrocyanide in acid solution to form ferric ferrocyanide or Prussian blue. Only a few exogenous minerals are important for the histochemical diagnosis. These include iron and calcium. Iron is recognized by the Prussian blue reaction (same as for haemosiderin) while calcium is recognized by the silver impregnation method.

Haemosiderin and iron stain

Haemosiderin is a golden brown granular pigment that is the product of the breakdown of haemoglobin and therefore occurs at the site of previous haemorrhage. The request for iron staining is in reality to check for the presence of haemosiderin in the section. Haemosiderin, however, should be differentiated from melanin, bile, formalin pigment and malaria pigment which do not contain iron. The iron-containing pigment (haemosiderin) reacts with potassium ferrocyanide in acid medium and yields a Prussian blue colour. This is called Perl reaction and is used to demonstrate ferric iron (and ferritin). It is one of the classic histochemical methods that were introduce by Perl in 1867.

Prussian blue stain

The principle of this method is that the reactive ferric iron, exemplified by haemosiderin, produces an intense and insoluble precipitate of Prussian blue that indicates the presence of iron. In this method a common artefact is the presence of blue granules, either on or around the section, following treatment with the hydrochloric-ferrocyanide mixture. This could be due to old ferrocyanide mixture or iron-contaminated water (rust). The simplest remedy is to have a suitably sized beaker containing distilled water to one side of the bath. The distilled water is maintained at the correct temperature and it is simple matter to float out sections to be stained by the Pearl's reaction.

Reagents

- *Aqueous potassium ferrocyanide (2%, w/v, aqueous)*: **POISON**
- *Hydrochloric acid (2%, v/v, aqueous).*
- *Neutral red (1%, w/v, aqueous)*

Procedure

1. Test sections and a control section to distilled water.
2. Mix equal parts of the hydrochloric acid and potassium ferrocyanide solutions and filter on to the sections. Leave for 30 min at room temperature, changing to a fresh solution after 15 min.
3. Wash for several minutes in water.
4. Counterstain with neutral red solution for 5 min.
5. Wash in water.
6. Dehydrate and differentiate in alcohol.
7. Clear and mount in a DPX-type mountant.

Result

Iron pigment (haemosiderin)—blue
Nuclei—red
Background—pale red

Von Kossa silver nitrate procedure for calcium

Insoluble inorganic calcium salts are normally found in bone and teeth. Calcium circulated in the blood in the free ionic form, which is not demonstrable histochemically. Abnormally, calcium is formed in tissue in hyperparathyroidism, necrosis (e.g. tuberculous caseation) and in association with some tumours such as myeloma.

Von Kossa's technique for the demonstration of the presence of calcium salts in tissue sections is oldest and widely used. It is a metal substitution method wherein silver is substituted for calcium forming a metallic salt with the anion of the calcium salt. The silver salt is then reduced to black metallic silver by light or photographic developer. Although not specific (melanin also tends to blacken) it remains the method of choice. As a rule, non-acidic fixation of tissue should be used, such as formalin or alcohol. Buffered neutral formalin is recommended. The method described here has omitted the post-silver hypo treatment as partial bleaching of the blackened calcium salts may occur.

Reagents

- *Silver nitrate (2%, w/v, aqueous)*: Store the solution in a brown bottle.
- *Counterstain*: Van Gieson's stain or 1% aqueous neutral red.

Procedure

All glassware should be rinsed with distilled water prior to use.
1. Sections to distilled water, two or three changes.
2. Transfer sections to a clear glass container (Coplin staining jar) containing the silver nitrate, or place on a slide rack and cover the section with the solution.
3. Expose the section to bright sunlight or high intensity light (a desk lamp with 60-watt bulb source) for 60 min. If exposed to sunlight the time may be less; check microscopically.
4. Wash in several changes of distilled water.
5. Wash well in tap water.
6. Counterstain as required, either in van Gieson or neutral red for 5 min.
7. Dehydrate, clear and mount in DPX.

Results

Calcium deposits—black
Background—according to counterstain used.
Cell nuclei are red and cytoplasm is pink with neutral red.

STAINS FOR MICROORGANISMS

Tissue sections are sometimes examined for the presence of certain microorganisms with special reference to bacteria and fungi (systemic). Many of these microorganisms can be seen in routine H&E stained sections; however, special stains are employed to make them easier to identify. Some of these micro-organisms may not pick up the routine stain, or they may be very few in numbers and are almost impossible to find without special stains. Only a few of the routinely used methods followed in Indian laboratories will be discussed here: Gram stain for bacteria, acid fast stain for mycobacterium (tuberculosis and leprosy), silver methenamine stain for fungi, and Giemsa stain for bacteria and blood parasites. A few commonly used histological stains to demonstrate the presence organisms in tissues are given in Table 37.3.

Table 37.3 Commonly used histological stains to demonstrate organisms in tissues

Stain	Organism	Example
Haematoxylin–eosin (H&E)	Viral, Toxoplasma, fungi (Aspergillus, Zygomycetes) Demonstrate cellular response	CMV, Herpes, Adenovirus, Toxoplasma
Gomori's methenamine silver nitrate (GMS)	Fungi (yeast and mycelial form)	Histoplasma, Candida, Aspergillus
Periodic acid Schiff (PAS)	Fungi, sporotrichosis, Blastomyces and Zygomycetes	Blastomyces Zygomycosis Coccidiodes
Acid fast	Mycobacteria, Nocardia	Mycobacteria
Gram	Bacteria, Actinomyces, fungi	Gram reacting bacteria, Actinomyces, Nocardia
Giemsa	Rickettsia, Pneumocystis (will stain internal structure), fungi	Histoplasma, Pneumocystis, Candida

General Purpose Stain

Giemsa stain

Giemsa stain is widely used as a bacterial stain, for the study of haematological elements, for bone marrow preparations, for blood parasites. Its use in histological specimen is a modified version of the original method that gives good results. Most acidophilic cells and eosinophils stain a similar colour. To achieve a good colour balance it is necessary to overstain initially with Giemsa, and then slightly overdifferentiate in weak acetic acid until there is a general pink cast to the cells. This offsets the loss of eosinophilia and gain in basophilia which results upon alcohol dehydration. Decalcification of tissue with strong acids should be avoided as it results in a poor colour balance. The only real disadvantage is the length of time required in staining.

Reagents

- *Giemsa stain*:
  This staining solution is readily available commercially but, to prepare a batch, the following formula may be use.
  Mix 7.36 g of Giemsa dry stain in 500 mL glycerol heated to 50°C in a water bath. Leave for 30 min at 50°C with periodic mixing. Allow to cool and add 500 mL methanol (the acetone content is immaterial). Mix and filter.
- *Acetic acid (differentiator)*:
  A convenient way of preparing the weak solution required in the staining procedure is to take 1 mL of 1% acetic acid solution (v/v, aqueous) and dilute with 99 mL of distilled water. This final solution is of 1 : 10,000 v/v strength of weak acetic acid.

Procedure

1. Section to distilled water.
2. Filter enough Giemsa stain into a Coplin jar filled with distilled water to render the solution a dark blue colour (0.5–1.0 mL).
3. Stain with the solution for at least 20 min at 56°C until the section is overall dark blue.

4. Rinse in distilled water and differentiate in weak acetic acid solution (1:10,000 v/v) until the section is predominantly pink in colour.
5. Rinse in distilled water, dehydrate, clear and mount as desired.

Result
Nuclei—purple
Azurophilic granules—blue
Red blood cells—yellow to pink
Eosinophil granules, red blood cells and other acidophil structures—pink

Bacteria

Gram staining of bacteria

Details of the Gram staining procedure are presented in the chapter on Bacteriology. The means by which some organisms retain the blue primary dye (gram-positive) and others (gram-negative) lose it upon differentiation is due to the action of iodine. The exact way in which iodine influences due fastness to differentiation is not clear. The traditional view is that iodine combines with the dye and gram-positive organisms as a type of mordant or trapping agent to form a solvent-resistant dye complex. Fixation is not important but initial freshness of tissue and the use of positive controls are, so that should test section be negative it is an indicator that the solutions and the skill of the operator are beyond reproach!

Special Note:
Both gram-positive and negative bacteria are demonstrated in the following technique. Although over differentiation with the acetone is possible, it is the method of choice for consistently good results. The technique for smears is similar in principle to that for sections and the points to remember are that they should either be heat-dried on a hot plate before staining, or wet-fixed smears through xylene and alcohols. Tissue which has been decalcified in strong acids (or too long in weak acids) will give inconsistent staining.

Reagents
- *Crystal violet stain*:
    A. Crystal violet solution (0.5%, w/v, in 25% alcohol)
    B. Sodium bicarbonate (5%, w/v, in water)
        Freshly mix 1 mL of solution A and 5 drops (0.25 mL) of solution B. Leave for 1 min.
- *Gram's iodine solution*:
    Add 1 g iodine in 2 g potassium iodide plus a few mL of distilled water in a mortar. Grind until dissolved and make up to a 300 mL volume. KI facilitates dissolving the iodine in aqueous medium)
- *Neutral red (1%, w/v, aqueous)*
- *Acetone*

Procedure
1. Sections to water.
2. Stain with crystal violet solution for 2 min.
3. Wash in water.
4. Treat with Gram's iodine solution for 2 min.
5. Wash, dehydrate quickly, clear and mount in DPX-type mount.

Result
Gram-positive bacteria, some fungi—blue
Gram-negative bacteria—red

Nuclei—red
Other tissues—yellow

Acid fast staining of bacteria

Mycobacteria such as tubercle bacilli have a lipid-rich cell wall capable of taking up strong phenol-dye solutions so that they retain the dye upon subsequent differentiation in acid or alcohol, that is, they are acid- and alcohol-fast. Most other organisms lose the dye and take up the counterstain. It has been shown that acid-fastness of mycobacterial stained with carbol fuchsin is due to the presence of carboxyl and hydroxyl groups on unsaturated lipids present in bacterial cells.

The Ziehl–Neelsen procedure is the traditional method of acid-fast staining and is reliable. The histological appearance in tuberculosis is usually (but not always) typical; even so, the demonstration of tubercle bacilli is a useful confirmatory procedure.

If potentially tuberculous unfixed material for cryostat sectioning is received, full aseptic procedure should be adopted, that is, use of gloves, gowns, etc. Following sectioning the slides should be fixed in 10% formalin for at least 10 min before staining, and all equipment including the cryostat interior should be thoroughly sterilized in either formalin or a glutaraldehyde solution.

Reagents

- *Carbol fuchsin solution*:
  Dissolve 1 g basic fuchsin (use the coarse granule, not the more purified type specified for Schiff's reagent) in 10 mL ethanol. Dissolve 5 g of phenol in 100 mL of distilled water. Mix the two solutions together. Store at room temperature and filter before use.
- *1% Acid–alcohol*:
  Conc. hydrochloric acid, (sp.gr. 1.19)   3 mL
  Alcohol, 70%   99 mL
- *Methylene blue solution* (0.2%, w/v, aqueous)

Procedure

1. Sections to water.
2. Filter on the carbol fuchsin and heat three times until the 'steam rises' (over a period of 10 min), or heat in a Coplin jar at 56°C for 30 min.
3. Wash well with water.
4. Differentiate in 1% acid–alcohol for 1–10 min.
5. Wash in water for 5–10 min.
6. Counterstain with the methylene blue solution for 30 sec.
7. Wash in water.
8. Differentiate and dehydrate in alcohol until the sections are a weak blue.
9. Clear and mount in a DPX-type mount.

Result

Tubercle bacilli—magenta.
Background—weak blue.
Erythrocytes—with slight reddish tint; these are a good index against over decolourization (yellowish orange).

Weak acid-fast staining

This method is recommended for delicate organisms such as *Mycobacterium leprae*. Compared with tubercle bacilli, the leprosy bacilli are much less acid- and alcohol-fast and their lipid envelope is more easily affected by fat solvents, diminishing the staining reaction. Initial dewaxing is done in a mixture of a vegetable oil and xylene. It is important not to over-stain with the methylene blue, as it will not be possible to remove the excess dye in alcohol.

Reagents
- *Carbol fuchsin solution*: as described before
- *Oil-xylene mixture*: One part vegetable oil (peanut oil or clove oil) and two parts xylene.
- *Acid–alcohol*:

Hydrochloric acid (concentrated, sp. gr. 1.19)	1 mL
Alcohol (70%)	100 mL

- *Methylene blue solution (0.2%, w/v, aqueous)*

Procedure
1. Warm the section and deparaffinise by placing in the oil mixture. Leave for at least 10 min.
2. Blot dry and wash in water. This step may be repeated, should any xylene-oil remain on the section.
3. Filter on the carbol fuchsin solution for 20 min at room temperature. Do not heat.
4. Wash. Differentiate in 1% acid–alcohol for 1 min.
5. Wash well in water and counterstain in weak (0.2%) methylene blue for 5–10 sec.
6. Wash, wipe edges, blot dry and clear in xylene. Repeat the blotting-xylene treatment until the section is clear. Air dry.
7. Mount in a DPX-type mountant.

Result
Leprosy bacilli, red blood cells—magenta
Background—pale blue

Fluorescence technique for tubercle bacilli and leprosy bacilli
Fluorescence demonstration of tubercle bacilli (and also leprosy bacilli) is superior to the acid-fast staining technique. But it requires special microscope and some expertise in its preparation. In this technique, background tissue fluorescence is masked by the potassium permanganate treatment. To stain for leprosy bacilli, avoid alcohol dehydration at the conclusion of the technique and de-wax initially in a vegetable oil–xylene mixture (as discussed earlier).

Reagents
- *Auramine—rhodamine solution*:
  Add 1.5 g of auramine O and 0.75 g rhodamine B to 50 mL of distilled water and 75 mL of glycerol. Mix and add 10 mL phenol liquefied by melting at 56°C. The solution will keep for up to 2 months. Filter before use.
- *Acid–alcohol solution*:
  - 0.5% hydrochloric acid in 70% alcohol for tubercle baciili
  - 0.5% aqueous hydrochloric acid for leprosy bacilli.
- *Potassium permanganate solution (0.5%, w/v, aqueous)*

Procedure
1. Section to water.
2. Treat the section with preheated (60°C) auramine-rhodamine mixture for 10 min.
3. Wash in water for 2 min.
4. Differentiate in either of the hydrochloric acid solutions for 2–3 min as appropriate.
5. Wash in water for 2 min.

6. Treat with the potassium permanganate solution for 1 min.
7. Wash in water for 2 min. Blot dry.
8. Dehydrate (omit for leprosy bacilli), clear and mount in a DPX-type mountant.

Demonstration of *Helicobacter*

Helicobacter pylori (formerly assigned to the Campylobacter group of organisms) are an organism that, since its recognition in 1984, has been firmly linked to gastritis and duodenal ulceration. It is gram-negative bacillus having the distinctive morphology of a stumpy cured rod. Staining by the conventional Gram staining gives indifferent results in histological materials. The use of Giemsa stains in the diagnosis of *Helicobacter pylori* infection in the gastric mucosa is time-consuming. The cresyl fast violet method, as described here, is simple and effective.

In gastric biopsies the organisms are normally found on the epithelial surface or in the mucosal glandular folds. It is recommended that a positive control slide is taken through, if possible, so that the relative colour balance of organisms to background can be assessed.

Cresyl fast violet technique

This is a popular technique and simple to do although differentiation of the due requires experience before good results are obtained.

Reagents

- *Cresyl fast (echt) violet (1%, w/v, aqueous)*
- *Alcohol*: 95% and absolute.

Procedure

1. Section to water.
2. Stain with the cresyl fast violet solution for 15 min.
3. Wash in water and differentiate in 95% alcohol until the organism can be recognized by its purple colour. Run a positive control for comparison.
4. Rinse in absolute alcohol, clear and mount as desired.

Result

Helicobacter—purple
Background—pale blue-purple

Staining of Fungi

Silver methenamine stain

Fungi have little affinity for Gram stain; only a few are acid-fast (e.g. Nocardia), and some of the fungi do not take the H&E routine stain. Gomori's methenamine–silver nitrate technique is routinely used in many laboratories as a general purpose fungal stain. The primary disadvantage is that the silver precipitation method causes fungi to stain black. In tissue containing black pigment from other sources such as the lung with carbon pigment, the organisms may go unidentified. Thus, in the case of lung and pulmonary lymph nodes, a modified PAS stain is used. When in doubt, both the methods can be adopted regardless of the type of tissue.

The Gomori's methenamine silver nitrate stain has been employed for the demonstration of glycogen and mucin. It is, however, widely used for the demonstration of certain fungi in tissue, more particularly the systemic fungi and opportunist fungi (*Aspergillus fumtgatus, Candida_albicans*). The method is not specific for fungi and is time-consuming but rarely fails to demonstrate any fungi present in tissue. A control should always be taken through to establish the efficacy of the reagents employed.

Special Note:
The connective tissue is blackened by over impregnation making fungal identification more difficult. Terminate treatment with the hexamine-silver when the fungi appear a dark brown colour and the background is still clear, that is, aim at slightly under-impregnating. The inclusion of the borate gives a final pH of approximately 8.0.

Reagents

- *Sodium metabisulphite solution (1%, w/v, aqueous)*
- *Chromium trioxide solution (chromic acid): 5%, w/v, aqueous.*
- *Silver nitrate–methenamine solution*
  Stock solution:
  To 100 mL of 3% aqueous hexamine add 5 mL of 5% aqueous silver nitrate. A white precipitate will form that dissolves on shaking. The solution keeps for 1–2 months at 4°C.
  Working solution:
  Dilute 2 mL of freshly prepared 5% aqueous sodium tetraborate solution with 25 mL of distilled water. Mix and add 25 mL of stock hexamine-silver.
- *Gold chloride solution (0.1%, w/v, aqueous):* This solution may be used repeatedly.
- *Sodium thiosulphate or hypo solution (5%, w/v, aqueous)*
- *Light green counterstain (0.2% in 0.2% acetic acid)*

Light green, S.F. (yellow)	0.2 g
Distilled water	100 mL
Glacial acetic acid	0.2 mL

Procedure

1. Test and positive control sections to water.
2. Treat with the chromic acid solution for 1 h. Wash in water.
3. Bleach in the metabisulphite solution for 1 min.
4. Wash in tap water for 5–10 min, then in several changes of distilled water.
5. The working hexamine solution should have been preheated to 56°C using a Coplin jar in a water bath. Treat the section in this solution at 56°C and examine after 10–20 min and after that at 3 min intervals until the fungi are blackened (read special note) but the background is clear. Use plastic forceps to hold the slides.
6. Wash in three changes of distilled water and tone in 0.1% aqueous gold chloride for 3 min.
7. Wash in water, fix in sodium thiosulphate for 5 min. Wash again.
8. Counterstain in light green for 1–2 min. Wash in water.
9. Dehydrate, clear and mount as desired.

Result

Fungi, cellulose, mucins, glycogen, starch—black
Background—pale green
Inner parts of micelle and hyphae—old rose

Tissue parasite demonstration

In developing countries with warmer climates, demonstration of the presence of tissue parasites in the sections helps in the diagnosis of parasitic infections. Although H&E preparation and Giemsa staining may be adequate but special technique may be applied to show the variegated structure of helminths and protozoa. The one that is particularly useful is the identification of Leishman-Donovan bodies for the diagnosis of *Leishmania donovani* infection (kalazar). These parasites are minute and not easily seen in H&E and conventional Romanowsky-type staining of tissue sections. Other methods have been discussed in Chapter 22 in Vol. II.

Reagents

- *Leishman stain*: This is commercially available from most laboratory suppliers. It is diluted with buffer (pH 4.7) before use.
  To prepare in the laboratory, rinse out a clean staining bottle with methanol. Add a few dry glass beads. Add 0.75 g of Leishman powder and 500 mL of methanol (CH_3OH). Mix well. Label with date. The stain is ready for use the following day. It is important to prevent moisture from entering the stain during its preparation and storage.
- *Weak solution of acetic acid (1 : 10,000, v/v)*: As described before (Giemsa).

Procedure

1. Take sections to distilled water.
2. Treat with diluted Leishman stain for 10 min or 1–2 h.
   Note: The staining time may need to be adjusted, especially when a new batch of stain is used or the stain has been stored for a long time.
3. Rinse in distilled water and differentiate in weak (1 in 10,000) acetic acid until the desired colour balance is achieved.
4. Rinse in distilled water and blot dry.
5. Dehydrate quickly, clear and mount as desired.

FROZEN SECTION TECHNIQUE

Sections can be prepared for histological examination in a few minutes by the frozen section technique. The principle involved is simple in comparison with paraffin wax embedding. The water in the tissue is frozen and as ice produces a firm block of tissue, the ice acts as the embedding medium. The consistency of frozen blocks is affected by the nature of the tissue and amount of water in the tissue. Tissues that have a low water content section better at colder temperatures; those with a higher content, being harder due to more ice crystals, section better at higher temperatures. It is possible to improve sectioning of frozen blocks in the cryostat by adjusting the temperature of the block tissue. For example, the optimum sectioning temperature of brain is –12°C while the adipose tissue of breast may require –35°C or lower. Fixed tissue of any nature is sectioned at –5 to –10°C.

The rapid development of the cryostat over the last three decades has made it possible to examine the 'urgent frozen sections'. It is now an indispensable technique for rapid diagnosis and intraoperative surgical consultation. In addition, many histochemical methods cannot be done without freezing microtomy because the drastic steps involved in paraffin sectioning destroy or lose the material sought.

Preparing frozen sections for histological studies has some disadvantages also. The structural details are distorted because of the lack of embedding material during cutting and handling. It is impossible to obtain serial sections in the case of cryostat sections and the staining is not as satisfactory in the case of unfixed frozen sections as seen in properly fixed material. The histopathologist will also find many freezing artefacts in the cryostat sections. Moreover, some of the finer details cannot be determined by this technique and certain special stains cannot be used.

We will try to describe here the general process of handling the freezing microtome (cryostat). However, because of the wide variations found between various microtomes we will leave to the reader the details of their operation available in the manufacturer's instruction booklet.

Tissue preparation: A suitable block of fresh tissue is selected and trimmed with a sharp scalpel so that its sides are parallel. The block should be about 5 mm thick. The tissue is directly taken for cryostat sectioning.

Freezing the tissue: Due to the water in the tissue it is advisable to freeze the tissue slowly to avoid tissue disruption. In most instances it will be wise to place the tissue on the freezing stage of cryostat and allow it to freeze. When the tissue is frozen, place the tissue block firmly on the microtome holder.

Freezing microtomy: Pull the stage holding knife forward to allow about 5 mm clearance between the subsequent down-travel of the block and the knife edge. Release the drive wheel lock and line up the tissue block to the knife to within 1–2 mm of the tissue with the frozen block parallel to the knife edge. When the face is almost in contact with the knife, release the ratchet from the micrometer wheel. Turn the wheel with the hand, a fraction of a turn at a time, to advance the tissue until the knife begins to cut the sections.

The cryostat cuts individual sections unlike the ribbons of sections with the paraffin preparations. Sections should be cut with a slow and even motion. If the adjustments are correct, the section will glide smoothly and flat beneath the antiroll plate. Some technicians use a camel-hair paint brush to start the section and to keep it flat as it glides out on the knife surface. Sectioning may be difficult in hot, humid weather.

The cutting of a frozen section requires experience and 'touch'. Start sectioning and continue until a complete section is obtained. Usually the block will have thawed to about the right consistency by this time. Do not freeze the tissues too hard or the sections may shatter. If this happens, allow the block to thaw slightly and try again. If it has become too soft the sections will also shatter or fracture. The technician will have to develop a proper feel for the correct temperature. Sometimes rubbing a finger across the block will give it the right consistency for good sections to be cut. Cut the sections slowly at about 5–10 μ thickness.

Mounting of frozen section: Mounting of the frozen section should be done carefully. The sections are not rigid like the paraffin sections and should be handled differently. The cryostat is provided with an antiroll plate which is flipped back after the section is cut. In practice, one edge of the glass slide is rested on the knife surface about 1 inch beyond the section and the other end is lowered gently until it is about 0.5–1.0 mm from the knife face, and the section will automatically transfer from the cold knife to the relatively warm slide. Never press the slide down on the section. A frost mark will remain where the section rested on the knife. This should be wiped away with soft gauze. The antiroll plate is re-positioned and another section may be cut.

No adhesive is needed to stick the section of unfixed tissue on the slide; air drying for about 30–60 sec will be good enough to hold the section.

Staining of Frozen Sections

The staining technique for frozen sections is basically the same as for paraffin sections. Since the major use of the cryostat is for rapid surgical diagnosis, time may be saved by using unfixed tissue. The latter will also adhere easily to the glass slide without the need for any adhesive mixture. Most often the sections are handled singly and they receive the top priority in the laboratory. In addition to the rapidity of diagnosis, there is another advantage of using unfixed frozen sections for histological studies. Freezing preserves the cellular enzymes and other substances that may be studied by histochemical techniques. If the tissues are fixed, they should be washed thoroughly before staining.

There are numerous methods of staining frozen sections, but for rapid surgical diagnosis two methods are widely used: H&E and polychrome methylene blue. Many workers also use toluidine blue with carbol fuchsin counterstain. There are many modifications of these but only the commonly used ones will be described here:

Haematoxylin–eosin for fresh cryostat sections

Although fixation prior to staining is not necessary, a brief 1–2 min immersion of the slide in 10 15% formalin will enhance the nuclear basophilia. Sections of certain material, for example, mucoid tumours may lift off the slides when placed in the formalin and this step should, therefore, be avoided and a dry section celloidinized instead.

The routine H&E staining method can be applied. It is a little more time-consuming, and in some laboratories a special staining row is set up just for frozen sections.

Reagents
Prepare the reagents as described earlier with routine staining.
- *Harris's haematoxylin (pre-filtered)*: Described earlier.
- *Acid alcohol (1%, v/v)*.
- *Sodium bicarbonate solution (2%, w/v, aqueous)*.
- *Eosin Yellow water soluble (1%, w/v, aqueous)*

Procedure
1. Wash section in water for 10–20 sec.
2. Stain with haematoxylin for 1 min.
3. Wash briefly in water; differentiate in acid–alcohol for 1–2 sec.
4. Wash briefly in water and 'blue' in sodium bicarbonate for 10 sec or so.
5. Wash in water 10–20 sec and, if time permits, check nuclear staining microscopically.
6. Stain with eosin for 30 sec.
7. Wash briefly, dehydrate, clear and mount as desired.

Polychrome methylene blue staining

The method of polychrome methylene blue staining is recommended for rapid diagnosis with frozen sections. Its use is, however, limited. Many laboratories use this as a preceding stain so that the pathologist could study the methylene blue-stained section whilst the comparatively slower H&E-stained section was completed. Touch or imprint smears of unfixed tumours, breast lumps or lymph nodes may also be stained to advantage with polychrome methylene blue. Polychroming of methylene blue is achieved by mixing with potassium carbonate when various azures are formed. The process is accentuated by ageing of the solution.

Reagents
- *Staining solution*:

Methylene blue	1 g
Potassium carbonate	1 g
Glacial acetic acid	3 mL
Distilled water	300 mL

Place the distilled water in a litre flask and add, with mixing, methylene blue and potassium carbonate. Boil for 10–15 min. While still hot add glacial acetic acid drop by drop, shaking vigorously until the formed precipitate is dissolved. Boil until the volume of fluid is reduced to 100 mL. Cool and filter. Allow to stand 4 weeks prior to use.

Procedure
1. Rinse frozen sections and imprint smears in water.
2. Stain with the polychrome methylene blue for about 30–60 sec.
3. Wash in water and blot dry.
4. Dehydrate in tertiary butyl alcohol; clear in xylene and mount in a DPX-type mountant (conventional ethanol dehydration will diminish the polychromasia).

Result
Nuclei—blue
Background—various shades of red-purple

HANDLING AND EMBEDDING OF SMALL TISSUE FRAGMENTS

Minute fragments of tissue (e.g. biopsy materials, bone marrow aspirate, endoscopy fragments and others) may require special handling to prevent loss during processing. One of the recommended ways is to wrap the fragments of tissues in lens paper for the processing through various reagents.

In the case of bone marrow aspirate, as soon as the smears have been made, whatever remains should be placed in fixative for 30–60 min. Allow the fragments to settle down, pour off the supernatant and transfer the marrow fragments into a Petri dish to fix in formalin for about 30 min and then process the marrow particles by wrapping in the lens paper.

Review Questions

1. What is the role of histology laboratory in clinical diagnosis?
2. What are the responsibilities of the histotechnician?
3. How is the specimen prepared for cutting sections?
4. Which fixative is considered ideal in the laboratories of developing countries? What are the problems of using formaldehyde as the fixative?
5. How would one remove the mercuric chloride deposits in sections?
6. Explain the steps of tissue processing? What are the advantages and disadvantages of using the automated tissue processor? How is it different from automated stainers?
7. What is the purpose of clearing? Which is the commonly used clearing agent?
8. Explain the process of 'take to water'. Why is it necessary?
9. Explain the process of dehydration.
10. Describe how you will prepare a biopsy specimen for the microscopic examination.
11. Why is Canada-balsam no longer used in histotechnology laboratory? Which are the popular mounting media currently used?
12. Why is fat treated differently in the staining process than other constituents of the body? State its clinical significance.
13. What are the stains used for amyloids?
14. Describe the way the frozen sections are handled in the laboratory.
15. What is the use of the cryostat?
16. How is rotary microtome different from sliding microtome?
17. State the principle of fluorescent microscope.
18. List the stains used in identifying bacteria, fungi and protozoan.

38

Laboratory Techniques in Diagnostic Exfoliative Cytology

◆

Krishna Mallik

Chapter Outline

- ◆ Collection of Specimens and its Clinical Significance
- ◆ Preparation of Specimens for Cytological Evaluation
  - Concentrating specimen by centrifugation
    - ❑ Thick specimen
    - ❑ Watery specimen
  - Preparation of smear
  - Fixation
    - ❑ Commonly used fixatives
      - ○ Ether–alcohol
      - ○ Schaudinn's fluid
      - ○ Carnoy's fluid
    - ❑ Fixation and mailing of smears
  - Cytological stains and staining techniques
    - ❑ Papanicolaou staining
    - ❑ Cresyl violet staining
    - ❑ Other staining procedures
- ◆ Identifying Characteristics of Benign and Malignant Cells
  - Normal non-malignant cells
- ◆ Review Questions

Human cells shed (exfoliate) into body fluids and secretions, providing materials for diagnosis. Exfoliative cytology is the microscopic examination of cells desquamated from a body surface or lesion as a means of detecting malignancy and other disorders. Thus the study of exfoliative cytology helps in the early detection of **cancer**. Such cells are obtained by aspiration, washing, smear or scraping.

There are two main techniques involved in the study of **exfoliative cytology**:
- The study of direct smears of the specimen without centrifugation.
- The study of concentrated cellular material (e.g. sediment).

Concentration is accomplished by centrifugation or membrane filtration. The latter is not as common in the laboratories of developing countries. Body fluids which are watery and dilute need to be concentrated. The use of cytocentrifuge has gained popularity in the past few decades. Concentration of cells in sputum presents special problems due to the viscous nature of the mucous material. The high viscosity prevents membrane filtration and normal centrifugation methods. Thus, mucolytic pre-treatments with various enzymes or chemical reagents can be used, with or without ultrasonic disintegration, followed by centrifugation. It is important that all specimen preparation is carried out in an approved safety cabinet and that appropriate protective clothing is worn.

In recent years fine needle aspiration (FNA) techniques have proved to be of increasing value. Cells from a variety of tissues such as breast, liver, thyroid and lymph nodes can be aspirated using fine bore needles. The aspirated material may be put in a fixative for subsequent concentration or placed directly on slides for fixation and staining.

Choice of a fixative is important and most cytological fixatives are based on the use of alcohol. Commonly used alcohol-based fixatives such as butanol–ethanol, ethanol–acetic and Carnoy's solution. They can be prepared in the laboratory or commercially available.

Smears that are made should be wet-fixed, i.e. the slide should be placed in the fixing solution before the smear dries. If the smear is allowed to dry, various artefacts occur. The most common of these artefacts are enlarged nuclei exhibiting ill-defined, weakly staining chromatin and indistinct cell outlines. It is also important to fix the sample as rapidly as possible. This applies particularly to serous effusions, as storage of the specimen even at 4°C will cause some cellular changes.

The techniques described in the following pages are used commonly use in clinical cytology laboratories, but it is important to remember that most histological demonstration techniques can also be used for cytological purposes. The difference is that dye uptake or reagent reaction times will be shorter when dealing with smears.

COLLECTION OF SPECIMENS AND ITS CLINICAL SIGNIFICANCE

Technicians are rarely involved in the collection of specimens. They should, however, be aware of the method of specimen collection and the sources of error. Some of the specimens are collected by the patient or attending nurse. These include urine, sputum and gastrointestinal specimens.

The majority of specimens for the study of exfoliative cytology are collected by the **attending physician** during physical examination. These include vaginal and cervical smears, breast secretions, urine and sputum. Uterine cancer is diagnosed from the study of vaginal secretions. Cancer of the urinary tract is diagnosed by the study of urine. Breast cancer can be diagnosed by evaluating breast secretions from the nipple. Prostatic carcinoma can be diagnosed by examining the secretions expressed from the prostate by massage (examine the urine simultaneously). The presence of malignant cells in any body cavity fluid indicates involvement of the **serous membrane** of that particular cavity, e.g. pleura, peritoneum.

In the physician's office, **smears should be made immediately following collection of the specimen** on clean pre-labelled slides (use a lead pencil for labelling on frosted slides). A cotton swab (dry or saline-dipped) may be used in preparing the smear. The swab is soaked in the exudates and then rolled over the slide. Special equipment may be used by the physician or attending nurse to obtain vaginal exudates and discharge from the cervical external orifice. Transfer a drop of the exudate onto the slide and prepare the smear. The mucus plug from the external cervical orifice is the vaginal pool material. It is most useful for detecting the presence of malignant cells when cervical cancer is present.

The **Pap test** is a simple procedure for the diagnosis of cervical cancer. After a speculum (the standard device used to examine the cervix) is placed in the vagina, cells are skimmed from the surface of the cervix with a cotton swab then smeared onto a glass slide. The cervix is the narrow neck of the uterus that opens into the vagina. The slide is delivered to a laboratory where a cytotechnologist (a professional who reviews Pap test slides), and when necessary, a pathologist (a health care professional who examines bodily tissue samples) examines the sample for any abnormalities. Each smear contains roughly 50,000–300,000 cells. Though not infallible, when performed properly the Pap test can detect a majority of cervical cancer. Early detection of cervical cancer increases the likelihood of a cure, according to the American Society of Clinical Pathologists.

Serous fluids (gastric and bronchial washings, exudates, peritoneal and pleural fluids) are occasionally collected. Add citrate solution to the fluids immediately to anticoagulate if the specimen is bloody. (See anticoagulate composition at end of this section for details.) If a delay is anticipated, refrigerate or add an equal amount of 10% formalin. If the specimens are delayed for an extended period, refrigerate the specimens until they can be pooled by centrifugation and fixative is added. Some technicians prefer to **fix** the specimens before centrifugation. The use of a refrigerated centrifuge is recommended. Gastric washings deteriorate fast, hence must be fixed promptly. A first morning urine specimen is most desirable for the study of exfoliative urinary cytology. This also undergoes fast deterioration.

Sputum specimens are examined for the diagnosis of lung cancer. Sputum originates deep in the lungs and can only be obtained by deep coughing. Saliva, however, is the watery fluid in the mouth occurring through spitting, and is not the desired material for the study of exfoliate cytology of bronchial secretions. A sputum specimen is collected in the early morning by deep coughing. The collected expectorate specimen must reach the laboratory within 1 hour, followed by prompt fixation. Sputum is preserved in 70% alcohol. Sputum is loosened (liquefy the mucus) by a high speed blender or by treatment with proteolytic enzymes or chemicals. Liquefied sputum is then centrifuged and this sediment is used for the preparation of a smear.

Other specimens are collected in the laboratory as **aspirates of body fluids**—spinal, serous, prostatic, bronchial, pulmonary and others. Whatever the specimen or method of collection, prepare the smear immediately, and dip the smear into the fixative while the smear is still moist. **Never let the smear dry**. A delay in fixation will result in an unreliable specimen due to the rapid decomposition, drying and distortion of exfoliated cells.

- *Anticoagulant composition*

Sodium citrate	25.5 g
Citric acid	8.0 g
Distilled water	100 mL

Keep the above solution in a refrigerator. Add 2 mL of the citrate solution to each 100 mL of body fluid.

PREPARATION OF SPECIMENS FOR CYTOLOGICAL EVALUATION

Smears are made either directly from the collected specimen or from a concentrated specimen. The latter is obtained by centrifugation or the use of a membrane filter. Specimens such as cervical smears, spinal fluid or breast secretions can be examined unconcentrated by making a direct smear followed by fixation and staining. Watery exudates such as urine, gastric, serous, pleural, ascites and others require concentration of the specimen prior to the making of a smear. Irrespective of the type of specimen, the smears must be promptly made and fixed; refrigeration is only effective for a short period.

Concentrating Specimen by Centrifugation

Thick specimen

Specimens with sufficient amounts of protein, such as mucus or albumin, need no additional adhesive agent for smear preparation. The following method is applicable for preparing the concentrated material (sediment) for cytological examination.

Preparation of Specimen
1. Fix the specimen by mixing it with an equal amount of 95% alcohol.
2. Place the fixed specimens in 50 mL centrifuge tubes. Balance the tubes and centrifuge at high speed (2500 rpm) for 20 min.
3. Decant the supernatant and re-suspend the sediment in a remaining drop of fluid. Pool the sediment, if necessary. The sediment is now ready for preparation of the smear.

Watery specimen

Watery specimens, such as urine and gastric fluids, are low in protein and require an additional adhesive agent, such as Meyer's albumin or pooled human serum or plasma. An ideal adhesive agent will allow the fixative and stain to pass through while not retaining the stain.

Procedure Transfer the specimen into centrifuge tubes as described in the previous procedure under 'Preparation of specimen'. Then add pooled human serum or plasma into the tubes. The serum or plasma will form a separate layer at the bottom of the centrifuge tube (serum is heavier than most body secretions). The volume of the serum (adhesive agent) should be greater than the expected volume of the sediment. During centrifugation the collecting sediment is coated with a film of the adhesive agent.

Alternative method: Add a drop of the adhesive agent (pooled serum or plasma or Meyer's albumin) on a clean slide. Put the specimen (with little or no protein) on the adhesive and then prepare the smear.

Preparation of Smear

The technical **quality of the smear** for cytological investigation greatly determines **accurate evaluation and diagnosis**. The skill of making good smears comes through experience. A good smear is thin, spread evenly and free from lumps. An adhesive agent is either added to the specimen before centrifugation or spread over the surface of the slide as described above. The addition of an adhesive agent prevents the cells from 'floating away' during processing.

Procedure
1. Transfer the fixed specimen (or sediment) onto a pre-labelled, clean microscope slide with a wire loop or an applicator stick. If necessary, prepare the slide with a coating of albumin.
2. Depending on the type of specimen, prepare the smear by one of the following ways:
   Streaking: Cover about 2/3 of the area of the slide. Try to keep the spreading uniform and do this fast enough so as not to allow the specimen to dry; it also helps in uniform spreading. Keep the spreading medium neither too thick nor too thin. The streaking method is used for the following types of specimens: mucoid secretions (e.g. vaginal secretion), sputum and gastric contents. The smears must be placed immediately into the fixative before any drying occurs.
   Spreading: Transfer the selected portion of the specimen to a clean glass slide. Excess material is removed with an applicator stick by 'sawing' out at the sharp glass edge. Spread a mucoid secretion over the slide using the teasing process. The film should be moderately thick. This method maintains the cellular interrelationship which is sometimes disturbed by the streaking technique. This procedure is recommended for sputum specimens and bronchial aspirates. (See Chapters 20 and 26 in Vol. II for further details.)

Pull-apart: This method is recommended for amucoid secretions such as urinary sediment, vaginal pool, breast secretions, serous fluids and others. It creates the most desirable smear for cytological examination since the cells are in one layer. Place a drop of the secretion in the middle of a clean slide. Place another clean slide over the drop of secretion but keep holding the edges of both the slides. The material will disperse evenly over the surfaces of the two slides. Slight movement of the two slides in opposite directions may be necessary to initiate flow of the material. The two slides are then pulled apart with a single uninterrupted motion and placed immediately in the fixative solution. The method is similar to the preparation of blood smear for differential count (Chapter 10 in Vol. I).

Fixation

In order to **prevent distortion** of cells as the smear dries up, the specimen must be immediately fixed while the smear is moist. In the following pages a number of fixatives will be discussed but the use of ether–alcohol (1:1) is recommended for most specimens.

Keep the fixative in a bottle or Coplin jar. Place each slide carefully in the fixative with a single uninterrupted motion to prevent rippling of the smeared material. Avoid the contact of the slide on the side of the container and make sure that the slide does not hit the bottom of the container hard. This may lead to the loss of valuable material by dislodging it. The level of the fixative should be above the level of the smear. Keep the smear in the fixative for at least 1 hour. Amucoid specimens (e.g. urinary sediment) need to be submerged in the fixative for only 30 minutes. The following points must be kept in mind while fixing the smear:

- Label the slide before making the smear.
- Open the bottle with fixative before making the smear.
- Fix the smear while it is moist.
- Use an appropriate holder (e.g. iron or stainless steel paper clips; do not use copper or brass clips) to hold the slide while they are transferred from one jar to the other.
- Give adequate time required for fixation. Prolonged fixation does not affect the smear.
- Fixed slides can be set aside for staining or can be left in the fixative until ready for staining.

Faulty fixation is perhaps the most frequent cause of unsatisfactory smears submitted for cytological examination. If staining is not done immediately the slides may be left in the fixative solution. Make sure the level of the fixative is above the level of the smear.

Commonly used fixatives

Ether–Alcohol This fixative is specially used with the Papanicolaou staining method but can be used for fixation of all types of cytological smears. It is easy to prepare and can be filtered and re-used. Extreme care must be taken, however, while handling this highly flammable fluid. In addition, the purchasing of ethyl alcohol without a tax-free permit becomes highly expensive for the laboratory. Ethyl alcohol may be substituted for methyl or isopropyl alcohol. Some laboratories use 95% ethyl alcohol or its substitutes (methyl or isopropyl alcohol) as fixatives without using ether. This makes the fluid less of a fire hazard. The omission of ether does not seem to alter the quality and effectiveness of fixation.

Absolute ethyl alcohol	50 mL
Ether	50 mL

Always use a covered jar with a tight stopper. Ether is highly volatile. After fixing the smear (30 minutes or longer), rinse in alcohol, followed by distilled water ('taking the smear to water') and proceed to stain by the selected procedure.

Schaudinn's Fluid This is a rapidly penetrating fixative used in diagnostic exfoliative cytology. It preserves smears which are to be stained by haematoxylin and eosin.

Mercuric chloride (saturated aqueous solution)	66 mL
Absolute alcohol	33 mL
Glacial acetic acid	1 mL

Fix the smears for 2 minutes or more. Wash in distilled water. Remove the mercuric chloride pigment (appears as black clumps) by adding a few drops of a saturated solution of alcohol–iodine. Rinse in water and proceed to stain by the selected procedure.

Carnoy's Fluid   This fixative is commonly used for urgent biopsies, but is also recommended for exfoliative cytology. Carnoy's fluid permits good nuclear staining. The fixation is done for 30 minutes to 3 hours. The solution is more expensive than ether–alcohol or 95% alcohol solution, and cannot be re-used effectively. The fixative is of particular value in fixing small pieces of tissue and is routinely used when rapid fixation and staining are required in the case of an urgent biopsy. The absolute alcohol helps in dehydration. Following fixation, the tissue is directly transferred to absolute alcohol. Many laboratories avoid using Carnoy's fluid for cytological work as the fixative tends to cause shrinkage and haemolysis of erythrocytes.

Absolute alcohol	60 mL
Chloroform	30 mL
Glacial acetic acid	10 mL

Fixation and mailing of smears

Often, the histology laboratory is not in close proximity to the physician's office. In such cases, the smear is fixed by ether–alcohol, air-dried after fixation, and mailed between two pieces of cardboard without further processing. Staining of fixed smears should be done upon arrival as early as possible.

If polyethylene glycol is available, fix the smear while it is still wet an in alcohol–ether–polyethylene glycol solution. This acts as a fixative as well as a protecting agent due to its waxy coating. Polyethylene glycol is water soluble and does not need to be removed prior to staining by the Papanicolaou method. This fixative is commercially available.

Ethyl alcohol	50 mL
Ether	50 mL
Polyethylene glycol	5 g

Note: Soften the polyethylene glycol at 56°C in an embedding oven before adding it to the ether–alcohol mixture. A clear stable solution is obtained after standing for several hours. Agitation expedites the process.

Cytological Stains and Staining Techniques

After fixing the smear, staining can be routinely done with haematoxylin and eosin, but staining with Papanicolaou stain is preferred.

Papanicolaou staining

The compound staining procedure developed by George Papanicolaou in 1942 has been the staining method of choice for the past eight decades. This method is highly reproducible and the stains are commercially available (Span Diagnostics, Surat, India). It is used for the demonstration of cellular components in smears of exfoliated cells.

Reagents

- Harris' alum haematoxylin (see Chapter 37 in this Volume for preparation).
- Acid alcohol (0.5%)

Concentrated HCl (sp. gr.1.19)	1 mL
Ethyl alcohol (70%)	200 mL

- Hydrochloric acid solution (0.5% and 0.25%): Same as above but use distilled water instead of alcohol. Diluting 0.5% HC1 with an equal volume of distilled water will yield 0.25% HCl.
- Orange G6 (OG6) and EA-36 or 50 (eosin-azure): These stains are commercially available (Ortho-Ethnor, Bombay, India; Span Diagnostics, Surat, India). They are ready for use following filtration and cannot be prepared in the laboratory.

Procedure

1. Fix the smear in equal parts of 95% alcohol and ether.
2. Hydrate the smear in decreasing concentrations of alcohol ('taking to water'): 80%–70%–50% (six dips in each).
3. Rinse gently in distilled water (rough handling may wash off the specimen from the slide).
4. Stain in diluted Harris' haematoxylin (without acetic acid, diluted with an equal amount of distilled water) for 6 minutes or for 2–3 minutes if full strength haematoxylin.
5. Gently rinse in distilled water.
6. Dip in 0.25% HC1 six times or in 0.5% HCl three times.
7. Place in running tap water for 5 minutes (run the water gently; be careful that cells do not wash off). This will thoroughly wash off the acid and stain the nuclei blue.
8. Check the slides under the microscope to see if the nuclei are adequately stained. If overstained, decolorize again in acid-alcohol. If understained (pale), return to haematoxylin stain. Continue the process until the nuclei are distinct, and the cytoplasm of the cells is clear and light blue in colour.
9. Dehydrate the slides by running through: Distilled water: 50%–70%–80%–95% alcohols (six dips in each).
10. Stain in OG 6 for 2 minutes.
11. Rinse in 95% alcohol for three changes (in three separate containers), six dips in each.
12. Stain in EA-36 or EA-50 for 2 minutes.
13. Rinse in 95% alcohol (three separate changes).
14. Dehydrate by passing through absolute alcohol (two changes).
15. Clear by rinsing in a mixture of absolute alcohol and xylene (six dips) followed by three changes in xylene (six dips).
16. *Note*: If the specimen is satisfactorily dehydrated and cleared, xylene will run off the slides in a smooth, clean sheet. If the clearing is not satisfactory, rivulets of liquid will show on the surface of the slide.
17. Mount in Permount or any satisfactory neutral medium.

Result

- *Nuclei*: blue with clear sharp details.
- *Cytoplasm*: varying shades of pink, blue, yellow, green-grey. If the contrast is unsatisfactory, decolorize in acid alcohol, wash thoroughly in tap water and repeat the staining procedure, increasing or decreasing the staining time as deemed appropriate.

Haematoxylin–eosin technique

H&E staining of smears follows the same broad pattern of staining as paraffin sections. The principle difference is that smears take up dyes more readily, as discussed earlier, thus staining times are shortened. There is no need to take smears through xylene before staining. This procedure uses Harris's haematoxylin, which provides improved results for general smear staining including imprint preparations. It is important the haematoxylin stain be filtered before use.

Reagents

- *Harris' haematoxylin*: As described earlier (Chapter 37 in this volume).
- *Acid–alcohol solution:* 1% hydrochloric acid in 70% alcohol.

Concentrated hydrochloric acid	1 mL
70% alcohol	99 mL

- *Sodium bicarbonate solution (2%, w/v, aqueous)*
- *Eosin–water solution (0.5%, w/v, aqueous)*

Procedure

1. Alcohol-fixed smears are washed thoroughly in water.
2. Stain with haematoxylin for 1 min.
3. Wash in water and differentiate in acid–alcohol until the nuclei are sharply stained and the background is relatively unstained. The length of this step depends on the type of material being stained, the fixative used, and more importantly, the avidity of the particular haematoxylin solution. An average differentiation time is from 2 to 6 seconds.
4. Wash in water, followed by the bicarbonate solution for 10–20 seconds.
5. Wash well in water.
6. Stain with eosin for 10–20 seconds.
7. Wash in water, dehydrate, clear and mount as desired.

Grunwald–Giemsa staining

Some laboratories prefer Romanowsky-type stains for examination of fine needle aspiration and serous fluid smears. Nuclear detail, the nucleoli in particular, is well-delineated but experience is still needed for accurate cell determination. With serous fluids, adenocarcinoma cells are distinguishable, especially if any intracytoplasmic vacuolation is present. For best results, smears should always be air dried, followed by fixation in methanol for 5–10 minutes.

Reagents

- *May-Grunwald solution*

    Stock solution

    Grind 0.3 g of the powdered May–Grunwald dye in a little amount of methanol. Decant, add more methanol and continue grinding until the dye is in solution and make up to a final volume of 100 mL. Filter.

    Working solution

    Dilute 20 parts of May–Grunwald solution with 30 parts of pH 6.8 phosphate buffer (see appendix).

- *Giemsa solution*

    Stock solution

Giemsa powder	1 g
Glycerine	66 mL
Absolute methyl alcohol	66 mL

    Mix Giemsa powder and glycerine and place in a 60 °C oven for 30 min to 2 h. Finally add 66 mL of absolute methyl alcohol.

    Working solution

Stock Giemsa solution	50 drops
Distilled water	50 mL

    Prepare solution at the time of use. Do not reuse.

Procedure

1. Stain fixed smears in the dilute May-Grunwald solution for 10 min.
2. Rinse in pH 6.8 buffer.
3. Stain in the diluted Giemsa solution for 30 min.
4. Wash and differentiate in pH 6.8 buffer for 5–20 min until the desired colour balance is achieved.
5. Allow smears to dry and mount in a DPX-type mount.

Results

Nuclei—purple
Cell cytoplasm—blue to mauve
Red blood cells—pink

Cresyl violet staining

Cresyl violet staining in exfoliative gynaecologic cytology is followed in many laboratories because of its simplicity and rapidity in addition to the clarity of morphologic cellular details.

Reagents

- Cresyl violet
- Acetic acid (1%)

Procedure

1. Prepare the smear and fix in an ether–alcohol fixative. Allow the ether–alcohol fixed slides to dry in air. The dry slides may be stored for an extended period until stained.
2. Hydrate the smear by dipping through 70% alcohol, followed by 50% alcohol, and then distilled water.
3. Immerse in 1% acetic acid for 30 sec, agitating gently.
4. Rinse in distilled water (two separate changes).
5. Stain in freshly filtered cresyl violet staining solution for 3 min, agitating gently during the first 15–30 seconds.
6. Drain and dehydrate by rinsing in acetone (two brief changes—10 and 5 seconds, respectively).
7. Clear in xylol, 5 min each.
8. Mount in balsam or Permount.

Other staining procedures

Several other staining procedures, described in staining tissue sections, are also followed in exfoliative cytological investigations. These include periodic acid-Schiff (PAS), silver stain method and Feulgen reaction.

IDENTIFYING CHARACTERISTICS OF BENIGN AND MALIGNANT CELLS

Although the histotechnician is not responsible for evaluating the stained smears, he should be able to differentiate between normal and abnormal cells. This knowledge enables evaluation of the specimen preparation for microscopic examination and if not satisfactory, the process can be repeated. Additionally, experienced technician can participate in the pre-screening of the slides and draw the attention of the cytopathologist to abnormal slides. It should be kept in mind that the limited training received by the technician, restricts his ability to confidently identify the types of malignant cells. The evaluation of the cytopathologist is essential.

Normal Non-malignant Cells

Epithelial cells line skin epidermis and the surface layer of mucous and serous membranes. The presence of various types of epithelial cells in the specimens submitted for exfoliative cytology is considered normal. The epithelial cells may or may not be nucleated, depending on the stage of development. In some normal specimens, reticuloendothelial cells and macrophages may also be present.

Epithelial malignant tumours (carcinomas) exhibit changes in the cellular structure of the exfoliated cells, including abnormalities in nuclear structure (increased diameter with dense chromatin) and increased nucleus. Cytoplasm ratio is one of the most important criteria of abnormal malignant cells. This is comparable to the presence of blast cells in circulating blood in patients with leukaemia. Another criterion that may identify the presence of malignant cells is their grouping. Epithelial cells often stay in groups, closely attached to each other. This adhesiveness decreases in malignant tumour cells, appearing as single cells or loosely attached groups of cells.

Review Questions

1. Discuss the clinical significance of cytological investigation.
2. What are the most commonly submitted specimens for the study of exfoliative cytology?
3. How are the specimens prepared for microscopic examination?
4. Which is the most commonly used fixative for cytological studies?
5. What is PAP smear? Describe the technique.
6. List some of the identifying characteristics of malignant cells.
7. Which is the most commonly used fixative for cytological specimens?
8. What is the difference between Schaudinn's fluid and Carnoy's fluid? Discuss the advantages of each of these fixatives.
9. How are watery specimens concentrated prior to their microscopic observations?
10. How are cytological specimens mailed to the reference laboratory?

Section IX

Section IX
Miscellaneous Information

Medical Terminology, Glossary of Technical Terms and Appendices

Rohini Chakravarthy and Kanai L. Mukherjee

PREFIXES COMMONLY USED IN MEDICAL TERMINOLOGY

Prefix is an affix attached to the beginning of a word.
Example: a or an means absent or deficient and when applied to the word anaemia, the latter means reduction of circulating red blood cells. See glossary for the use of prefixes.

Prefix	Meaning	Prefix	Meaning
a, an	absent, deficient	iso	equal
ab	away from	macr(o)	large
aniso	unequal	mal	bad, abnormal
ante	before	mega	huge, great
anti(i)	against	meta	after, next
auto	self	micro	small
baso	blue	necro	dead
bi	two	neo	new
co, com, con	with, together	neutro	neutral
contra	against	olig	few
di	two	pan	all
dipl(o)	double	peri	around
dis	apart, away from	phago	to eat
dys	bad, difficult, painful	poly	many
		post	after
e, ecto, ex	out from	pre, pro	before
end (o)	inside, within	pseudo	false
enter(o)	intestine	py(o)	pus
epi	upon, after	quad(r)	four
hyper	above, excessive	sub	under
hypo	under, deficient	super, supra	above
inter	among	tetra	four
intra	within	trans	through

SUFFIXES COMMONLY USED IN MEDICAL TERMINOLOGY

Suffix is an "affix" attached to the end of a word.
Example: algia, means pain and when applied to the word neuralgia, the latter means severe sharp pain along the course of a nerve.

Suffix	Meaning	Application (example)
aemia	in the or of the blood	bilirubinaemia
algia	Pain	neuralgia
blast	primitive, germ	erythroblast
centesis	puncture, aspiration	amniocentesis
cide	death, killer	bacteriocide
ectomy	excision, cut out	gastrectomy
ferent	carry	afferent
genie	origin, producing	pyogenic
itis	inflammation	pharyngitis
lysis	free, breaking down	haemolysis
oma	Tumour	hepatoma
opathy	disease	adenopathy
osis	state or increase	leukocytosis
otomy	cut into	phlebotomy
paenia	lack of	leukopaenia
troph(y)	nourishment	hypertrophy

GLOSSARY OF TECHNICAL TERMS

A

ABO blood group: The basic blood group system in humans, which is determined by the antigenic characters of red cells. The cells agglutinate when mixed with corresponding antibody.
Abscess: A localized collection of pus in a cavity produced by the breakdown of tissues.
Absorbance: Applied in photometry; it expresses the amount of light absorbed by a solution; also called optical density (O.D.); it is related to Beer's Law (an optical phenomenon).
Absorption: Applied in the blood bank; it implies the removal of specific antibodies present in the serum with their specific antigen present on red cells.
ACD: The abbreviated form of acid-citrate-dextrose, an anticoagulant used in the blood bank.
Accuracy: A measure of how close a determined value is to the true value.
Acetone: An organic metabolite coming from Incomplete degradation of fat; found in the blood and urine in diabetic patients; bears a characteristic fruity smell; one of the components of ketone bodies.
Acquired immunodeficiency syndrome (AIDS): A form of severe immunodeficiency caused by infection with the human immunodeficiency virus (HIV).
Acid: A sour substance like lemon juice (citric acid); it neutralizes bases (alkali), turns litmus paper red; carries hydrogen ions (H) and the pH is below 7.0. Common laboratory acids are hydrochloric acid, sulphuric acid and nitric acid. These are highly corrosive.

Acid fast: Not decolorised easily by acids after staining. It pertains to acid fast bacteria like *Mycobacterium* spp. that retain the red dye after acid-alcohol treatment. Other bacteria lose the colour and picks up the blue colour of the counterstain (methylene blue).
Acidophilic: Staining readily with acid dyes, for example, methylene blue.
Acidosis: When the pH of the blood tends to fall below pH 7.4; related to respiratory problem (respiratory acidosis), or metabolic or kidney disorders (metabolic acidosis).
Acute: Having severe symptoms and a short course.
Acute phase proteins: Proteins that increase rapidly in serum during acute infection, inflammation, or following tissue injury.
Adhesion: The act of two parts of surfaces sticking together.
Adsorption: It is a loose adherence on the surface as distinct from absorption which penetrates deeper.
Aerobe: A micro-organism that lives and grows in the presence of free oxygen.
Aerobic: Requiring oxygen.
Aerosol: A colloidal system in which solid or liquid particles are suspended in a gas, especially a suspension of a drug or other substances to be dispensed in a fine spray or mist.
Agar: A gelatinous colloidal extraction of a sea alga, used especially in culture media for growing micro-organisms.
Agglutination: The clumping or aggregation of particulate antigens due to reaction with a specific antibody.
Agglutination inhibition: Interference with, or prevention of, agglutination.
Agglutinin: An antibody in serum that brings about agglutination of cells (red cells or bacteria). Example; anti-A and anti-B
Agglutinogen: An antigen which will react with a specific antiserum and will show agglutination, for example, A and B antigens.
Aggregate: The total substances making up a mass; a cluster or clump of particle.
Aggregation: The collecting of separate objects into one mass.
Alanine aminotransferase (ALT): An enzyme present in high concentration in liver tissue and that is measured to assess liver function; also called SGPT.
Albumin: A water soluble protein found in blood plasma and serum.
Alimentary tract: The digestive tube from the mouth to the anus.
Alkali: A substance with caustic characters; when in solution it has OH ions; pH more than 7.0; reacts with acid and forms salt; also called base, for example, sodium hydroxide.
Alkaline phosphatase (ALP or AP): An enzyme widely distributed in the body, especially in the liver and bone.
Alkalosis: When the pH of blood tends to rise above 7.4 due to respiratory or metabolic (or kidney) problems.
Alkaptonuria: Presence of alkaptone bodies (homogentisic acid) in urine, which causes the urine to turn dark on standing or with addition of alkali.
Allele: One of two or more different genes containing specific inheritable characteristics tfeafe occupy corresponding positions (loci) on paired chromosomes. For example the genes for blood types A, B and 0 are at the same position on alleles.
Allergy: A condition resulting from an exaggerated immune response; hypersensitivity.
Amoeba: A minute unicellular protozoon, for example, *Entamoeba histolytica* causes amoebic dysentery.
Amorphous: Without visible differentiation of structure.
Amperometry: The technology that uses electrodes and electrode potential to measure electron generation.
Ampoule: Small glass container capable of being sealed to preserve the contents in a sterile condition.
Amyloid disease: A pathologic condition in which liver spleen and kidney tissue is replaced by an amorphous (without shape) wax-like material.

Amylopsin: enzyme of pancreas which hydrolyses complex carbohydrates into soluble sugars.
Anaemia: It is a pathological condition caused by reduction in circulating red cells.
Anaerobe: An organism that lives and grows in the absence of molecular oxygen.
Anaerobic: Growing in the absence of oxygen.
Analyte: A chemical substance that is the subject of chemical analysis.
Analytical grade reagents: Pure chemicals of known composition.
Anaemia: A condition in which the red blood cell count or haemoglobin level is below normal; a condition resulting in decreased oxygen-carrying capacity of the blood.
Anamnestic response: Rapid increase in blood immunoglobulins following a second exposure to an antigen; booster response or secondary response.
Anhydride: A form of a substance where the water molecule is chemically removed.
Anhydrous: The chemical form of a salt without water molecule. **Example:** copper sulphate–anhydrous form, $CuSO_4$ and hydrated form, $CUSO_4.7H_2O$.
Anion: Negatively charged ion attracted to the anode during electrolysis.
Anisocytosis: Marked variation in the sizes of erythrocytes when observed on a peripheral blood smear.
Anopheles: The genus of mosquito that is the definitive host for the human malaria parasite (genus *Plasmodium*) and is capable of transmitting the organism to humans.
Anterior: Situated in the frontal part.
Antibiotic: A chemical substance produced by a micro-organism which has the capacity to inhibit the growth of or to kill other micro-organisms. The general term 'antimicrobial substance' may not come from another organism.
Antibiotic sensitivity: Refers to the sensitivity of a micro-organism towards an antimicrobial agent. The test is done in the bacteriology laboratory.
Antibiotic susceptibility testing: Determining the susceptibility of bacteria to specific antibiotics.
Antibody: Serum protein that is induced by, and reacts specifically with, a foreign substance (antigen); immunolglobulin.
Antibodies: Proteins that react with the specific antigens that stimulated their production; present in the plasma; produced by lymphocytes and plasma cells.
Anticoagulant: A chemical that prevents blood coagulation.
Antigens: A foreign substance that induces an immune response by causing production of antibodies and/or sensitized lymphocytes that react specifically with that substance; immunogen.
Antiseptic: A chemical used on living tissues to control the growth of infectious agents.
Antiserum: Serum that contains antibodies.
Antistreptolysin-O test (ASO): Antibody that opposes the action of strepto-lysin, a haemolysin produced by streptococci. The ASO test is a serological test done in the diagnosis of streptococcal infection.
Antitoxin: A substance that will neutralize toxins.
Anuria: Absence of urine production.
Apheresis: The process of removing a specific component, such as platelets, from donor blood and returning the blood to donor circulation.
Aplastic: When the marrow stops making blood cells it is said to be aplastic.
Aqueous: Watery, especially with reference to solutions having water as solvent.
Arteriosclerosis: A term applied to a number of pathological conditions in which there is thickening, hardening and loss of elasticity of the walls of arteries. *Atherosclerosis* is a form of arteriosclerosis which is often attributed to hypertension, increased blood lipid levels (especially cholesterol and triglycerides), physical inactivity and other risk factors.
Artery: A blood vessel that carries oxygenated blood from the heart to the tissues.

Artefact: Anything artificially produced; in microscopy, structures and features produced by the technique and not occurring naturally (optical effect) (also spelt as artifact).
Arthritis: Inflammation of the joints.
Ascitic fluid: Serous fluid accumulated in the abdominal cavity.
Asepsis: Freedom from infection.
Aseptic: Without infection.
Aseptic technique: Work practices used to prevent contamination when working with micro-organisms.
Aspiration: Act of inhaling. Also means removal of fluids or gases from a cavity by suction.
Assimilation: The absorption and utilization of digested food stuffs by the tissue cells.
Atherosclerosis: A form of *arterioscloreosis* in which lipids, calcium, cholesterol and other substances deposit on the inner walls of the arteries.
Atrial: Of or relating to a body cavity.
Atypical: Not conformable to the type; in microbiology the term is specifically applied towards strains of unusual type.
Aüer body: A cellular inclusion body found in granulocytes (neutrophils) as needle-like red-coloured objects in case of acute granulocytic leukaemia.
Auto-agglutinin: An antibody present in serum capable of causing agglutination of its own red cells.
Autoantibody: An antibody directed against the self (one's own tissues).
Autoclave: Equipment that sterilize materials by steam under pressure.
Autoimmunity: Immunologic reaction of the body towards its own protein (auto-antigen). Systemic erythematosus is an *autoimmune disease*.
Autotrophic: Self-nourishing; usually pertains to green plants.
Average: The sum of a set of values divided by the number of values; the mean.
Azurophilic: Staining readily with azure dye (bluish).

B

B lymphocytes (B cells): The type of lymphocyte primarily responsible for the humoral immune response.
Bacillary dysentery: Dysentery caused by bacterial infection; *Shigella* is most often the infectious agent causing shigellosis. It is a bad form of diarrhoea with blood in stool.
Bacillus: A rod-shaped micro-organism; (plural: bacilli).
Bacteria: Minute, unicellular organism; (singular: bacterium).
Bacterial meningitis: Inflammation of membranes of spinal cord or brain (meninges) due to bacterial infection.
Band cell: Non-segmented neutrophils; immature neutrophils.
Basopaenia: Decrease in number of basophil cells as seen on differential count.
Basophil: Any structure, cell or histologic element staining readily with basic dyes. In haematology, basophils take the dark colour of methylene blue, a basic dye.
Basophilia: Abnormal increase in the number of basophils.
Basophilic stippling: Dark purple-coloured inclusion bodies (Wright's stain) found in erythrocytes, often associated with lead poisoning and other blood-related disorders. They are the remnants of RNA and other nuclear materials remaining inside the red cells after the nucleus is lost from the cell.
Beer's law: A mathematical relationship that demonstrates the linear relationship of concentration to absorbance and that forms the basis for spectrophotometric analysis.
Bence-Jones protein: A protein found in the urine of patients with multiple myeloma. When urine samples are heated to 50°–60°C a precipitate forms. This disappears when the urine is boiled and re-appears when the urine cools.

Benign: Not malignant or progressive, not recurring, favourable for recovery.
Bile: A thick yellow-green fluid made by the liver, the concentrated in the gall bladder, excreted into the intestine to assist in the emulsification of fats.
Bile obstruction: That which is due to an impediment to the flow of bile from the liver to the intestine (duodenum).
Bile pigment: The same as bilirubin.
Bilirubin: A non-haeme pigment derived from haemoglobin breakdown whose accumulation in the body leads to jaundice. It is formed in the liver.
Biopsy: A diagnostic microscopic examination of tissue removed from the living body.
Biohazard: Risk or hazard to health or the environment from biological agents.
Blank: Commonly applied in photometry or any other analytic procedure, which represents the zero value of the analyte. In colorimetry a cuvette is filled with water ("water blank") or the reagent ("reagent blank") and this blank is used for the "zero setting" (absorbance = 0, transmittance = 100%) of the colorimeter before reading the absorbance of the unknown or test specimen.
Blast cell: An immature blood cell normally found only in the bone marrow.
Blind sample: An assayed sample that is sent as an unknown to laboratories participating in proficiency testing programs.
Blood bank: Clinical laboratory department where blood components are tested and stored until needed for transfusion; immunohaematology department; transfusion services; also the refrigerated unit used for storing blood components.
Bloodbourne pathogen (BBP): Pathogens that can be present in human blood (and blood-contaminated body fluids) and that cause disease.
Blood coagulation: A sequential process by which fibrinogen is converted to fibrin through the mediation of various coagulation factors. The result is the formation of a "blood clot".
Blood group antibody: A serum protein (immunoglobulin); that reacts specifically with a blood group antigen.
Blood group antigen: A substance or structure on the red blood cell membrane that stimulates antibody formation and reacts with that antibody.
Blood grouping: Finding a person's blood group by the appropriate procedure followed in the blood bank.
Blood groups: The different blood groups (A, B, AB and 0) found in humans and designated by the antigenic character of the red cells. The blood group is determined by reacting (haemagglutination) with the corresponding antibody.
Blood incompatibility: Blood not compatible between the donor and the recipient. This is tested by the procedure of cross-matching.
Blood transfusion: A procedure by which blood is taken from a healthy person or donor and given to the patient or recipient.
Blood urea nitrogen (BUN): An expression of the urea concentration in blood; its rise in blood reflects kidney failure.
Bovine albumin: One of the plasma proteins of the cow; used in cross-matching
Bowman's capsule: A component of a nephron present in the kidney; it functions as a filter in the formation of urine.
Bright field microscope: Common light microscope with lighted background of magnified darker objects.
Budding: Asexual reproduction by division into two parts, the larger parent body and smaller bud, for example, in yeast.
Buffer solution: A solution that resists change of pH.
Buffy coat: the layer of white cells and platelets between the red cells and the supernatant plasma of centrifuged blood.
BUN: Blood urea nitrogen; a test measuring urea in blood.

C

Cabot's ring: A cytoplasmic inclusion body found in erythrocytes in case of various anaemias; it has a ring-like appearance.
Calculus: An abnormal concretion of mineral salts formed within the body, for example renal calculus.
Calibration: The process of checking, standardization, or adjusting a method or instrument so that it yields accurate results.
Calorie: Amount of heat required to raise the temperature of 1 g of water to 1°C.
Capillaries: Very small blood vessels joining arteries.
Capillary puncture: Puncture of the capillary to obtain blood, for example, skin puncture.
Capillary tube: A slender glass or plastic tube used for laboratory procedures.
Carcinogen: A substance with the potential to produce cancer in human or animals.
Cardiopulmonary circulation: The system of blood vessels that circulates blood from the heart to the lungs and back to the heart.
Capsule: A sheath of continuous enclosure around an organ or structure; also called capsula (little box).
Cardiac: Related to the heart.
Cardiolipin: A lipid-like substance obtained from fresh beef heart which has a non-specific antigenic character and reacts with "reagin" (also called, Wassermann antibody). Cardiolipln is used as an antigen in non-treponemal serodiagnosis of syphilis.
Carrier: A person who harbours an organism, has no symptoms or signs of disease, but is capable of spreading the organism to others.
Cast: A gelled protein formed in renal tubules; its presence in a urine sample is related to renal failure.
Catalyst: A substance that alters the rate of chemical reaction without apparently participating in it; it is needed in small quantity
Catheterization: Use or passage of a catheter (a tube used to withdraw fluids). Catheterization of urinary bladder is a standard technique to draw uncontaminated urine specimen; the catheter is Introduced through the urethra into the bladder.
Cation: Positively charged ion, which is attracted to the cathode in electrolysis.
Caustic: A chemical substance having the ability to burn or destroy tissue
Cell diluting fluid: A solution used to dilute blood for cell counts
Cell-mediated immunity: Immunity provided by T lymphocytes and cytokines
Celsius (C) scale: Temperature scale having the freezing point of water at zero (0°) and the boiling point at 100°
Centi-: A prefix denoting 1/100 part; **Example:** a centimetre is 1/100 of a meter
Centrifuge: An instrument with a rotor that rotates at high speeds, in a closed chamber
Cerebrospinal fluid (CSF): The fluid that is present around the brain and in the spinal cord
Cestode: Belongs to the phylum *Platyhelminthes*, which includes tapeworms; member of Cestoda family
Cholesterol: A monohydric solid alcohol; a widely distributed sterol in animal tissues. It can be synthesized in the liver and is a normal constituent of bile. It is the principal constituent of most gallstones. It is important in metabolism, serving as a precursor of various steroid hormones, for example, sex hormones and adrenal corticoids.
Chromogen: A substance that becomes coloured when it undergoes a chemical change
Chronic: Persisting for a long time, not acute
Chyle: Milky looking fluid of lymph and emulsified fat absorbed into the intestine after the digestion of food
Clean catch: A midstream urine sample collected after the urethral opening and surrounding tissues have been cleansed.

Clot: A semisolidifled mass of coagulum as of blood; blood clots because of the coagulation process

Clue cells: Vaginal epithelial cells covered with tiny, Gram-variable bacteria and seen in vaginal secretions of patients with bacterial vaginosis

Coagulase test: A test to differentiate between *Staphylococcus aureus* and other *Staphylococcus* sp.

Coagulation: Formation of a clot; most often related to blood clotting and formation of fibrin from fibrinogen

Coagulaton factors: A group of plasma proteins (and the mineral calcium) involved in blood clotting

Coarse adjustment: Control that adjusts position of microscope objective and is used to initially bring objects into focus

Cocci (s., coccus): A round-shaped bacterium, look like balls. **Example:** *Staphylococcus* spp., *Streptococcus* spp.

Codominant: In genetics, a gene that is expressed in the heterozygoue state, that is, in the presence of a different allelic gene

Coefficient of variance: A calculated value that compares the relative variability between different sets of data

Coenzyme: An organic enzyme component necessary for the function of the holoenzyme which consists of coenzyme and apoenzyme. **Example:** NAD (nicotinamide adenine dinucleotide)

Coliform bacteria: This group includes *Aerobacter aerogenes* and *Escherichia coli*. Their presence in water, especially *E. coli*, is presumptive evidence of faecal contamination.

Collagen: A protein connective tissue found in skin, bone, ligaments and cartilage

Colony: A defined mass of bacteria, localised, assumed to have grown from a single organism

Colony count: An estimation of the number of organisms in urine by counting the colonies on a urine culture plate

Commensal: An organism that lives with, on, or in another, with out injury to either

Communicable: Able to be transmitted directly or indirectly from one individual to another.

Complement: A thermolabile protein formed in normal blood serum. It participates in the coagulation process and is deliberately added to the system in case of complement fixation tests. Because of its interference in most serological tests (other than complement fixation), it is removed by heating the serum (56°C/20 min) before performing the test.

Confluent growth: Bacterial growth in which colonies overlap each other and cannot be successfully picked out individually for subculture.

Congenital: Existing at the time of birth or born with the defect

Contaminant: Any substance or biologic agent whose presence results in other substances or biologic agents being impure, i.e. foreign organisms developing accidentally in a pure culture.

Convalescent: Stage of disease in which the patient is on the way to recovery.

Counterstain: A stain that follows the main stain in order to colour the cells or tissues differently. **Example:** safranin in Gram stain or methylene blue in acid fast stain.

Counting chamber: A special piece of equipment for counting cells; also called a haemocytometer.

C-reactive protein (CRP): A special protein found in patients with inflammatory disorders that reacts with anti-CRP.

Creatinine: The end product of creatine metabolism, following hydrolysis. It is one of the important non-protein constituents of blood, and a rise in the creatinine concentration of serum indicates renal failure.

Creatinine kinase (CK): An enzyme present in large amounts in the brain tissue and in heart and skeletal muscle and that is measured to aid in diagnosing heart attack

Crenated cell: With a notched or toothed edge; shrivelled up; **Example:** crenated red blood cells as an abnormal morphology

Crisis: A time during the illness when the patient becomes very ill indeed

Critical measurements: Measurements made when the accuracy of a solution's concentration is important; measurement made using glassware manufactured to strict standards
Cross-matching: A way of testing the compatibility of donor's blood with recipient's blood prior to transfusion
Cryoprecipitate: The precipitate that results from the cooling of fresh plasma; it is rich in factor VIII (coagulation factor) and used in the treatment of haemophilia.
Crystals: A naturally produced angular solid of definite form; crystals are found in urine, synovial fluid and in other specimens; may have diagnostic significance.
CSF: See cerebrospinal fluid
Culture: Growth of micro-organisms in a special medium; the process of growing micro-organisms in the laboratory
Culture medium: A substance used as the substrate on which micro-organisms may grow. Those most commonly used are agar-based solid medium and broth (liquid medium).
Cutaneous: Relating to the skin
Cuvette: A small transparent glass container, which holds liquids for photometric measurements
Cyst: The resting or inactive state of a protozoon
Cystitis: Inflammation of the urinary bladder
Cytokine: Any of various non-antibody proteins secreted by cells of the immune system and that help regulate the immune response; lymphokinase
Cytology: The study of cells

D

D-dimer: One of the products formed from the breakdown of fibrin by plasmin
Deci: Prefix used to indicate one-tenth of a unit.
Definitive host: The host in which the sexual phase of the parasite is seen
Deionized water: Water that has had most of it mineral ions removed
Deoxyhaemoglobin: The haemoglobin formed when oxyhaemoglobin releases oxygen to tissues
Dermatology: The medical speciality concerned with the diagnosis and treatment of skin diseases.
Dextrose: A simple sugar of the monosaccharide group, also known as grape sugar or glucose.
Diabetes: Usually refers to **Diabetes mellitus**, a disorder of carbohydrate metabolism, characterized by increased blood sugar, (hyperglycaemia) and glucose discharge in urine (glucosuria). Diabetes mellitus is caused by inadequate production or utilization of insulin. **Diabetes insipidus**, on the other hand, is caused by inadequate secretion of vasopressin or antidiuretic hormone (ADH). The disease is characterized by polyuria and polydipsia.
Diarrhoea: Frequent passage of abnormally watery bowel movements. It is a frequent symptom of gastrointestinal disturbances. Acute diarrhoea is characterized by sudden onset.
Diastase: An enzyme that converts starches into sugars.
Differential count: A determination of the relative numbers of each type of leukocyte on stained blood smear; white blood cell differential count; leukocyte differential count;
Differential media: These are the culture media capable of differentiating bacteria, when grown on them, by their morphological features, for example, McConkey agar, Eosine-methylene blue (EMB) agar.
Differential stain: Like Wright stain can differentiate various blood cells by its colour reaction.
Diluent: A liquid added to a solution to make it less concentrated
Dilution: A solution made less concentrated by adding a diluent; the act of making a dilute solution; the degree to which a solution is made less concentrated
Dilution factor: Reciprocal of the dilution

Diplococcal (singular; diplococcus): Any of various spherical bacteria appearing in pairs. **Example:** *Streptococcus pneumoniae*
Disaccharide: Sugar that yields two monosaccharides after hydrolysis; **Example:** sucrose.
Disinfectant: A chemical used on inanimate objects to kill or inactivate microbes
Disseminated intravascular coagulation (DIC): A bleeding disorder characterized by widespread thrombotic and secondary fibrinolytic reactions
Dissemination: Scattering or distribution
Distilled water: The condensate collected from steam after water has been boiled
Diuretic: A substance which when taken into the body, promotes the secretion of urine
Diurnal: Having a daily cycle
DNA: The nucleic acid that carries genetic information and that is found primarily in the nucleus of all living cells; deoxyribonucleic acid
Döhle body: An inclusion body found in neutrophils in severe infections. Also called *Amato body*
Donor: A person who gives blood or an organ to be used in another body (recipient). A universal donor is the one whose blood is of group 0 and whose blood is therefore usually compatible with most other blood types. In actual practice this compatibility rarely occurs because of the many factors other than the major blood antigens (A, B, AB) which determine blood compatibility.
Drabkin's reagent: A haemoglobin diluting reagent that contains iron, potassium, cyanide and sodium bicarbonate
D^u antigen: An antigen found as weak Rh-positive (Rh-variant) and recognized by reacting with anti-D with heat followed by anti-human globulin reaction (indirect Coombs).
Dysentery: Stomach disorder marked by inflammation of the intestine, with abdominal pain and frequent stools containing blood and mucus.
Dysfunction: Impaired or abnormal function

E

Ectparasite: A parasite that lives on the outer surface of a host
Ectopic pregnancy: Development of foetus outside the uterus, extrauterine pregnancy
EDTA: Ethylenediaminetetraacetic acid; an anticoagulant commonly used in haematology
Eggs (ova): The product of the sexual life cycle; refers to parasite eggs in the clinical laboratory.
EIA: Enzyme immunoassay
Electrolytes: Substances that dissociate into ions when in solution, for example, Na^+, Cl^- ; they conduct electricity through the solution.
Electrolyte solution: A solution that conducts an electrical current
Elephantiasis: A chronic infectious condition characterized by pronounced swelling at distal parts of the body specially the leg, which looks like an elephant foot (causal agent: *Wuchereria bancrofti*).
Elliptocyte: Elongated, cigar-shaped red blood cell
Embolus (pl., emboli): A mass (clot) of blood or foreign matter carried in the circulation
Endemic: Recurring in a specific location or population
Endogenous: Produced within; growing from within
Enrichment medium: A culture medium that encourages the growth of some organisms over others (commensals). **Example:** GN broth favours the growth of *Salmonella* and *Shigella*; faecal specimen is inoculated in the broth for overnight growth (18 h) and then plated on a selective primary plate (e.g. **Salmonella-Shigella** agar) for further isolation

Enzyme: A special protein produced by living cells, which acts as a catalyst, accelerating biochemical reactions.
   Example: Amylase (an enzyme) converts starch into glucose.
Enzyme immunoassay (EIA): An assay that uses an enzyme-labelled antibody as a reactant
Eosinopenia: Fall of eosinophil count, opposite of eoslnophilia.
Eosinophil: A granular leukocyte that takes the eosin stain when the blood smear is stained with the polychromic Romanowsky stain.
Eosinophilia: Abnormal increase in eosinophil count in the blood
Epidemic: Disease affecting many persons at the same time, spreading from person-to-person and occurring in an area where the disease is not prevalent
Epidemiology: The study of the factors that cause disease and determine disease frequency and distribution
Epithelial cells: The surface cells of the body found in many body fluids (urine, peritoneal fluid). Their increased presence may indicate pathologic condition.
Epithelium: The layer of cells forming the epidermis of the skin or the surface layer, inside or outside, of an organ
Erythroblast: A nucleated red cell prior to the mature non-nucleated erythro-cyte; its presence in the blood circulation indicates blood-related disorders.
Erythroblastosis foetalis: Haemolytic anaemia of the foetus due to incompatibility of mother's blood with her offspring. This is also called the haemolytic disease of newborn or HDN.
Erythrocyte: Another name for a red blood cell; contains haemoglobin and functions in the transport of gases (oxygen and carbon dioxide) between the lungs, tissues and cells.
Erythrocyte sedimentation rate (ESR): A haematological test that gives the rate of fall of blood sediment (red cells) due to gravity when a blood column in a tube is left undisturbed.
Erythrocytosis: Abnormal excess of red blood cells in the peripheral blood; some times called polycythemia
Ester: A compound formed from an alcohol and an acid by removal of water. Fat is an ester of glycerol (alcohol) and fatty acids.
Ethics: A system of conduct or behaviour; rules of professional conduct
Euglobins: A globulin that is insoluble in water but soluble in saline solutions
Eye piece: Component of the microscope, ocular
Exchange transfusion: A process of blood transfusion in which the entire blood is exchanged. It is a therapeutic measure to treat haemolytic disease of the newborn.
Exo-: Prefix indicating without or outside of. **Example:** exotoxin is the toxin produced by a micro-organism (e.g. diphtheria, tetanus) and excreted into its surrounding medium.
Expectoration: Clearing of secretions from the respiratory tract by coughing
Exudate: An abnormal fluid formed by a tissue, which accumulates in a cavity, or matter that penetrates through vessel walls into adjoining tissue, or the passing out of pus or serum. In comparison to a transudate, there are more cells, protein and solid material in an exudate.
Exudation: Morbid oozing of fluids, usually the result of inflammatory conditions

F

Facultative anaerobe: Organism that prefers to live as an anaerobe but will adapt to aerobic conditions of growth
Faeces: The waste from the bowel or gut discharged by way of the anus; also called stool, excreta. It is the body waste such as food residue, bacteria, epithelium and mucus.
Fahrenheit (F) scale: Temperature scale having the freezing point of water at 32° and the boiling point at 212°

False positive report: A report, which is sent out positive when it should be negative
Fastidious bacteria: Bacteria that require special nutritional factors to survive
Fat: An organic compound, necessary for the body nutrition; insoluble in water but soluble in organic solvents (ether, alcohol); an ester of glycerol with fatty acids and grouped under lipids
Febrile: Pertaining to a fever (feverish). *Febrile agglutination* is a serological test where agglutination of bacterial cells is seen. *Febrile transfusion reaction* is the reaction seen in a recipient following blood transfusion that results in fever and chill
Femtolitre (fL): A unit of volume; 10^{15} L
Fibrin: An insoluble protein that forms from fibrinogen (present in plasma) because of blood clotting
Fibrin degradation products (FDP): Degradation products formed when plasmin cleaves fibrin or fibrinogen; formerly fibrin split products
Fibrinogen: A plasma protein produced in the liver and converted to fibrin through the action of thrombin
Fibrinolysis: Enzymatic breakdown of a fibrin clot
Field diaphragm: Adjustable aperture attached to microscope base
Field of view: the view through the eyepiece of the microscope or any other optical instrument
Filariae: Nematode worms, which live in the tissues. **Example:** *Wuchereria bancrofti.*
Filariasis: A chronic disease due to one of the filariae species.
Film: A thin layer of blood or other material spread on a slide or coverslip and meant for microscopic observation.
Filtration: The process of filtering or passing of a fluid through a filter (e.g. filter paper) to separate fluids from suspending solids. The fluid is called the filtrate and the solid is called the precipitate or residue.
Fine adjustment: Control that adjusts position of microscope objectives and is used to sharpen focus.
Fix, Fixation, Fixative: To fix a tissue is to kill it and to keep it looking just as it did when it was alive. It is commonly applied in histology. The goal of fixing is to permit accurate and undistorted microscopic - visualization of the tissues. A fixative is a substance that serves tJ fix or preserve pathological specimens. The process is known as fixation.
Flaccid: Soft, flabby, not firm.
Flagellate: A protozoon, which moves with the help of flagella. **Example:** *Trichomonas vaginalis.*
Flagellum (pl., Flagella): Slender, lash-like appendage that serves as organ of locomotion for sperm cells and some protozoa
Flammable: Very easily burnt (also inflammable).
Flocculation: A flaky precipitation.
Fluorescent: Having the property of emitting light of one wavelength when exposed to light of another wavelength
Fluke: A parasitic worm belonging to the class Trematoda, phylum Platyhelminthes. Most flukes have complex life cycles which include asexual forms that live in a snail (mollusc). **Example:** Blood fluke, liver fluke.
Folic acid: A member of the B vitamin complex
Fungi: A class of organisms macroscopic or microscopic, mostly saprophytes, which may be parasitic and possess plant-like characters but lack chlorophyll; filamentous (mould form) or yeast-like; parasitic fungi-mycotic agents
Fluorescence: A property of certain substances to emit light when exposed to certain types of light radiation, usually ultraviolet. It is caused by the absorption of high energy shorter wavelengths of light (below 400 nm) and emits simultaneously longer wavelengths of light (yellowish-green).

Fluorescent antibody (FA): An antibody, which has been stained or marked by a fluorescent dye that glows under ultraviolet light; emitting a yellowish-green colour under fluorescent microscope when ultraviolet light is the illumination source
Formula weight (FW): Weight of the entity represented by a chemical formula; molecular weight
Forward grouping: The use of known antisera (antibodies) to identify unknown antigens on a patient's cells; forward typing; direct grouping

G

Gamma globulin: A kind of plasma globulin that may originate from immunologic reaction or other pathologic conditions (gammaglobinopathies); produced by lymphocytes and plasma cells; several kinds of immunogammaglobulins—IgG, IgM and others
Gamma glutamyl transferase (GGT): An enzyme that is present in liver, kidney, pancreas and prostrate, and that is measured to assess liver function
Gastric: Belonging to the stomach
Gastric juice: The digestive juice of the gastric glands of the stomach
Gauge: A measure of the diameter of a needle
Genes: Segments of DVA that code for specific proteins or enzymes and that are the structural units of heredity
Genotype: The allelic genes that are responsible for a trait; blood group genotypes AA and AO appear as A by the haemagglutination reaction with anti-A; so called phenotype A
Gaussian curve: A graph plotting the distribution of values around the mean; normal frequency curve
Giardiasis: The disease caused by *Giardia lamblia*
Giemsa stain: A polychromatic stain used for staining blood cells and blood parasites
Gland: An organ capable of secretion
Globin: The protein portion of the haemoglobin molecule
Globulins: One of the plasma proteins; the others are albumin and fibrinogen. It is more soluble in saline than in water.
Glomerular filtration rate (GFR): The rate by which the glomerulus is filtering blood in the nephron, the functional unit of kidney. The GFR falls in case of renal failure.
Glomerulonephritis: Inflammation of the glomeruli
Glucose: The important sugar in the body. It is the only source of energy for most body cells and is particularly needed for brain cells and erythrocytes. Glucose is also known as dextrose and grape sugar.
Glucose dehydrogenase: Enzyme that converts glucose to gluconolactone and is used in glucose analytical methods
Glucose oxidase: An enzyme that converts glucose to gluconic acid and that is used in glucose analytical methods
Glycolated haemoglobin (GHb): See Haemoglobin A1c
Glycogen: The storage form of glucose found in high concentration in the liver
Glycogenesis: The process of conversion of glucose to glycogen; the process is insulin dependent.
Glycolysis: Energy production mechanism as a result of metabolic breakdown of glucose
Glucosuria: The presence of sugar in the urine
Gonococcus: Another name for *Neisseria gonorrhoeae*, the causal agent of gonorrhoea
Gonorrhoea: A contagious infection spread by sexual contact and caused by *Neisseria gonorrhoeae*
Gout: A painful condition in which blood uric acid is elevated and urates precipitate in joints
Gravimetric analysis: Analysis based on weight
Gram (g): The basic unit of mass in the metric system
Gram-formula weight: The weight in grams of the entity represented by a chemical formula

Gram negative: Designation for bacteria that lose the crystal violet (purple stain) and retain the safranin (red stain) in the Gram stain procedure
Gram positive: Designation for bacteria that retain the crystal violet (purple stain) in the Gram stain procedure
Gram staining: A procedure for staining of bacteria, which are then classified as gram negative or gram positive
Granulocytes: A special group of leukocytes, which has granulation in the cytoplasm; includes neutrophils, eosinophils and basophils
Granulocytic leukaemia: Leukaemia caused by the increase of granulocytes.
Gut: The entire system that joins the mouth to the anus; stomach and intestines are part of this system

H

Haemacytometry: The technique of counting blood cells in a glass chamber with grids, by means of a microscope.
Haeme-: A prefix meaning pertaining to blood; the iron-containing portion of the haemoglobin molecule
Haemagglutination: Agglutination of red blood cells.
Haematocrit (Hct): Is also called packed cell volume or PCV. It is determined by centrifuging anticoagulated (whole) blood for a specific time and with specified centrifugal force. It is expressed in per cent of packed red cell volume out of the whole blood volume.
Haematology: The study of blood and blood-forming tissues
Haematoma: A clinical condition indicating localized collection of extravascular blood
Haematopoiesis: The formation and development of blood cells.
Haematuria: Presence of blood in urine
Haemoconcentration: Increase in the concentration of cellular elements in the blood
Haemoglobin: The red substance inside red blood cells; a conjugated protein with haeme (iron + porphyrin) and globin; carries oxygen from the lungs to the tissues
Haemoglobin A 1c: Haemoglobin modified by the binding of glucose to the beta globin chains of haemoglobin; also called glycated or glycosylated haemoglobin
Haemoglobinuria: Presence of haemoglobin in urine
Haemolysis: Rupture or destruction of red blood cells resulting in the release of haemoglobin
Haemolytic anaemia: A type of anaemia due to destruction of red blood cells
Haemolytic disease of the newborn (HDN): Occurs in the newborn baby with jaundice, caused by the transfer of immune antibody from the mother to the foetus; also called erythroblastosis foetalis
Haemophilia: A bleeding disorder resulting from a hereditary coagulation factor deficiency or dysfunction
Hemopoiesis: The process of blood cell formation and development; haematopoiesis
Haemosiderin: An insoluble form of tissue storage iron, which can be seen under the microscope following special staining with Prussian blue stain; presence in urine may indicate possible haemolytic reaction within the body; presence in bone marrow may indicate non-utilization of iron in haemoglobin synthesis
Haemostasis: The arrest of bleeding either by vasoconstriction or by coagulation
Haemorrhage: Uncontrolled bleeding
Ham's test: A haematological test that indicates whether the erythrocytes of the patient can stand the acid condition; diagnoses paroxysmal nocturnal haemoglobinuria (PNH)
Heinz bodies: Abnormal red cell inclusion bodies found in haemolytic anaemia and other blood disorders
Helminth: A group of parasitic worms, multicellular; most members have a clearly defined sexual life cycle
HEPA filter: High-efficiency particulate air filter used in hiological safety cabinets
Heparin: A natural anticoagulant, which is basically a mucopolysaccharide, used in exchange transfusion

Hepatic: Pertaining to the liver
Hepatitis: Inflammation of the liver
Hepatitis B virus (HBV): The virus that causes hepatitis B infection and is transmitted by contact with infected blood or other body fluids
Hepatitis C virus (HCV): The virus that causes hepatitis C infection and is transmitted by contact with infected blood or other body fluids
Heterophile antibodies: Antibodies that are increased in infectious mononucleosis
Hexokinase: An enzyme that converts glucose to glucose-6-phosphate and that is used in glucose analytical methods
Histamine: Found in all body tissues, related to vasoconstriction (stoppage of bleeding) and allergic reactions
Histology: The study of the structure of the tissues
Histocompatibility testing: Performacne of assays to determine if donor and recipient tissue are compatible
Histogram: A graph that illustrates the size and frequency of occurrence of articles being studied
HIV: Human immunodeficiency virus, a retrovirus that has been identified as the cause of acquired immunodeficiency syndrome (AIDS)
Homeostasis: The tendency toward steady state or equilibrium of body processes
Homo: Prefix denoting the same; for example, homozygous
Homogentisic acid: An acid in the urine due to incomplete oxidation of tyrosine; presence in urine is abnormal; if found in infant's urine, may lead to mental disorders unless properly treated; also called alkaptone
Hookworm: A small worm that lives in the small gut; a nematode
Hormone: A chemical substance found in the body that has a regulatory function; as an example, insulin is a hormone that regulates carbohydrate metabolism
Host: An organism that harbours or nourishes another organism
Howell-Jolly bodies: Abnormal inclusion bodies found in erythrocytes in case of erythrocyte-related disorders
HPF (high power field): It is the objective of the microscope with 40× magnification; also called high-dry
Human chorionic gonadotrophin (hCG): The hormone of pregnancy, produced by the placenta; also called uterine chorionic gonadotropin, uCG
Human immunodeficiency virus (HIV): The retrovirus that has been identified as the cause of AIDS
Human leukocyte antigen (HLA): Any of several antigens present on leukocytes and other body cells that are important in transplant rejection
Humoral immunity: Immunity present in the body fluid (in circulating blood); provided by B lymphocytes and antibodics; cellular immunity, on the other hand, is limited to the cells only
Hyaline: Glass-like, transparent, pale
Hydrolysis: A biochemical reaction in which water molecules are taken in during the decomposition process; for example, starch hydrolysed to sugar
Hygroscopic: Absorbs moisture from the environment (air); used as a desiccant; for example, Calcium chloride.
Hyper-: Denoting over or above; for example, hyperglycaemia
Hyperglycaemia: Blood glucose levels above normal
Hyperkalaemia: Blood potassium levels above normal
Hyperlipidaemia: Excessive amount of fat in blood
Hypernatraemia: Blood sodium levels above normal
Hypersensitivity: State of reactivity in which the body reacts to a foreign agent more strongly than normal
Hypertonic: Having a greater salt concentration that the cell cytoplasm
Hyphae: Filaments of fungi that give rise to mycelium; as found in mould
Hypo-: Prefix denoting under or below, opposite of hyper-, for example, Hypoglycaemia; hypokalaemia, hypolidiaemia, hyponatraemia
Hypochromic: Staining less intensely than normal, more commonly applied to describe "poor coloured"

(low haemoglobin) erythrocytes; common in iron deficiency anaemia
Hypoglycaemia: Blood sugar levels below normal
Hypothyroidism: Thyroid function deficiency
Hypotonic: Having a smaller salt concentration than the cell cytoplasm
Hypovolaemia: Abnormally decreased volume of circulating blood

I

Icterus index: A scale to indicate the yellow colour of the body fluid (urine, plasma) under conditions of jaundice
Immune antibodies: Antibodies formed after birth with known stimulation; opposite of natural antibody; for example, anti-D (immune) and anti-A (natural)
Immunity: Defence against infection.
Immunization: The process of producing immunity to an antigen
Immunize: To render immune
Immunoassay: A diagnostic laboratory procedure using antigen–antibody reactions
Immunocompetent: Capable of producing a normal immune response
Immunocompromised: Having reduced ability or inability to produce a normal immune response
Immunoglobulins (Ig): Antibodies; serum proteins that are induced by and react specifically with antigens (immunogens)
Immunohaematology: The study of the human blood groups; also called blood banking or transfusion services
Immunologic reaction: Antigen and antibody reaction
Immunology: The branch of medicine encompassing the study of the immune processes and immunity; also known as serology
Immunosuppression: Suprssion of the immune response by physical, chemical, or biological means
Incompatible blood: A term used in the blood bank when the donor's blood does not match with the recipient's blood
Incubation: The interval between exposure to infection and the appearance of the first symptom; in microbiology, it refers to the warm environment of the culture medium
Infection: A pathological condition caused by growth of micro-organisms in the host
Infectious disease: Disease due to infection by pathogenic micro-organism—viruses, bacteria, mycotic agents or intestinal parasites
Infectious mononucleosis: A contagious viral disease caused by Epstein-Barr virus
Inflammation: A non-specific protective response to tissue injury brought about primarily by release of chemicals such as histamine and serotonin and action of phagocytic cells
Inoculation: Process of transferring a population of micro-organisms to a growth medium
Inoculum: The substance used in inoculation, a small amount of micro-organisms taken on an inoculating loop or needle for transfer
Insecticide: A chemical to kill insects
Inspissation: A special process of sterilization with low heat; applied to serum of such substances, which deteriorate by heat
Insulin: A pancreatic hormone; related to glucose metabolism; deficiency leads to diabetes mellitus
Inter-: A prefix denoting between or among.
Example: Intercellular, means between cells.
Intermediate host: The host in which the asexual, immature, or larval form of the parasite is found; for example, in the tapeworm, the pig is the intermediate host
Intoxication: Poisoning

Intra-: Prefix meaning within; intracellular, means within the cell
Intravascular: Within the blood vessels
Intrinsic factor: Related to a factor present within the stomach, the absence of which leads to poor absorption of vitamin B_{12} or folic acid and results in pernicious anaemia
Ion: A charged atom
Ionized calcium: In the body, a mineral that plays an important role in hemostasis
Ion-selective electrode: An electrode manufactured to respond to the concentration of a specific ion
Iris diaphragm: Part of the condenser of a microscope, which opens and closes to alter the light reaching the object
Iso-: Prefix denoting equal; for example isotonic solution, meaning equal osmotic pressure
Isoagglutinin: An antibody, which will agglutinate all red blood cells of the same species
Isoantibody: An antibody produced by one individual that reacts with isoantigens of another individual of the same species; for example, anti-A reacting with antigen A
Isoenzyme: The variants of the same enzyme like lactic dehydrogenase isoenzyme–LD_1, LD_2 and others. These are often separated by electrophoresis and their location on the electrophoretogram is located by reacting with their common substrate (e.g. lactic acid or pyruvic acid for LD).
Isolation technique (as applied to microbiology): Obtaining bacteria in pure culture by subculturing discrete colonies
Isotonic: Having the same salt concentration as the cell cytoplasm.
Isotonic solution: A solution that has the same concentration of dissolved particles as the solution or cell with which it is compared; for example, 0.85% sodium chloride has the same osmotic pressure as red blood cells; also called *"physiological saline"*
In vitro: Within laboratory
In vivo: Within the living body

J

Jaffe reaction: Reaction of creatinine with alkaline sodium picrate.
Jaundice: Yellow discoloration of skin due to an excess of bilirubin in the blood. Hepatic jaundice, due to liver disorder; haemolytic jaundice, due to increased destruction of red cells; obstructive jaundice due to mechanical impediment in the flow of bile from the liver to the duodenum.

K

Kala azar: Highly fatal infectious disease caused by *Leishmania donovani*, a blood parasite
Ketone bodies: Acetone, acetoacetic acid and betahydroxybutyric acid; products of increased fat metabolism; grouped together as ketone bodies or ketones; related to ketosis, metabolic acidosis, increased anion gap and diabetic acidosis
Ketonuria: Presence of ketones in urine
Ketosis: Excessive amount of ketone bodies accumulating in blood
Kilo: Prefix used to indicate one thousand (10^3) units
Kirby-Bauer A method related to antibiotic sensitivity test where the diameter of zone of inhibition is measured in mm

L

Lactate dehydrogenase (LD or LDH): An enzyme widely distributed in the body that is measured to assess liver function
Lancet: A sterile, sharp-pointed blade used to perform a capillary puncture
Larva: Immature stage of an invertebrate
Latent: Dormant; in an inactive or hidden phase
LDL cholesterol: Low density lipoprotein fraction of blood cholesterol; "bad" cholesterol
LE factor: A factor (antibody) that develops in patients with lupus erythematosus (an autoimmune disease); directed towards the protein from connective tissue (due to degeneration) and the nucleus of polymdrphonuclear cells
Lectins: A group of haemagglutinating proteins, with antibody like character that comes from plant seeds; anti-A is an example
Leprosy: A chronic disease due to infection with *Mycobacterium leprae*
Leukaemia: A malignant blood disease in which there are too many white cells in the blood; blood cancer
Leukocyte: White blood cells, ("leuko" means white)
Leukocytosis: A clinical condition where the total white cell count is more than normal
Leukopaenia: A clinical condition where the total white cell count is less than normal
Leukopoiesis: Production of leukocytes, a component of haematopoiesis
Levey-Jennings chart: A quality control chart used to record daily quality control values
Lipaemic: Having a cloudy appearance due to excess lipid content; lipaemic serum after meal
Lipase: Enzyme that splits fat; produced by the pancreas as a digestive enzyme
Lipid: A fat-like substance easily stored in the body as reserve fuel; fat is a lipid
Lipoprotein: A complex lipid in conjugation with protein; the form in which lipids are transported in blood
Litre (L): Basic metric unit of volume equivalent to 1000 mL and weighs 1 kg
Loop: A ring or circle of wire or string; used as an easily sterilizable spoon to transfer small quantities (inoculum) of specimens in bacteriology
Lumbar puncture: Putting a needle into the lower part of the arachnoid space to obtain cerebrospinal fluid (CSF)
Lymph: A transparent, alkaline fluid that comes out of the capillaries and is taken back to the blood through the lymphatic vessels
Lymph nodes: Bean-shaped organs in the groins and in many other parts of the body where lymph is filtered and in which lymphocytes are made
Lymphoblast: The immature nucleated precursor of the mature lymphocyte
Lymphocyte: A kind of white blood cell; lymphocytes and plasma cells produce globulins (including immunoglobulins)
Lymphocytosis: An increase above the normal number of lymphocytes in the blood
Lymphoma: A neoplastic disorder of lymphoid tissue
Lyophilize: Remove water from a frozen solution under vacuum; freeze-dry
Lyse: To burst and break open to dissolve
Lysis: A breaking up or dissolution; for example, haemolysis is the disintegration of red blood cells

M

Macro-: Prefix indicating large; opposite of micro
Macrocytic: Having a larger-than-normal cell size

Macrocytic anaemia: A type of anaemia in which abnormally large red cells are seen in the blood; seen in pernicious anaemia

Macrophages: A large mononuclear phagocytic cell, which is able to "eat" bacteria and other small particles

Malaria: A disease caused by a blood parasite (protozoa) of the *Plasmodium* genus

Malignant: Cancerous; progressive; not benign

Marrow: Short form of bone marrow

Mean: The sum of a set of values divided by the number of values; the average

Mean cell haemoglobin (MCH): Mean corpuscular haemoglobin; average red blood cell haemoglobin; expressed in picograms (pg)

Mean cell haemoglobin concentration (MCHC): Mean corpuscular haemoglobin concentration; comparison of the weight of haemoglobin in a red blood cell to the size of the cell expressed in percentage or g/dL

Mean cell volume (MCV): Mean corpuscular volume; average red blood cell volume; in a blood sample, expressed in femtolitres (fL) or cubic microns (μ^3)

Media (s., Medium): The substrates on which the microbes are cultured in the laboratory

Medullary: Pertaining to bone marrow

Medical Technology: Clinical laboratory science

Medical Laboratory Technician (MLT): Clinical Laboratory technician

Medical Technologist (MT): Clinical laboratory scientist

Megakaryocytes: Large cells in the bone marrow from which platelets are derived

Megaloblast: An abnormal type of immature red cell

Megaloblastic anaemia: An anaemia in which megaloblasts (immature red cells) are seen in circulation; they are bigger in size than the normal red cells; also called macrocytic anaemia; pernicious anaemia

Melaena: A stool, which is black or tarry-coloured because it contains blood that become dark by acidic gastric juice

Melanin: A dark pigment of skin, hair and certain tumours

Meningitis: Inflammation of the meninges, the covering of the brain

Meningococcus: Another name for *Neisseria meningitidis*

Meniscus: The curved upper surface of a liquid in a container

Metre (M): Basic metric unit of length or distance

Metric system: A widely accepted system of measurement that recognizes the litre (volume), gram (weight) and degrees Celsius (temperature)

MIC: Minimum inhibitory concentration

Micro-: Prefix meaning small; for example, microcytic, or small red blood cells; also used as prefix to indicate one-millionth (10^{-6}) of a unit

Microaerophilic: Preferring a low concentration of oxygen

Microcytic anaemia: Anaemia in which small red cells are produced. **Example:** Iron deficiency anaemia.

Microhaematocrit: A haematocrit performed in capillary tubes using a small quantity of blood; packed cell volume (PCV)

Microhaematocrit centrifuge: An instrument that spins capillary tubes at a high speed to rapidly separate cellular components of the blood from the liquid portion of the blood

Micrometer: A ruled device for measuring small objects

Micron (μ): Lengthwise it is the thousandth part of a millimetre or a millionth part of a metre (μm); millimicron or 10^{-9} m (old expression) is now replaced by the term nanometre (nm)

Micro-organism: A small living microscopic organism; for example, Virus, bacteria

Microscope arm: The portion of the microscope that connects the lenses to the base

Microscope base: The portion of the microscope that rests on the table and supports the microscope

Microtomy: The process of cutting thin sections of tissues by means of a microtome in order to facilitate the microscopic observation of their internal structure

Midstream urine: A urine sample collected from the mid-portion of a urine stream

Mili-: Prefix used to indicate one-thousandth (10^{-3}) of a unit

Millilitre: (mL or ml); one thousandth part of a litre or $1\ mL = 10^{-3}\ L$

Minimum inhibitory concentration (MIC): The minimum concentration of an antibiotic required to inhibit the growth of a micro-organism

Molar solution: Solution containing one mole of solute per litre of solution

Mole: Molecular weight in gram; millimole is the molecular weight in milligrams

Molecular weight (MW): Weight of a molecule, when expressed in gram, it is called gram molecular weight or GMW or mole. It is the total of the atomic weights of all elements. **Example:** molecular weight of water or H_2O is $1 + 1 + 16 = 18$

Mono-: Prefix meaning one. **Example:** mononuclear, with one nucleus

Monochromator: A device that isolates a narrow portion of the light spectrum

Monoclonal: Of one kind

Monoclonal antibody: Antibody derived from a single cell line or clone

Monocyte: A kind of white blood cell; largest with a single nucleus; convoluted or horse-shoe-shaped nucleus

Monomorphic: With a single morphological structure as against dimorphic, with two morphological structures. This is more commonly referred to with mycotic agents. **Example:** Dermatophytes or moulds are found only as filamentous form (monomorphic).

Monosaccharide A simple sugar, like glucose, which cannot be further broken down into other sugars.

Mordant: A substance that fixes a dye or stain to an object; for example, iodine in Gram staining

Morphology: The form and structure of cells, tissues and organs

Mucoprotein: A substance present in all connective and supportive tissues; a protein combined with carbohydrate

Mucus: A sticky white substance made by some epithelial cells

Mutagen: A substance with the potential to make a stable change in a gene that then can be passed on to offspring

Mycelia (s., mycelium): A mass of hyphae (hair-like) that makes up the vegetative body of moulds

Mycobacteria: The genus of bacteria causing tuberculosis (*Mycobacterium tuberculosis*) and leprosy (*Mycobacterium leprae*); acid fast staining is their characteristic feature

Mycology: The study of fungi

Mycosis: Infection caused by fungi

Mycoplasma: The smallest free-living group of bacteria that lack a cell wall and grow in the absence of oxygen.

Myeloblast: A kind of very young white cell, which will grow to become a granulocyte (neutrophil, basophil or eosinophil)

Myelocyte: An immature white cell of the myelocytic series; a granulocyte

Myoglobin: A pigmented, oxygen-carrying protein found in muscle tissue

Multiple myeloma: A disease also known as plasmocytic leukaemia where the plasma cells are more in circulation; characterized by the presence of Bence-Jones protein in urine and increased globulin concentration of serum

N

Necrosis: Death of areas of tissue or bone surrounded by healthy cells; commonly applied to bone
Nematode: A roundworm
Neo-: A prefix meaning new growth. **Example:** neoplasm (cancer)
Nephritis: Inflammation of the kidney
Nephro-: Prefix denoting kidney
Nephron:. Functional unit of kidney that consists of the glomerulus, tubules and collecting ducts for the urine which passes to the urinary bladder
Neurology: Study of the nervous system
Neutral: Neither acidic nor alkaline but between them both. **Example:** Distilled water is neutral (pH 7.0).
Neutrophil: A neutral-staining leukocytes; also called polymorphonuclear cells (PMN); usually the first line of defense against infection
Nodule: A small lump
Non-protein nitrogen (NPN): sum of all non-protein nitrogenous constituent of blood; urea, creatinine, ammonia are some of the examples
Normal flora: Micro-organisms that are normally present at a specific site
Normoblast: A young red cell with nucleus
Normochromic: Having normal colour
Normocytic: Having normal cell size
Nosepiece: Revolving unit to which microscope objectives are attached
Nosocomial infection: An infection acquired in a hospital or health care facility
Nucleated red blood cell (NRBC): A red blood cell that has not yet lost its nucleus
Nucleus (pl., nuclei): The central structure of a cell that contains DNA and controls cell growth and function

O

Objective: Magnifying lens closest to the object being viewed with a microscope
Occult: Concealed or hidden
Ocular: Eyepiece of the microscope that contains a magnifying lens
Ocular micrometer: Micrometer that fits in microscope eyepiece and that is used to measure microscopic objects
Oedema: Excessive fluid in the tissues causing them to swell
Oliguria: Decreased production of urine
Opportunistic parasite: An organism that causes disease only in immunocompromised hosts
Oncotic: Pertaining to swelling
Osmosis: a process whereby liquids of different concentrations, separated by a semi-permeable membrane percolate and mix until their concentrations are equal
Osmolality: Solute concentration of a fluid measured in terms of osmotic pressure, which increases with increased solute concentration
Osmotic fragility: Bursting of erythrocytes due to osmotic pressure following endosmosis or drawing in of water due to higher solute concentration inside the cell
Ovum (pl., ova): An egg
Oxidation: Combination with oxygen or removal of hydrogen
Oxyhaemoglobin: The form of haemoglobin that binds and transports oxygen

P

Packed cell volume (PCV): The percentage volume occupied by the packed red cells in whole blood when the latter is centrifuged. It is also called haematocrit or, in short, crit.

Pancreas: A gland situated behind the stomach, between the spleen and duodenum that secretes digestive enzymes (external secretions) into the digestive tract and insulin (internal secretion) into the circulation.

Pancytopaenia: Abnormal depression of all cellular elements; common in case of aplastic anaemia.

Pandemic: Widespread disease transmitted person-to-person and occurring over an entire country, continent, or even worldwide

Parallax: A shift in the apparent position of an object due to a change in position of the observer. Parallax error is introduced at the time of taking readings from pipettes and burettes unless the eye is kept at the level of the fluid.

Parasite: An organism that lives in or on another species and the expense of that species

Parasitology: The study of parasites; often it only means the study of worms and protozoa infecting the intestinal tract.

Parfocal: Having objectives (of microscope) that can be interchanged without varying the instrument's focus

Paroxysm(s): The cycles of chills and fever associated with malaria and that occur 36–72 h apart, depending on the *Plasmodium* spp.

Partial thromboplastin: The lipid portion of thromboplastin, available as a commercial preparation; formerly cephaloplastin

Pathogen: Any disease-producing organism

Pathogenic: Capable of causing damage or injury to the host

Pathologist: A physician specially trained in the nature and cause of disease; associated with clinical diagnosis by laboratory methods

Pathology: Science dealing with changes in body tissues, organs and body fluids due to diseased conditions

Pepsin: A gastric proteolytic enzyme which converts proteins into peptone in an acid medium

Percent solution: A solution made by adding units of solute needed per 100 units of solution

Percent transmittance: The percentage of light that passes through a solution

Percardial fluid: Fluid within the pericardial cavity

Peritoneum: The membrane lining the abdominal cavity and the organs contained within it

Peroxidase: The enzyme that converts hydrogen peroxide to water and oxygen

Petechiae: Small, purplish haemorrhagic spots on the skin

Petri dish: A shallow covered dish made of plastic or glass; used in microbial culture

pH: A measurement of the hydrogen ion concentration expressing the degree of acidity or alkalinity of a solution

Phagocyte: A cell capable of ingesting micro-organisms and other substances. The process is called **phagocytosis**

Phenotype: The character that is exhibited or shown as against the real genetic set up; in blood banking, the blood type determined by blood typing tests; for example, red cells of blood groups AA and AO (genotypes) will agglutinate with anti-A (phenotype)

Phlebotomy: Venipuncture; entry of a vein with a needle; the venipuncturist is called **phlebotomist**

Photometry: Measurement of the intensity of light; as seen in colorimetry

Physiological saline: 0.85% sodium chloride solution (0.15M)

Pico: Prefix used to indicate 10^{-12}

Picogram (pg): Micromicrogram; 1×10^{-12} g

Pinworm: *Enterobius vermicularis*, a small parasitic nematode; also called seatworm

Pipette, pipet: A glass tube for holding or measuring volumes of liquid
Plasma: The fluid portion of whole or anticoagulated blood
Plasma cell: A differentiated B lymphocyte that produces antibodies
Plasmin: An enzyme that binds to fibrin and initiates breakdown of the fibrin clot (fibrinolysis)
Platelets: Small non-nucleated cells found in the blood; also called thrombocytes that function in blood coagulation
Pleomorphic: Having varied shapes
Pleural fluid: The fluid in the space between the pleural membrane of the lung and the inner chest wall
Pneumonia: Inflammation of lungs with exudation and consolidation
Poikilocytosis: Abnormally shaped red cells
Point-of-care testing (POCT): Testing outside the traditional laboratory setting; bedside testing
Poly-: Prefix denoting many
Polychromasia: Multicoloured red cells
Polymorph: A polymorphonuclear leukocyte
Polyclonal antibodies: Antibodies derived from more than one cell line
Polycythemia: An excess of red blood cells in the peripheral blood
Polyuria: Excessive secretion of urine
Porphyria: A disturbance of porphyrin metabolism characterized by increase in formation and excretion of porphyrins or their precursors
Porphyrin: An organic compound with iron; when the iron is attached to protein, it is called protoporphyrin (haeme) which is a component of haemoglobin
Positive: Present, opposite to negative
Postprandial: After meal
Precision: Reproducibility of results; the closeness of obtained values to each other
Prefix: Modifying word or syllable(s) placed at the beginning of a word
Primary medium: A medium that provides nutritional requirements for an organism and is used to recover the organism from infectious material
Proglottids: Segments of the tapeworm
Promyelocyte: A young white cell, which will mature into a polymorphonuclear cell (PMN)
Prostatic: Related to prostate, a gland surrounding the neck of the bladder and urethra in the Male; contributes to the secretion of semen
Protein: Characteristic constituent of animal and plant tissues formed by the linkage of amino acids
Proteinuria: Protein present in urine
Proteolytic: Having the power to hydrolyse protein (digestion)
Prothrombin: Coagulation factor II; precursor of thrombin
Prothrombin time (PT): A coagulation-screening test used to monitor oral anticoagulant therapy
Protoporphyrin: Porphyrin attached to protein; when combined with iron, it forms haeme, a component of haemoglobin
Protozoa: A single-celled micro-organism with a nucleus like *Trichomonas vaginalis*
Prozone effect: This is seen due to excess of antibody where a positive reaction with antigen occurs at higher dilutions
Purulent: Like pus
Pus: A thick, usually yellowish liquid made of millions of dying polymorphs (neutrophils). A pus cell is a polymorphonuclear cell
PVA (Polyvinyl alcohol): A preservative used for faecal specimens
Pyogenic: Pus producing
Pyuria: Pus in urine; the urine is turbid, foul smelling and loaded with white blood cells and bacteria

Q

Quadrant: One-fourth of a circle; one-fourth of an agar plate (in petri dish)
Qualitative analysis: General screening and not quantitative
Quality control: A system that verifies the reliability of analytical test results through the use of standards, controls and statistical analysis
Quantitative analysis: The determination of the amount of substances present in measurable terms
Quantitative transfer: Transfer of a pre-weighed substance without any loss; a term commonly used in preparing solutions
Quellung reaction: An immunologic reaction with an apparent swelling of the capsule; for example swelling of *Pneumococcus* with the addition of antisera as seen under the microscope

R

Radioactive: Capable of emitting radiant energy
Radioimmunoassay (RIA): An immunological assay that uses radioisotopes
Radioisotope: Radioactive form of an element
Random urine specimen: A urine specimen collected at any time, without regard to diet or time of day
Reagin: A non-specific antibody that reacts with cardiolipin; also called Wassermann antibody; produced during syphilis infection and in other pathologic conditions
Recipient: A patient to whom blood is given
Reciprocal: Inverse; one of a pair of numbers (as 2/3 and 3/2) that has a product of one
Red blood cell indices: Calculated values that compare the size and
Reducing agent: A substance that loses electrons easily, hence causing other substances to be reduced
Reduction: A type of reaction in chemistry in which oxygen is removed, or hydrogen added or the substance which is reduced gains electrons (positive valence decreased)
Reference laboratory: An independent regional laboratory that offers routine and specialized testing services to hospitals and physicians
Reflectance photometer: An instrument that measures the light reflected from a coloured reaction product
Refractometers: An instrument used for measuring the refractive index of a substance; used in measuring the specific gravity of urine
Renal threshold: The blood concentration above which a substance not normally excreted by the kidneys appears in the urine
Reservoir host: The host, other than the usual host, in which the parasite lives and is infectious
Reticulocyte: An immature red blood cell that takes up brilliant cresyl blue or new methylene blue stain by the supravital staining process
Reticulocytosis: An increase above the normal number of reticulocytes in the circulating blood
Reticular: A network
Reticuloendothelial system: Involves a number of organs (bone marrow, liver, spleen and others) related to blood cell production
RF (Rheumatoid factor): Autoantibodies that are directed against human IgG and are often present in the serum of rheumatoid arthritis patients
Rh blood group system: One of the systems of blood groups that is responsible for producing the immune antibody, anti-D
Rh (D) immune globulin (RhIG): A concentrated purified solution of human anti-D antibody used for injection; RhoGam

Rickettsia: a micro-organism transmitted by lice, fleas, ticks; cannot be cultured in the laboratory; causal agents of Rockey Mountain spotted fever and Q-fever
RNA (Ribonucleic acid): The nucleic acid that is important in protein synthesis and that is found in all living cells
Rouleau(x): Red blood cells piled on top of one another like a stack of coins or dishes (plural rouleaux)

S

Sahli pipette: A pipette used in measuring small quantities of specimens (20 µL) and is used in haemoglobin determination; blood pipette
Saline: A solution of salt in water (0.85% sodium chloride)
Sample: In statistics, a subgroup of a population
Saprophytes: Organisms like moulds and fungi, which live on dead matter.
Satellitism: The phenomenon in which certain bacterial species, like, *Haemophilus influenzae* grow more vigorously in the immediate vicinity of the colonies of other unrelated species (*Staphylococcus aureus*)
Saturated solution: A solution containing as much of the solute as can be dissolved
Schistocytes: Fragments of erythrocytes
Schistosomiasis: Infection with schistosoma worms
Scolex: The attachment organ of a tapeworm; the head
Scurvy: A disease due to deficiency of vitamin C, marked by anaemia, spongy gums and haemorrhage, caused by a vascular defect
Sedimentation: The process of solid particles settling to the bottom of a liquid
Segmented neutrophils: Mature neutrophils with nuclei divided in several segments (normally 3 to 5); polymorphonuclear cells (PMN); often abbreviated as seg.
Selective medium: A bacteriological medium that allows growth of some organisms while inhibiting the growth of others
Semen or seminal fluid: Fluid discharged at ejaculation in the male, consisting of secretion of glands (prostrate) associated with the urogenital tract and containing spermatozoa
Sensitize: To render more reactive
Sepsis: Poisoning that is caused by the products of activity pathogenic micro-organisms
Septicaemia: Morbid condition resulting from the presence of pathogenic bacteria and their associated toxins in the blood
Sequestrene: An anticoagulant chemically known as ethylene diamine tetra-acetate (EDTA), commonly used in haematological studies
Serology: The study of antigens and antibodies in serum using immunological methods; laboratory testing based on the immunological properties of serum
Serum: The liquid obtained from blood that has been allowed to clot
Sickle cell anaemia: Inherited blood disorder in which the red cells can deform to sickle shape (drepanocyte) due to the presensce of the abnormal haemoglobin (HbS)
Sideroblast: Immature nucleated red blood cell with iron granules, recognized by Prussian-blue staining. Siderocytes are mature red blood cells without nucleus. The iron granules (ferritin) are due to their lack of utilization in the formation of haemoglobin. Their presence in bone marrow (sideroblasts) and in circulation (siderocytes) is considered as abnormal.
Slant culture: Bacterial culture in a test tube where the medium is solidified in a slant. This provides more surface; like TSI.
Sleeping sickness: An acute infectious disease caused by *Trypanosoma* infection (trypanosomiasis); prevalent in Africa

Slide method: Applied in blood grouping when the testing is done on a microscope slide
Smear: A specimen spread thinly on a slide
Smudge cells: White blood cells, which are smudged in appearance on the smear; also called basket cells. Increased number of smudge cells may indicate chronic lymphocytic leukaemia
Solid chemistry: An analytical method in which the sample is added to a strip or slide containing, in dried form, all the reagents for the procedure
Solubility: The extent to which a solute will dissolve in a solvent; the substance in solution is called the solute and the liquid in which the solute is dissolved is called the solvent
Solute: The substance dissolved in a given solution
Specific gravity: The ratio of the mass of a given substance to the mass of an equal volume of water; a measurement of density
Specimen: In the clinical laboratory it refers to some thing (e.g. urine) taken out of a person as a sample to examine.
Spectrum: Collection of sequentially arranged bands of different wavelengths of light; the visible spectrum ranges between 400–700 nm (violet to red)
Sperm: Short for spermatozoon (plural: spermatozoa) mature male germ cell present in semen which impregnates the ovum (female germ cell) in sexual reproduction.
Spherocytes: A small, globular, completely haemoglobinized red blood cell without a paler region in the centre
Spirochaetes: Motile, helical, or spiral bacterial of the family Spirochaeta
Sputum: Matter ejected from the trachea, bronchi and lungs through the mouth
Stab culture: A technique of bacterial culture in which organisms are introduced into a solid agar medium with a wire or needle; also refers to band neutrophils
Standard: A chemical solution of a known concentration that can be used as reference or calibration substance
Standard deviation: A term used in statistics and quality control; a commonly used measure of dispersion or variability in a distribution; a measure of the spread of a population of values around the mean
Starch: Carbohydrate stored by certain plants. It is a polysaccharide that turns the iodine colour to blue
Stat: Immediately; stat procedure calls for immediate, attention, like handling of CSF specimens; also known as emergency procedure
Steatorrhoea: Diarrhoea with much undigested fat in the stool
Stem cell: An undifferentiated cell
Sterile: Free from living organisms
Sterilization: Complete elimination of all living micro-organisms from an article or area
Steroid and sterol: A group of organic compounds with special chemical structure. It includes many hormones and also cholesterol
Stippling: A spotted condition of red blood cells, known as basophllic stippling, Is seen under certain pathological condition like lead poisoning
Streaking: Making lines or stripes; in bacteriology streaking it done on the primary plate for isolation of organisms
Sub-: A prefix denoting beneath or under
Sucrose: A disaccharide; cane sugar
Suffix: Modifying word or syllable(s) placed at the end of a word
Supernatant: The liquid above a solid deposit after centrifugation
Supravital staining: A dye that stains living cells or tissues
Suspension: Solid particles hanging in a liquid
Swab: A piece of cotton wool or gauze rolled on the tip of a plastic or wooden stick; used to apply antiseptic on the skin or for collection of specimens (throat swab, stool swab)

Symbiosis: An association between two different organisms, which is of mutual benefit
Symptom: Any subjective evidence of disease or of a patient's condition
Synovial fluid: Viscous fluid secreted by membranes lining the joints
Systemic lupus erythematosus (SLE): An autoimmune disease; a connective tissue disorder

T

Target cell: Abnormal red blood cell with a darker region in the middle
TC: Marking on pipettes indicating "to contain"; these pipettes are washed out; Sahli pipette is a TC pipette
TD: A marking on pipettes indicating "To deliver"; all volumetric pipettes are TD pipettes; it is not necessary to wash them out
Thalassaemia: A hereditary haemolytic anaemia marked by poor synthesis of normal haemoglobin (HbA) while foetal haemoglobin (HbF) continues to form in the body
Therapeutic agent: Substance administered in the treatment of a disease
Thermolabile: Easily altered or decomposed by heat (thermo-). **Example:** Factor VIII (cryoprecipltate).
Thermostable: Not easily affected by heat.
Thoma pipette: A pipette meant for dilution and not for dispensing specific volume
Thrombin: A protein formed from prothrombin by the action of thromboplastin and other factors in the presence of calcium ions; factor II
Thrombocyte: Another name for platelet
Thrombocytopaenia: Denotes too few platelets in the blood circulation
Thrombocytosis: Abnormal increase in the number of platelets in the blood
Thrombosis: The formation, development or existence of a blood clot or thrombus within the vascular system
Thrombus (pl. thrombi): A blood clot that obstructs a blood vessel
Titre: In serology, the reciprocal of the highest dilution that gives the desired reaction; the concentration of a substance determined by titration
Tlymphocytes: The type of lymphocyte responsible for the cell-mediated immune response
Todd unit: Expresses the titre of antistreptolysin-O (ASO), produced by a patient infected with *Streptococcus pyogenes*
Tourniquet: A band used to constrict blood flow
Transferrin: A serum globulin that binds and transports iron.
Transfusion: Taking blood from one person (donor) and giving it to another person (recipient).
Transport medium: A medium that provides the proper environment for organisms during transport
Trematode: A class of flatworms commonly called **flukes** belonging to the phylum *Platyhelminthes*.
Trend: An indication of error in the analysis, detected by increasing or decreasing values in the control sample
Treponema: A genus of spirochaetes, *Treponema pallidum* is the causal agent of syphilis
Trichomoniasis: A sexually transmitted genitourinary infection caused by the parasitic protozoan, *Trichomonas vaginalis*
Trichrome stain: A stain commonly used to identify parasites in faecal smears
Trophozoites: The motile, active and reproductive phase of protozoa
Tuberculosis: An infectious disease caused by the tubercle bacillus, *Mycobacterium tuberculosis*
Typhoid fever: An acute infectious disease accompanied by fever, headache and abdominal pain. The causal agent is *Salmonella Typhi*
Typhus: An infectious disease caused by rickettsial organisms, transmitted through ticks.

U

Ulcer: Wound
Universal donor: A person of blood group O whose blood can be given to anyone
Universal recipient: A person of blood group AB who can be the recipient for any of the other blood groups as donor blood A, B, or O
Uraemia: A pathologic condition due to the accumulation of urea in blood
Urea: The nitrogenous constituent of urine; final product of protein metabolism; synthesized in the liver; formed by combination of ammonia and carbon dioxide, $CO(NH_2)_2$
Urease: An enzyme, which breaks down urea
Urethra: The canal through which urine is discharged from the urinary bladder
Uric acid: Breakdown product of nucleic acids
Urine: The fluid excreted by the kidney stored in the bladder and discharged through the urethra
Urinary tract: The parts of the body through which the urine flows—the kidneys, ureters, bladder and urethra
Urinometer: A device to determine the specific gravity of urine
Urinalysis or urine analysis: Analysis of urine through physical examination, microscopic examination of sediment and chemical screening
Urobilinogen: A breakdown product of bilirubin formed by the action of intestinal bacteria
Urochrome: The yellow pigment that gives urine its colour

V

Vacuole: A membrane-bound compartment in cell cytoplasm
Vasoconstriction: A narrowing of the diameter of a blood vessel
VDRL: Short form of Venereal Disease Research Laboratory test, which is a screening serodiagnostic test for syphilis
Vector: An agent that transports a pathogen from an infected host to a non-infected host
Vein: A blood vessel that carries deoxygenated blood from the tissues to the heart
Venereal: Disease spread through sexual contact; like, syphilis
Venipuncture: Introduction of a needle into a vein for the withdrawal of blood or injection of a fluid; phlebotomy
Virology: Th study of viruses
Virulent: Highly infectious
Visible spectrum: Wavelengths of light that are visible to the eye in the form of colours; ranges between 700 and 400 nm
Vitamins: Accessory food factors necessary for a well balanced diet (e.g. B_{12})
Vitamin B_{12}: A vitamin essential to the proper maturation of blood cells and other cells in the body
Vitamin K: A vitamin essential for the production of coagulation factors II, VII, IX and X
Viviparous organism: Parasites giving birth to living young which develop within the maternal Body; ova (eggs) are not seen (e.g. *Trichinella*)
von Willebrand's disease: A bleeding disorder known as vascular haemophilia caused by vascular defect along with factor VIII deficiency

W

Wassermann antibody: An antibody that reacts with cardiolipin. It is also called reagin
Weil-Felix reaction: A serological method based on the principle of febrile agglutination and applied in the diagnosis of rickettsial diseases.
Westergren method: A technique applied in the determination of erythrocyte sedimentation rate (ESR)
White blood cells (WBC): Blood cells that function in immunity; leukocytes
Wintrobe method: A technique applied in the determination of erythrocyte sedimentation rate
Working distance: Distance between the microscope objective and the microscope slide when the object is in sharp focus
World Health Organization (WHO): The United Nations Agency concerned with g;pbal public health; active in developing countries
Wright's stain: A polychromic stain (produces multicolour effect on cells) with eosin and methylene blue used for staining blood smears.

X

Xanthoehromic: Having a yellow colour
XDP: Fibrin-degradation products that contain the D-dimer cross-linked region

Y

Yeast : Plant-like micro-organisms related to fungi; budding (fission) is the characteristic feature of its asexual reproduction.

Z

Zone of inhibition: In the antibiotic susceptibility test, the area around an antibiotic disk that contains no bacterial growth
Zoonotic: Infection or disease that can be transmitted from vertebrate animals to humans

APPENDICES

APPENDIX A: SOURCES OF INFORMATION AND READINGS

GENERAL

Baker, F. J. et al (2001). *Baker and Silverstone's introduction to medical laboratory technology* (7th ed.). Oxford University Press.

Basham, A. L, (1976). *The practice of medicine in ancient and medieval India. In: Asian medical systems: A comparative study* (Ed. C. M. Leslie.). University of California Press.

Bauer, J. D. (1982). *Clinical laboratory methods.* C.V. Mosby.

Bharucha, C. et al. (1970). *Handbook of medical laboratory technology.* Christian Medical College, Vellore, India.

Burtis, C.A., et al. (Eds.) (1998). *Tietz's textbook of clinical chemistry* (3rd ed.). W.B. Saunders Company.

Doucette L. J. (1997). *Mathematics for the Clinical Laboratory.* W.B. Saunders.

Frankel, S., et al. (1970). *Gradwohl's clinical laboratory methods and diagnosis* (7th ed.). C.V. Mosby.

Harr, R. R. (2006). *Clinical laboratory science review* (3rd ed.). F. A. Davis.

Henry, J. B. (2006). *Clinical diagnosis and management by laboratory methods.* W.B. Saunders.

Hepler, O. E. (1949). *Manual of clinical laboratory methods* (4th ed.). Charles C. Thomas.

Leslie, C. M. (Ed.) (1976). *Asian medical systems; A comparative study.* University of California Press.

Johnson, C. W., et al. (2002). *Essential laboratory mathematics: Concepts and applications for the chemical and clinical laboratory technician.* Delmar Cengage Learning.

Lindh, W. Q., et al. (2002). *Comprehensive medical assisting* (2nd ed.). Thomson Delmar Learning.

Linne, J. J. and Ringsrud, K. M. (1999). *Clinical laboratory sciences: the basics and routine techniques* (4th ed.). C.V. Mosby.

MacFate, R. P. (1972). *Introduction to the clinical laboratory.* Year Book Medical Publishers Inc.

Maurice, K. (1973). *A medical laboratory for developing countries.* The English Language Book Society and Oxford University Press.

Mukherjee, K. L. (1979). *Review of clinical laboratory methods.* C.V. Mosby.

Mukherjee, K. L. (1979). *Introductory mathematics for the clinical laboratory.* American Medical Association (American Society of Clinical Pathology).

Oppenheim, I. A. (1981). *Textbook for laboratory assistants.* C.V. Mosby.

Polansky, V. D. (2002). *Medical laboratory technology: pearls of wisdom* (2nd ed.). Boston Medical Publishing.

Raphael, S. S. (Ed.) (1983). *Lynch's medical laboratory technology.* W.B. Saunders.

Ravel, R. (1995). *Clinical laboratory medicine: Clinical application of laboratory data* (6th ed.). C.V. Mosby.

Taub, H. (1974). *Laboratory skill for allied health occupations.* Rinehart Press.

Turgeon, M. L. et al. (2007). *Clinical laboratory science: The basics and routine techniques* (5th ed.). C.V. Mosby.

Westgard. J. O. (2002). *Basic QC practices* (2nd ed.). AACC Press, Washington, DC.

Widman, F. K. (1979). *Clinical interpretation of laboratory tests.* F.A. Davis Co.

Wittman, K. S. and Thomas, J. C. (1977). *Medical laboratory skill.* McGraw-Hill.

World Health Organization (WHO) (2003). *Manual of basic techniques for a health laboratory* (2nd ed.).

World Health Organization (WHO). (2005). *Laboratory biosafety manual.*

PHLEBOTOMY

Garza, D. and Becan-Mc-Bride, K. (2004). *Phlebotomy handbook: blood collection essentials* (7th ed.). Prentice-Hall.
Hoeltke, L. B. (2006). *The complete textbook of phlebotomy* (3rd ed.). Thompson Delmar Learning.
Kalanick, K. (2004). *Phlebotomy technician specialist*. Thomson Delmar Learning.
McCall, R..E. and Tankersley, C. M. (2007). *Phlebotomy essentials* (4th ed.). Lippincott Williams & Wilkins.
Turgeon, M. L. (1999). *Clinical haematology theory and procedures* (3rd ed.). Lippincott Williams & Wilkins.

HAEMATOLOGY

Bernadette, F. R. et al. (2007). *Hematology: clinical principles and applications* (3rd ed.). W.B. Saunders.
Brown, B. A. (1980) *Hematology: principles and procedures* (3rd ed.). Lea & Febiger.
Carr, J.H. and Rodak, B.F. (1999). *Clinical hematology atlas* (3rd ed.). W.B. Saunders.
Dacie, J. V. and Lewis, S. M. (1975). *Practical haematology* (5th ed.). Churchill-Livingstone.
Lamberg, S. L. (1978). *Laboratory manual of hematology and urinalysis*. AVI Publishing Co.
McKenzie, S. B. (2006). *Clinical laboratory hematology*. Prentice-Hall.
Seiverd.C. E. (1973). *Haematology for medical technologists*. Lea & Febiger.

COAGULATION

Biggs, R. (1972). *Human blood coagulation, haemostasia and thrombosis*. Blackwell Scientific Publications.
Bloom, A. L. and Thomas, D. P. (1981). *Haemostasia and thrombosis*, Churchill-Livingstone.
Thompson, A. R. and Marker L.A. (1983). *Manual of hemostasis and thrombosis* (3rd ed.). F.A. Davis.

BLOOD BANK (IMMUNOHAEMATOLOGY)

Blaney, K. D. and Howard, P. R. (2008). Basic and applied concepts of immunohematology (2nd ed.). C.V. Mosby.
Bowley. C. C., et al. (1971). Blood transfusion: a guide to the formation and operation of a transfusion service. World Health Organization.
Bryant, N. J. (1994). An Introduction to Immunohematology (3rd ed.). W. B. Saunders.
Erskine, A. G. and Socha W.W. (1978). The principles and practice of blood grouping (2nd ed.). C.V. Mosby.
Harmening, D. M. (2005). Modern blood banking and transfusion practices (5th ed.). F. A. Davis.
Mollison, P. L. (1979). Blood transfusion in clinical medicine (6th ed.). Blackwell Scientific Publications.
Ortho Technical Manual (1960). Blood group antigens and antibodies. Ortho Pharmaceutical Corp.
Rudmann, S. V. (2005). Textbook of blood banking and transfusion medicine (2nd ed.). W.B. Saunders.
Technical manual (1981). American association of blood banks (8th ed.). Washington, D.C.
Williams, H. B. (1978). Laboratory manual of serology, immunology and blood banking. AVI Publishing Co.
Zmijewski. C. M. (1978). Immunohematology (3rd ed.). Appleton-Century-Crofts.
Zmijewskij, C. M. and Haesler, W. E., Jr. (1982). Textbook of blood banking science. Appleton-Century-Crofts.

MICROBIOLOGY

Adams. A. R. D. and Maegraith, B.G. (1976). *Clinical tropical diseases* (6th ed.). Blackwell Scientific Publications.

Bartelt, M. A. (1999). Diagnostic bacteriology: A study guide. F. A. Davis.
BBL (1968). Manual of products and laboratory procedures. Becton, Dickinson.
Buchanan, R. E. and Gibbons, N. E. (Eds.) (1974). Bergey's manual of determinative bacteriology (8th ed.). Williams and Wilkins.
Cruickshank, R., et al. (Eds.). (1975). Medical microbiology. Churchill-Livingstone.
Forbes, B. A., et al. (2007). Bailey and Scott's Diagnostic Microbiology (12th ed.). Mosby.
Garcia, L. S. (2007). Diagnostic Medical Parasitology (5th ed.). American Society for Microbiology. Washington DC.
Kern, M. E and Blevins, K. S. (1997). Medical mycology: a self-instructional text (2nd ed.). F. A. Davis.
Lennette. E. H., et al. (Eds.). (1985). Manual of clinical microbiology (4th ed.) American Society for Microbiology, Washington, D.C.
Levanthal R. and Cheadle, R. F. (2002) Medical parasitology: a self-instructional text (5th ed.). F. A. Davis.
Mahon, C. R., et al. (2006) Textbook of diagnostic microbiology (3rd ed.). Saunders.
Melvin. D. M. and Brook, M. M. (1974). Laboratory procedures for the diagnosis of intestinal parasites. US Government Printing Press, Washington, D.C.
Myers, R. M. and Koshi, G. (1982). Diagnostic procedures in medical microbiology and immunology/serology. Christian Medical College, Vellore, India,
Paik, G. (1980). Reagents, stains, and miscellaneous test procedures. *In* Lenette, E.H., et al. (Eds.). Manual of clinical microbiology (3rd ed.). American Society for Microbiology, Washington, D.C.
Roberts, L. and Janovy, J., Jr. (2008). Foundations of parasitology (8th ed.). McGraw-Hill.
Stokes, E. J. and Ridgway, G. L. (1980). Clinical bacteriology (5th ed.). Edward Arnold.
Washington, J. A. II. (Ed) (1985). Laboratory procedures in clinical microbiology (2nd ed.). Springer-Verlag.
Zeibig, E. A. (1997) Clinical parasitology: a practical approach. W.B. Saunders.

IMMUNOLOGY

Abbas, L. (2009). Basic Immunology (3rd ed.). W.B. Saunders
Doan, T., et al. (2007). Immunology. Lippincott Williams & Wilkins.
Male, D. M., et al. (2007). Immunology (7th ed.). C.V. Mosby.
Turgeon, M. L. (2008). Immunology and serology in laboratory medicine (4th ed.). Elsevier Health Sciences.

CLINICAL PATHOLOGY

Brunzel, N. A. (2004). Fundamentals of urine and body analysis (2nd ed.). W.B. Saunders.
Graff, S.L. (1983). A handbook of routine urinalysis. Lippincott Williams & Wilkens.
Strasinger, S. K. and Di Lorenzo, M. S. (2009). Urinalysis and body fluids (5th ed.). F.A. Davis.

CLINICAL BIOCHEMISTRY

Arneson, W. L. and Brickell, J. M. (2007). Clinical chemistry: a laboratory perspective. F.A. Davis.
Anderson, S. C. (2002). Clinical chemistry: concepts and applications. McGraw-Hill Medical.
Bishop, M. L., et al. (Eds.) (2004). Clinical chemistry: principles, procedures, correlations (5th ed.). Lippincott Williams & Wilkins.
Blick, K. E. and.Liles, S. M (1985). Principles of clinical chemistry. John Wiley & Sons.
Burtis, C. A., et al. (2007). Tietz fundamentals of clinical chemistry (6th ed.). W.B. Saunders.

Kaplan.L. A. and Pesce A. J. (1984). Clinical chemistry. C.V. Mosby.
Wootton, I. D. P. (1964). Microanalysis in medical biochemistry. J. A.Churchill Ltd.

HISTOLOGY AND CYTOLOGY

Armed forces institute of pathology (1960). Manual of histologic and special staining technics. McGraw-Hill.
Baker, J. R. (1966). Cytological technique: the principles underlying routine methods. Methuen.
Bancroft, J. D. and Gamble, M. (2007). Theory and practice of histological techniques (6th ed.). Churchill-Livingstone.
Bitensky, J. R. and Chayen, J. (1979). Quantitative cytochemistry and its applications. Academic Press.
Carson, F. L. (1997). Histotechnology: a self-assessment workbook (2nd ed.). American Society of Clinical Pathology.
Chayen, J., et al. (1991). A guide to practical histochemistry (2nd ed.). John Wiley.
Cibas, E. S. and Ducatman, B. S. (2009). Cytology: diagnostic principles and clinical correlates (3rd ed.). W.B. Saunders.
Culling, C. F. A. (1974). Handbook of histopathological and histochemical techniques (3rd ed.). Butterworth.
Drury, R. A. B. and Wallington E. A. (1967). Carleton's histological technique (4th ed.). Oxford University Press.
Gray, P. (1964). Handbook of basic microtechnique (3rd ed.). McGraw-Hill.
Gridley, M. F. (1960). Manual of histologic and special staining technics. McGraw-Hill.
Lillie, R. D. (1977). H. J. Conn's biologicl stains: a handbook on the nature and uses of the dyes employed in the biological laboratory (9th ed.). Williams & Wilkins.
Lillie, R. D. and Fullmer, H. M. (1976). Histopathologic technic and practical histochemistry (4th ed.). McGraw-Hill.
Kiernan J. A. (2008). Histological and histochemical methods: theory and practice (4th ed.). Cold Spring Harbon Laboratory Press.
Ramzy, I. (2000). Clinical cytopathology and aspiration biopsy (2nd ed.). McGraw-Hill Professional.
Thompson, S. W. (1974). Selected histochemical and histopathological methods. C. C. Thomas.
Wick, M. R. (Ed.). (2008). Diagnostic histochemistry. Cambridge University Press.
Young, B., et al. (2006). Wheater's functional histology: a text and colour atlas (5th ed.). Churchill-Livingstone.

MEDICAL TERMINOLOGY AND LABORATORY DATA

Brooker, C. (2003). Churchill livingstone pocket medical dictionary (15th ed.). Churchill-Livingstone.
Chabner, D. (2007). The language of medicine (8th ed.). W.B. Saunders.
Dennerll, J. T., et al. (2002). Medical terminology made easy (3rd ed.). Thomson Delmar Learning.
William. A. N. (2007). Dorland's illustrated medical dictionary (30th ed.). W.B. Saunders.
Ehrlich, A. and Schroeder, C. L. (2000). Medical terminology for health professions (4th ed.). Thomson Delmar Learning.
Faulkner, W. R. and King, J. W. (1970). Handbook of clinical laboratory data, CRC (2nd ed.). Chemical Rubber Co. Press.
Medical Laboratory Observer (1984). Clinical laboratory reference. Medical Economics Co.
Sormunen, C. (2003). Terminology for allied health professionals (6th ed.). Thomson Delmar Learning.
Venes, D., et al. (Eds.). (2005). Taber's cyclopedic medical dictionary (20th ed.). F.A. Davis.

INTERNET LINKS

http://www.highbeam.com/Medical+Laboratory+Observer/publications.aspx?
http://www.encyclopedia.com/doc/1G1-94777974.html
http://www.who.int/en/
http://www.who.int/publications/en/
http://www.google.com/
http://www.labce.com/?gclid=CJLKoNrvk5kCFaCT7QodzBy9Zw
http://www.austincc.edu/kotrla/phb_links.htm
http://www.bd.com/vacutainer/products/venous/
http://www.dml.co.nz/clin_handbook.asp

APPENDIX B: COMMENTS ON REPORTING OF TEST RESULTS

The technician must know the **normal or reference value** of the test. A list of these values is given in this appendix. One should bear in mind that the normal values and reference range may vary from laboratory to laboratory as well as on the methodology used. The method of specimen collection may also influence these results. The laboratory must specify its own normal ranges.

The technician should have the knowledge to recognize **abnormal test results** and its trend. Just getting some numerical figures without a meaningful conclusion is wasteful. Abnormal test patterns or trends can sometimes provide more useful information than single test outcome deviations. Conversely, single test results can be normal in patients with a proven disease or illness. While studying the result one must take into consideration the **biocultural normal variation**. Thus low haemoglobin level in Asiatic Indians and high haemoglobin concentration in Mexican Americans are common observations.

Panic test results must be immediately communicated to the physician. Time-critical information is of limited value if it is delayed or not received. Even though computerized communication technologies contribute to faster information delivery, clinicians are often left waiting for crucial laboratory data. The wireless networks can expedite the reporting of vital patient data to the health care provider so that treatment can begin without delay.

Medical laboratory personnel must be able to recognize **margins of error**. For example, if a patient has a battery of chemistry tests, the possibility exists that some tests will be abnormal owing purely to chance. This occurs because a significant margin of error arises from the arbitrary setting of limits. Thus if the patient has a group of tests performed on one blood sample, the possibility that some of the tests will "read abnormal" due purely to chance is not uncommon.

NORMAL VALUES

Laboratory Reference Values

While referring to the normal or laboratory reference values, one should bear in mind that they vary from laboratory to laboratory, different populations and the methodology used. The laboratory must specify its own normal ranges.

Haematology

TEST/Method	Groups/Details	Normal range (conventional unit)	Special comments
Haemoglobin	Children	10–14 g/dL	Use EDTA anticoagulated blood and complete the test within 8 h.
	Adult male	13–17 g/dL	
	Adult female	12–15 g/dL	
Micrhaematocrit	Children	32–38%	
	Adult male	42–52%	
	Adult female	36–48%	
WBC count	Children		Use EDTA anticoagulated blood and complete the test within 4 h
	Adults		
WBC differential count	Neutros (seg)	40–75%	
	Lymph	20–45%	
	Mono	2–10%	
	EOS	1–6%	
	Baso	0–1%	
	Band neutros	3–6%	
Reticulocyte count		0.5–1.5%	Use EDTA anticoagulated blood and complete the test within 2 h
ESR/Wintrobe	Adult male	0–9 mm/h	Use EDTA anticoagulated blood and complete test within 2 h
	Adult female	0–20 mm/h	
RBC Indices	MCV	82–92 fl	Same as Haemoglobin Haematocrit
	MCH	27–32 pg	
	MCHC	32–36%	
Platelet count		$15–40 \times 10^4/\mu L$	EDTA anticoagulated blood and complete test within 1–2 h

Coagulation

TEST/Method	Normal range (conventional unit)	Special comments
PT	10–14 sec	Citrated plasma. Complete the test promptly
APTT	31–39 sec	
Bleeding time/Ivy	2–5 min	Done on patient
Bleeding time/Duke	1–3 min	
Clotting time/ Lee-white	5–11 min	No anticoagulant

Clinical Biochemistry

TEST (serum analysis)	Normal range (conventional unit)	Special comments
Alkaline aminotransferase (ALT)	7–30 U/L	
Albumin	3.3–5.3 g/dL	
Alkaline phosphatase (ALP)	70–150 U/L	

(Contd)

TEST (serum analysis)	Normal range (conventional unit)	Special comments
Aspartate aminotransferase (AST)	12–30 U/L	
Bicarbonate (HCO_3^-)	22–28 mEq/L	
Bilirubin, Total	0.2–1.3 mg/dL	
Bilirubin, Direct	0.1–0.4 mg/dL	
BUN	15–45 mg/dL	
Calcium	8.5–10.5 mg/dL	
Chloride	98–109 mEq/L	
Cholesterol	150–250 mg/dL	
Creatinine	0.5–1.5 mg/dL	
Creatinine kinase (CK)	10–120 U/L	
Globulin	1.8–3.3 g/dL	
Gamma glutamyl transferase (GGT)	3–40 U/L	
Glucose	70–110 mg/dL	
Iron	65–165 µg/dL	
Lactate dehydrogenase	95–200 U/L	
Phosphorus	2.5–4.8 mg/dL	
Potassium	3.5–5.5 mEq/L	
Sodium	135–145 mEq/L	
TSH	0.35–5.0 µIU/mL	
Total protein	6.0–8.0 g/dL	
Triglycerides	50–150 mg/dL	
Uric acid	2.1–7.4 mg/dL	

Other Body Fluids

Test	Normal range (conventional unit)	Special comments
24-Hour Urinary Discharge		
Calcium	100–300 mg/day	Varies with body weight
Creatinine	1.5–2.0 g/day	
Protein	10–100 mg/day	
Urobilinogen	0.4–1.0 mg/day	Protect specimen from light
Clearance Study		
Creatinine clearance	Male 113–167 mL/min	Serum and urine specimens required
	Female 117–135 mL/min	
Urea clearance	41–68 mL/min	
CSF		
Glucose	40–80 mg/dL	
Protein	20–40 mg/dL	

APPENDIX C: MSCELLANEOUS INFORMATION

Concentrations of Common Acids and Bases

Acid or base (concentrated)	M.W.	Sp.Gr.	Percentage (%)	Normality N	Amount of acid/base required to make 1 L of 1 N solution (mL)
HCl (Hydrochloric acid)	36.46	1.19	36.0	11.7	95.5 mL
HNO_3 (Nitric acid)	63.02	1.42	69.5	15.6	64.0 mL
H_2SO_4 (Sulphuric acid)	98.08	1.84	96.0	35.9	28.4 mL
NH_4OH (Ammonium hydroxide)	35.04	0.90	58.6	15.1	66.5 mL

Acid-base Indicators

Indicator	Approximate pH range	Colour change	Preparation
Methyl orange	3.4–4.8	red to yellow	0.05–0.2% aqueous or aqueous ethanol
Methyl red	4.8–6.0	red to yellow	0.02 g in 60 mL ethanol and 40 mL water
Phenol red	6.6–8.0	yellow to red	0.1 g in 28.2 mL of 0.01 N NaOH and 221.8 mL water
Phenolphthalein	8.2–10.0	no colour to pink	0.05 g in 50 mL ethanol and 50 mL water

Preparation of Phosphate Buffers

Phosphate buffers are generally useful, since the range of the mixtures is from pH 5 to 8.
Reagents
A. **Monobasic potassium phosphate (0.066 M)**:
   Dissolve 9.0727 g of KH_2PO_4 in distilled water and dilute to 1000 mL in a volumetric flask. The solution must be absolutely clear and should yield no test for chloride or sulphates (Chapter 4 in Vol. I). Keep the solution in refrigerator.
B. **Dibasic sodium phosphate (0.066 M)**:
   Dissolve 11.867 g of $Na_2HPO_4.2H_2O$ in distilled water and dilute to 1000 mL in a volumetric flask. *Note:* If the dibasic sodium phosphate has 12 moles of water of crystallization, expose the salt to the ordinary atmosphere for two weeks; it will then contain 2 moles of water of crystallization). The solution should be absolutely clear and free from chloride or sulphates. Keep in the refrigerator.

Procedure
Mix the solutions (A) and (B) in the following proportions in order to obtain the desired pH.

Desired pH	Solution A	Solution B
5.288	9.7	0.2
5.589	9.5	0.5
5.906	9.0	1.0
6.239	8.0	2.0
6.468	7.0	3.0
6.643	6.0	4.0
6.813	5.0	5.0
6.979	4.0	6.0
7.168	3.0	7.0
7.381	2.0	8.0
7.731	1.0	9.0
8.043	0.5	9.5

APPENDIX D: CONVERSION OF CONVENTIONAL UNITS TO INTERNATIONAL (SI) UNITS

Test	Conventional units	Conversion factor	SI units
Albumin	g/dL	154	µmol/L
Bicarbonate	mEq/L	1	mmol/L
Bilirubin	mg/dL	17.1	µmol/L
Calcium	mg/dL	0.25	mmol/L
Chloride	mEq/L	1	mmol/L
Cholesterol	mg/dL	0.026	mmol/L
Creatinine	mg/dL	88.4	µmol/L
Creatinine clearance	mL/min	0.0167	mL/s
Glucose	mg/dL	0.0556	mmol/L
Haematocrit	%	0.01	ratio
Haemoglobin	g/dL	0.621	mmol/L
MCH	pg	0.0155	fmol
MCHC	%	0.01	ratio
MCV	μ^3 (cu.µ)	1	fL
PCO_2	mmHg	0.133	kPa
pH	none	antilog	nmol/L
Phosphate (as P)	mg/dL	0.323	mmol/L
Platelet count	$10^3/mm^3$	10^6	$10^9/L$
Potassium	mEq/L	1	mmol/L
Protein (total)	g/dL	10	g/L
RBC count	$10^6/mm^3$	10^6	$10^{12}/L$
Sodium	mEq/L	1	mmol/L
Triglyceride (as triolein)	mg/dL	0.0113	mmol/L
Urea nitrogen	mg/dL	0.357	mmol/L
Uric acid	mg/dL	0.0598	mmol/L
WBC count	$10^3/mm^3$	10^6	$10^9/L$

APPENDIX E: TABLE OF PANIC VALUES

Test	Low	Possible effect	High	Possible effect
PCV (HCt)	<15%	Heart failure anoxaemia	None	
Hb	<5 g/dL	Anoxaemia	None	
Platelet Ct	<30,000/µL	Haemorrhage	None	
PT	None		>40 s	Haemorrhage
Bleeding time	None		>15 m	Haemorrhage
Clotting time	None		>15 m	Haemorrhage
APTT	None		>125 s	Haemorrhage
Bilirubin total (newborn)	None		>18 mg/dL	Brain damage
Serum glucose	<40 mg/dL	Brain damage	>700 mg/dL	Diabetic coma
Serum phosphate	<1 mg/dL	Seizures and coma	None	
Serum potassium	<2.5 mEq/L	Muscle weakness, paralysis, cardiac problems	>6.5 mEq/L	Cardiac problems
Serum sodium	<120 mEq/L	Oedema, heart failure	>160 mEq/L	Oedema, heart failure
Serum bicarbonate	<10 mEq/L	Acid-base imbalance, anoxaemia	>40 mEq/L	Acid-base imbalance, anoxaemia
PCO_2	<20 mmHg	Anoxaemia	>70 mmHg	Anoxaemia
Blood pH	<7.2	Anoxaemia	>7.6	Anoxaemia
Blood PO_2	<40 mmHg	Anoxaemia	None	Anoxaemia

Microbiology

Laboratory observation	Clinical condition
Positive blood culture	Worsening sepsis
Positive CSF Gram stain	Bacterial meningitis
Positive CSF culture	Bacterial meningitis
Positive India ink preparation of CSF	Mycotic meningitis

Spinal fluid

	Low critical value	High critical value
Total protein	Low -None	>45 mg/dL (>450 mg/dL)
Glucose	<80% of blood level	
Microsocopy: WBC	Low-None	>20 Segmented neutrophils
Microsocpy: Blasts or malignant cells	Low-None	>10/mm^3

Urinalysis

	Low ciritical value	High critical value
Urine microscopy	None	Presence of pathologic crystals, RBC
Urine glucose	None	>1000 mg/dL glucose (>55 mmol/L)
Urine ketone	None	Strongly positive

Blood Bank

Test	Result
Antibody identification	Positive
Coombs	Positive direct Coombs

APPENDIX F: DIAGNOSTIC TEST PANELS

Disorder	Laboratory test
General health	Glucose, BUN/creatinine, cholesterol, TGL, GOT (AST), ALP, uric acid, total protein, albumin, total bilirubin, LD, Ca, Na, K
Anaemia	Complete blood count (CBC), reticulocyte count. *Hypochromic microcytic*: serum iron and iron binding capacity. *Macrocytic*: B_{12} and folate analysis
Bone-related and joint	Uric acid, Ca, P, ALP, total protein, albumin
Cardiac injury	LD and CPK; isoenzymes (LD, CPK)
Cardiac risk	Cholesterol, TGL, glucose, HDL cholesterol
Bleeding disorder	Bleeding time, clotting time, PT and APTT
Collagen disease and arthritis	ESR, RF, uric acid, ANA test/anti-DNA (for LE) and CRP
Diabetes	Glucose (blood and urine), glucose tolerance test, Na, K, Cl, cholesterol, TGL
Electrolyte imbalance	Na, K, pH, blood gases, BUN
Hypertension	BUN/creatinine, Na, K, Cl, thyroxine, urinary vanillyl mandelic acid, urine analysis, urinary free cortisol
Hepatic	GOT (AST), GPT (ALT), ALP, gamma-glutamyl transpeptidase (GGT), bilirubin (total and conjugated), albumin, prothrombin time
Neoplasm	Alpha foetoprotein (AFP), carcinoembryonic antigen (CEA), PSA, LD, ALP
Pancreatic	Amylase, lipase, glucose, Ca
Parathyroid	Ca, P, Mg, urinary Ca, total protein, albumin, ALP
Renal	BUN, creatine, creatinine clearance, total protein, albumin, Na, K, Cl

Note: All analyses are with serum (or plasma) unless otherwise stated for urine

APPENDIX G: PROFESSIONAL ORGANIZATIONS CONNECTED WITH INDIAN CLINICAL LABORATORIES

All India Medical Laboratory Technologists' Association

Registered Office:
L 1/249B, DDA Flats, Kalkaji
New Delhi 110019, INDIA
Head Office:
Room No. 404, Capitol Tower,
Block A, 4th Floor, Fraser Road,
Patna 800001, Bihar, INDIA

Indian Association of Pathologists and Microbiologists

Dr Niranjan Rout, Honorary Secretary (2008),
Department of Oncopathology
A. H. Regional Cancer Center,
Cuttack 753007, INDIA
E-mail:secretaryiapm@gmail.com

World Health Organization

Regional Office for South East Asia
World Health House, New Delhi 110002, INDIA

International Association of Medical Laboratory Technologists (IAMLT)

Adolf Fredriks Kyrkogata 11
S-111 37 Stockholm, SWEDEN
Contact person: Margareta Haag, Executive Director
Website: http://www.iamlt.se

APPENDIX H: SUPPLIERS OF CLINICAL LABORATORY PRODUCTS

Indian Manufacturers and Suppliers Directory

Provides the directory of various manufacturers and suppliers of laboratory equipment.
Internet contact: JimTrade.com

India Mart

Maintains and provides the names of manufacturers and suppliers in India for various laboratory equipment
Internet contact: indiamart.com/

C/O Eperium Business Solutions India Pvt. Ltd.

They maintain the directory of the suppliers for the diagnostic laboratories in India.

3rd Floor, NSIC-STP Extn., Administrative Block,
NTS Okhla Industrial Estate, Phase III,
New Delhi, 110020; INDIA
Intenet contact: trademart.in

Indian Industry
Provides the directory of qualified manufacturers and suppliers of clinical laboratory diagnostic kits
Internet contact: http://www.indianindustry.com/

Clinical laboratory equipment, supplies and reagents

Adair, Dutt & Co. (India) Private Ltd.
Importers and dealers of laboratory equipment with the brand name ADCO. .
H.O. Power Tools Bhavan, 2, BBD Bag East
Kolkata, 700001, West Bengal, INDIA

Abbott Healthcare Pvt. Ltd
Diagnostic kits, reagents and supplies
404-Business Point Plot No. 349
Western Express Highway
Andheri (East),
Mumbai, 400069, INDIA

J.T.Baker Chemical Co.
A worldwide company that supplies high purity reagents and speciality chemicals. The products are stocked by the local distributors in India.
Head Office
222 Red School Lane
Phllipsburg, New Jersey 08865, USA

Bayer Healthcare Diagnostic Division
Instrument for quick diagnostic tests, A_1C assay, tests for diabetes and others. Pharmaceutical and laboratory products
Kolshet Road, Thane 400607
Maharashtra, INDIA

Beckman Coulter (U.K.) Limited
Manufacturer of laboratory equipment
Oakley Court
Kingsmead Business Park
London Road, High Wycombe
Buckinghamshire HP11 1JU

BDH (British Drug House) and Glaxo Laboratories Ltd.
Leading suppliers of laboratory chemicals and diagnostic reagents in India
Dr. Annie Besant Road,
Mumbai 400025, INDIA

Becton Dickinson and Co. (BD)
Manufacturer and distributor of hospital and laboratory equipment and supplies
6th Floor Signature Tower - B
South City I, NH 8
Gurgaon 122001, Haryana, INDIA

Bharat Laboratories
Bharat Laboratories is one of the oldest suppliers of clinical laboratory products in India. Laboratory chemicals, reagent strips, blood bank reagents are its specialities.
Road 27, Wagle Estate
Thane 400604
Maharashtra, INDIA

Bio/Data Corporation
Supplier of equipment and reagents for haematological tests and equipment used in physician's office (point of care).
Horsham, PA, USA

Biodata Corporation
Best Instruments, INDIA (Distributor)
bestinst@dataone.in

bioMérieux India Pvt. Ltd.
Specialized in the laboratory supplies of microbiology and blood bank
A-32, Mohan Cooperative, Industrial Estate
New Delhi 110044, INDIA
http://www.biomerieux-diagnostics.com

Bioscience Corporation
Suppliers of laboratory glasswares and plastic wares; microtitre plates and automatic pipettes
6/67 Hanuman Society
Paranjpe "B" scheme Road No. 1
Vile Parle (East)
Mumbai 400057, INDIA

Biosite, Inc.
Specialist in D-dimer and various other diagnostic test equipment in physician's office Asia
Level 3, Three Pacific Place
1 Queen's Road East, Hong Kong
Unit 22, Ormeau Business Park
Cromac Avenue, Belfast, BT7 1JA, UK

BioTek Instruments Pvt. Ltd.
Leader in microplate and other laboratory equipment and supplies
Unit 223, Linkway Estate
New Link Road, Malad (West)
Mumbai 400064, INDIA
www.biotek.in

Blue Dot Ltd.
New Delhi, INDIA
Distributors of Technicon products.

Boehringer Ingelheim India Pvt. Ltd.
Laboratory supplies and equipment. Some of its products are sold through Roche Diagnostics.
1st floor, Alexandra
St. Sebastin Road, Bandra West
Mumbai 400050, INDIA

Borosil Glass Works Ltd.
Borosil Glass Works Ltd. is associated with the Corning Glass Works of the United States. They supply volumetric glassware of highest precision.
Mumbai 400018, INDIA

Fisher Scientific
Remel Products
Mumbai 400022, INDIA
suhas.ghogre@thermofisher.com

HemoCue Inc.
Medical supplies, Point of care (POC) equipment and reagents for haematological tests
40 Empire Drive, Lake Forest, CA 92630, USA

Hycor Biomedical Ltd.
Equipment and supplies for hospitals, laboratories and doctor's office
Pentlands Science Park
Bush Loan, Penicuik
Edinburgh EH26 OPL, UK

Decruz Corporation
Decruz is the agent and distributors of various diagnostic reagents and products used in clinical laboratories and blood banking.
44 Cawasji Patel Street
Mumbai 400023, INDIA

Diatek (P) Ltd.
The Diatek company sells various kits used in routine blood chemistry. Most of the methods are based on colorimetric procedures.
109, Microwave Road, M.Q.
Trichur 680001, Kerala, INDIA

E. Merck (India) Ltd.
Worldwide supplier of reliable laboratory chemicals and reagents.
Shiv Sagar Estate A
Dr. Annie Basant Road, Worli,
Mumbai 400018, INDIA

Glaxo-Wellcome-SmithKline Consumer Healthcare
Leading supplier of pharmaceutical products and clinical laboratory test kits.
DLF Plaza Tower,
DLF Phase I, Gurgaon 122002 Haryana, INDIA.

ITC Infotech India Ltd.
Virginia House
37, J.L Nehru Road
Kolkata 700071, INDIA

J.M. Parekh Co.
J.M.Parekh Company market their products under the brand name of Microaid. They are the suppliers of laboratory apparatus and hospital appliances.
Amersi Road,
P.O. Malad,
Mumbai 400064, INDIA

J. Mitra and Bros
Supplier of Medical Equipment; importers and distributors of laboratory instruments for corning and other leading companies.
20, Double Storey Market,
New Rajinder Nagar, New Delhi 110060, INDIA

New India Chemical Enterprises
Sell their products under the brand name of NICE. Supplier of chemicals, laboratory reagents and supplies.
Cochin 682024, INDIA

Nova Biomedical India
Hospital supplies and pharmaceutical products; specialized in diabetes; works in collaboration with Abbott (India).
307, Apra Plaza II
Plot No.14, Sector 10
Dwarka, New Delhi 110075, INDIA
novabio@nde.vsnl.net.in

Ortho Diagnostics (Johnson and Johnson) Division of Ethnor Limited
Supplier of blood bank reagents, Rhogam and routine chemistry kits and blood bank products
Registered Office
Johnson & Johnson Ltd.
30 Jorjett Street
Mumbai 400036, INDIA

Pasteur Biological Laboratory (India)
Supplier of various laboratory products.
1-7 P.C. GIDC Estate,
Umbergam (W.R.)
Gujarat 396171, INDIA

Quidel Corporation
Brand names microVue, TECOmedical; distribute rapid diagnostic supplies, pharmaceutical products; works in collaboration with bioMérieux India Pvt. Ltd
A-32, Mohan Cooperative Ind. Estate
New Delhi 110024, INDIA

Remel, Inc.
Diagnostic test kits, clinical laboratory supplies; Associated with Fisher Scientific (Thermofisher)
Mumbai 400022, INDIA
suhas.ghogre@thermofisher.com

Remi Group
Supplier and importer of various laboratory equipment
52, Mittal Court "A"
Nariman Point,
Mumbai 400021, INDIA

Roche Scientific Company (India) Pvt. Ltd.
Pharmaceuticals Division
"The View", 2nd Floor
165, Dr. Annie Besant Road, Worli,
Mumbai 400018, INDIA
girish.telang@roche.com

Roche Diagnostics (India) Pvt. Ltd.
761, Solitaire Corporate Park,
167 Har Govind Ji Marg,
Chakala, Andheri (East)
Mumbai 400093, INDIA

Sarabhai Chemicals
Manufacturer and importers of a variety of chemicals.
P.O. Box 80, Baroda, INDIA

Scientific Instrument Co. Ltd.
Markets its products under the brand of SICO. It is one of the leading suppliers of instruments and laboratory appliances in India and other developing countries. It has repair facilities in Delhi, Calcutta, Mumbai (Bombay) and Hyderabad.
6 Tej Bahadur Sapru Road,
Allahabad 211001, INDIA

Solco Basle Ltd.
Primarily deals with products for "coagulation time" determinations. Also, pharmaceutical products.
Belco Pharma
515, Modern Industrial Estate
Bahadurgarh, 124507, Haryana, INDIA

Span Diagnostics Ltd.
Manufacturer of laboratory products, equipment, diagnostic kits, blood bank reagents, laboratory chemicals and many more.
173-B, New Industrial Estate,
Udhna, Surat 394210, INDIA.
Regional Office
Town Center #303,
Andheri Kurla Road, Marol,
Andheri (East), Mumbai 400059, INDIA

Sysmex India Pvt., Ltd.
Sysmex is a market leader in the field of clinical laboratory testing and health information technology.
308, Ascot Centre, 3rd Floor,
Next to Hotel Le Royal Meridian,
Sahar Airport Road, Andheri (East),
Mumbai 400099, INDIA

Systronics Ltd.,
Hospital and laboratory equipment; civil engineers.
88-92 Indl Area, Naroda,
Gujarat 382330, INDIA

Techno Instrument Division
Manufacturer and distributor of laboratory equipment, precision instruments.
V.N. Ourav Marg,
Chembur,
Mumbai 400071, INDIA
Registered Office:
199 Churchgate Reclamation,
Mumbai 400020, INDIA
Blue Dot Ltd., INDIA, are the distributors of Techno products.

Wellcome Research Laboratories
Wellcome now merged with Glaxo-SmithKline.
Supplies laboratory test reagents with special reference to serologic testing. Some of their products are: Thrombo-Wellcotest; rapid latex test for the detection of FDP.
DLF Plaza Tower,
DLF Phase I, Gurgaon 122002, Haryana, INDIA

Wesix Enterprises
Wesix Enterprises is a small firm that distributes various analytical reagents and chemicals to local hospitals and laboratories. It also markets kits for diagnostic chemical tests.
44, Bachibabu Naidu Street, Triplicane,
Chennai 600005, INDIA

Index

Acid–base balance and blood gases, 945–951
   acidosis and alkalosis, 947(t)
   anion gap, 948
   bicarbonate determination, 949
   buffer system of body, 946
   definitions, 945
   determination of blood gases, 948
   Siggaard Andersen nomogram, 948, 948(f)
Analytes commonly tested in chemistry, 953–955, 954(t))
   albumin, 953
   A/G ratio, 955
   Glucose, 953
   Protein, 953
   total serum protein, 953
Analytical approach in toxicology, 973–979
   microdiffusion analysis, 973, 973(f)
      chemical oxidation of ethanol (and acetone), 974
      general screening for ethanol and acetone, 974
   specimens, 973
   volatile toxic substances, 974(t)–979
      carbon monoxide, 976
      cyanide, 977
      ethanol (enzymatic oxidation), 974
      ethanol and acetone (dichromate), 974
      methanol, isopropanol, formaldehyde, 978
Application of analytical techniques, 852
   photometry, 853–861
      absorption photometry, 855, 855(f)
         Beer's law, 855, 856(f)
            principles, 855, 855 (f)
      colorimeters and spectrophotometers, 856
         basic technique of colorimetry, 857
         components, 854(f), 856
         preparation of calibration curve, 858
         significance, 859, 859(f)
         some commonly used terms, 858
         taking of colorimeter readings, 858
      complementary filter, 854(t), 856(f)
      light source, 854
      physical properties of light, 853(f)
      quality of light, 854
      reflectance photometry, 860
         solid phase technology, 861
      turbidometry and nephelometry, 861, 861(f)
   titrimetry, 852
Automated analysersin developing countries, 885–891
   Auto Pacer, 890, 891(f)
      components, 890
   Autoanalyzers, 885
      components, 885, 886(f)
   Clinical Corona, 887, 887(f)
      components, 888, 888(f)
   historical background, 885
   SEAC (Ames), 891
Automation in developing countries, 892
Automation, introductory remarks, 873

Basic analytical techniques, 851
   calculation of result, 851
   chemical reaction, 851
   specimen processing, 851
   standard to compare, 851
Basic clinical biochemistry, 834–835
   chemistry profiles, 830(f), 834
   reference (normal) ranges, 834, 835(t)
   types of specimens for chemical analyses, 834
   units of measure in clinical chemistry, 834
Basic physiology and biochemistry, 822, 822(f)
   amino acids, 825
   bilirubin, 825, 826(f)
   carbohydrate, 823, 824(f)
   digestive system, 823
   endocrine glands, 823
   lipids, 826, 827(f)
      triglycerides, 827
   nucleic acid, 825–826
   ormothine cycle, 825(f)
   protein, 824, 824(f)
   steroids, 828(f)
   sterols, 827
   urea, 825, 825(f)
Basic steps in analytical chemistry, 851
Basic terminologies in histology and cytology, 993
Biochemical tests, introduction, 895
   normal values, 896(t)
   routine tests, 895, 896(t)

I.2 Index

collection of blood specimen, 842, 842(f)
patient preparation, 841
preparation of protein free filtrates, 845, 846(f)
    Folin-Wu method, 846
    Somogyi method, 846
    TCA (trichloroacetic acid) method, 846
preparation of serum, 844(f), 845
safety precautions, 847
separation of blood components,
special problems with blood specimen, 843
    haemoconcentration, 843
    haemolysis, 844
    over centrifugation, 844
specimen preservation, 843
specimen transport, 843
timing of specimen collection, 841
unacceptable specimen for testing, 844
Blood specimen for biochemical analysis, 841–847

Carbohydrate metabolism, 960
Cardiac function tests, 958
Cerebrospinal fluid, 848
    clinical significance, 848
    specimen handling, 848
Chemistry profile, 953
    biochemical test profile, 954(t)
Classification of automated systems, 873–874
    centrifugal analysis, 874
    continuous flow analysis, 873
    discrete analysis, 874
Clinical significance of glucose in circulation, 904–905
    diabetes and diabetes management, 904
    HbA1c (glycated haemoglobin), 905
Computers in the clinical laboratory, 878-884
    challenges of computerization, 879
    computer application in clinical laboratories, 878
    computerization of laboratory instruments, 883
        computer housing, 884
        concluding remarks, 884
        machine failure, 884
    conclusion, 884
    glossary of terms, 879
    operation of a computer, 881, 882(f)
        hardware, 881
            central processing unit (CPU), 882,
            components and primary parts, 882(f)
        input/Output (I/O), 882
            memory/storage unit, 883
            software, 883

Determination of bilirubin, 916–919
    Jendrassik and Grof method, 917–919
        direct, 918
        indirect, 918
    total, 918
Determination of blood glucose, 896–905
    clinical significance, 904
    glucose oxidase method, 900
    o-toluidine method, 897
    quick screen of blood glucose, 903
Determination of blood urea, 911
    diacetyl monoxime method, 911
Determination of creatinine clearance, 916
Determination of creatinine, 914
    alkaline picrate method, 914
Determination of serum protein, 906–911
    determination of serum albumin, 909
    determination of total protein in serum, 906
    Biuret method, 906
Diabetes and diabetes management, 905
Diagnostic biochemical profiles, 834-838
    cardiac function panel, 837
    electrolytes, 835
    kidney function panel, 836
        BUN (blood urea nitrogen), 836
        creatinine, 836
        uric acid, 836
    lipid profile, 838
    liver function panel, 836–837
        bilirubin, 836
        direct, 836
        indirect, 837
        total, 837
    diagnostic enzyme assay, 836
    protein, 836
    mineral metabolism, 838
        iron, 838
        phosphorus, 838
    protein, 835
    thyroid function profile, 838
Diagnostic enzymology, 919–935
    NAD-NADH system, 919
    principle of enzyme reaction, 919
    routine analysis of diagnostic enzymes, 921
        alkaline phosphatase, 921
            p-nitrophenylphosphate method, 921
        amylase, 933
        creatinine kinase (CK), 928
        lactic dehydrogenase (LD), 930
        transaminases, 924
            ALT and AST, 924
Drug screening, 980–985

acetaminophen, 980
barbiturates, 983
cannabinoids, 984
chloral hydrate, halogenated hydrocarbons, 981
cocaine, 984
cyclic antidepressants, 984
date-rape and knockout drugs, 985
imipramine, 982
opioids, 984
phenothiazine derivates, 980
salicylates, 982
sympathomimetic drugs, 985

Electrochemical technology, 868
Electrochemistry, 861–863
    ion-selective electrode, 862
    pH meter, 862(f)
    potentiometry, 861, 862(f)
Electrolytes, 939–944
    calcium, 940
        cresolphthalein complexone method, 941
    chloride, 943
        ion selective electrode, 944
        colorimetric method, 944
    sodium and potassium, 940
        ion selective electrode, 940
Electrolytes, 955, 862–863
Electrophoresis, 869–871, 870(f)
    electrophoretogram chart reader, 870(f)
    electrophoretogram chart, 870(f)
    haemoglobin electrophoresis, 871
Exfoliate cytology, 1054-1062
    clinical significance, 1054
    collection of specimens, 1055
    preparation of smear, 1057
        fixation and commonly used fixatives, 1058
            Carnoy's fluid, 1059
            ether-alcohol, 1058
            Schaudinn's fluid, 1058
        fixation and mailing of smears, 1059
    preparation of specimens, 1056
        concentrating specimen, 1957
            thick specimen, 1057
            watery specimen, 1057
    stains and staining techniques, 1059-1062
        cresyl violet staining, 1062
        Grunwald-Giemsa, 1061
        Haematoxylin-eosin, 1060
        other staining procedures, 1062
        Papanicolaou staining, 1059

Frozen section technique, 1050
    staining of frozen sections, 1051
Functions of various organs, 823(f)
    brain, 832
    endocrine glands, 831
    heart, 831
    kidney, 831
    liver, 829, 826(f)
    lung, 832
    pancreas, 831

Gastric function tests, 962–965
    clinical significance, 963
    laboratory investigation, 963
        acidity, 964-965
        chemical screening, 963
        physical examination, 963
        test for blood, 964
    normal value, 963
    specimen, 963
Glycated haemoglobin, HbA1c, 905

Haemoglobin degradation, 826(f)
Handling of small tissue fragments, 1053
Heavy metal poisoning, 985–987
    iron overdose, 986
    Reinsch screening test, 985
    specific test for mercury, 986
Histology and cytology laboratories, 991–993
    exfoliate cytology, 992
    role, 991
    specimen, 992
Hyperlipidemia, 959

Identifying characteristics of abnormal cells, 1062
    benign and malignant cells, 1063
    normal non-malignant cells, 1062
Immunochemistry, 863–868
    enzyme immunoassay (EIA), 865. 865(f)
    fluorescent antibody (FA) technique, 866, 868(f)
    labelled antibody techniques, 864
    nephelometry, 864
    radial immunodiffusion (RID), 863, 864(f)
    radioimmunoassay (RIA), 865, 866(f), 867(f)
        liquid phse, 867(f)
        solid phase, 866(f)
    visible immunologic reactions, 864(f)
Interrelated metabolic processes, 823, 823(f), 828, 829(f)

Kidney (renal) function tests, 956–957
    blood electrolytes, 956

blood urea nitrogen, 956
glomerular filtration rate (GFR), 956
serum creatinine, 956
uric acid, 957

Laboratory equipment and reagents, 994–1002
  reagent, 994
  use and care of equipment, 996–999
    embedding equipment, 997
    floating bath, 1000, 1000(f)
    freezers and refrigerators, 1002
    incubators, 1002
    microscope, 996
    microtome, use and care, 997–1000, 998(f)
      cryostat, 998, 999, 998(f),
      freezing microtome, 998(f), 999
      rocking microtome, 998
      rotary microtome, 998
      sliding microtome, 998
    paraffin oven, 997, 997(f)
    slide warmer, 1001, 1001(f)
    tissue processor and stainer, 1001
    vacuum embedding oven, 996–997
  use and care of laboratory supplies, 995(f), 1002
    containers for specimens, 1003
    microscope slides and cover slips, 1002
    mounting media, 1003
Lipid metabolism, 959
  cholesterol, 959
  triglycerides, 959
Lipid profile, 935-938
  desirable limits, 936
  liporoteins–HDL and LDL, 938
  serum triglycerides, 938
  specimen, 935
  total cholesterol, 935
Liver function tests, 957-959
  bilirubin in urine, 957
  biochemical profile, 959(t)
  liver enzymes, 957, 958
    alkaline phosphatase, 958
    aminotransferases (ALT, AST), 958
    gamma glutamyl transferase, 958
    lactic dehydrogenase, 958
  prothrombin time, 957
  serum albumin, 957
  serum bilirubin, 957
    direct, 957
    indirect, 957
  serum total cholesterol, 957
  serum total protein, 957
  urobilinogen in urine, 957
Logging in of specimens, 1008

Mineral metabolism, 955
  calcium, 955
  iron, 955
  phosphorus, 955

Normal and abnormal biochemical processes, 821

Other tests of organ function, 960–961
  creatinine clearance for kidney, 960
    body surface, 960, 961(f)
    calculation of clearance rate, 960
      corrected, 960
      uncorrected, 960

Pancreatic function tests, 965–967
  blood tests, 965
  faecal test, 965
  laboratory investigation of pancreatic juice, 966
    chemical screening, 966
    physical examination, 966
Pathological biochemistry, 832–834
  diabetes mellitus, 833(f)
Point of care testing: A new approach, 891
Preparation of reagent solutions, 1004
  dilutions from stock solutions, 1004
Preparation of sections, 1021–1025
  section cutting, 1022,
    attaching paraffin block to microtome, 1022
    attaching section to slide, 1021(f), 1023
    cutting the section, 1022, 1023(f)
    problems in section cutting, 1024
    storage of paraffin blocks, 1024
Preparation of stock solution, 898(f)
Preparation of tissues, 1009–1015
  decalcification, 1013
  detecting the end point, 1014
  fixation, 1009, 1010(f)
  preparation of fixatives, 1010
    routine fixatives, 1010
    special fixatives, 1011
  removal of fixatives, 1011(f)
Processing of tissues, 1015–1020, 1015(t)
  automatic tissue processor, 1017(f),
    timer devices, 1018(f), 1019(f)
  clearing, 1016
  dehydration, 1016
  embedding, 1018–1020, 1020(f)
  infiltration (impregnation), 1016

tissue processing, 1016, 1017(t)

Reference values in clinical chemistry, 835(t)
Ringing, 845
Role of toxicology laboratory, 972
Routine haematoxylin-eosin staining (H&E), 1028
   morphology of some cells, 1030(f)
Routine staining procedure in histology, 1025–1030
   basic information, 1025
   post-staining procedures, 1027
      mounting, 1027(f), 1028
   preparation for staining, 1026
   pre-staining treatments, 1025
   staining, 1026, 1026(f)

Significance of specimen in biochemical analyses, 840
Special stains and staining techniques, 1030–1050
   connective tissue stains, 1031
      collagen and collagen fibres, 1031
         elastic fibres, 1034
         reticulin, 1033
      stains for particular substances, 1037–1043
         amyloids, 1038
         carbohydrate, 1037
         lipids, 1040
         pigments and minerals, 1041
   stains for microorganisms, 1043–1050
      bacteria, 1045
      acid fast staining, 1046
      common histological stains, 1044(t)
      demonstration of helicobacter, 1048
      fluorescence technique, 1047
      fungi, 1048
      general purpose stain, 1044
      Gram staining, 1045
      tissue parasite, 1049
      weak acid fast staining, 1046
Stains in histology, 1008–1052
   acid fast stain, 1046
   alkaline congo red, 1038
   congo-red stain, 1038
   cresyl fast violet, 1048
   Giemsa stain, 1044
   Gram stain, 1045

   Haematoxylin and eosin, 1028
   Masson's trichome stain, 1032
   oil red O stain, 1040
   periodic acid-schiff (PAS), 1037
   polychrome methylene blue staining, 1052
   Prussian blue stain, 1042
   silver methenamine stain, 1048
   Sudan black stain, 1041
   toluidine blue stain, 1039
   van Gieson's stain, 1031
   Verhoeff's stain, 1036
   Von Kossa silver nitrate procedure, 1043
   Wiegert's resorcin-fuchsin stain, 1035
Steps of automation, 874–877
   automated "stat" testing, 877
   calculation of results, 877
   overcoming interference, 875
   quality control and preventing maintenance, 877
   reaction conditions, 876
      dry chemistry, 876
      liquid chemistry, 876
      use of ion selective electrode, 876
   reaction measurement, 876–877
      sensing the end point, 877
   sample handling and measurement, 874
   transport and delivery of specimen, 875
      reagent handling, 875
Structures of important organic compounds, 822(f), 824(f)

Tests for malabsorption, 967
   D-xylose absorption test, 967
      patient preparation and after care, 967
      specimen collection, 967
   test procedure, 967
Thyroid function tests, 960
Time saving devices and kits, 892
Transferrin, 838
True glucose, 900

Urine spcimen, 847-848
   collection of 24-h urine, 848(t)
   procedure of specimen collection, 848
   types of urine specimens, 847